Panic Disorder:
Clinical Diagnosis,
Management and Mechanisms

PANIC DISORDER: CLINICAL DIAGNOSIS, MANAGEMENT AND MECHANISMS

Edited by

David J Nutt, MD, MRCP, FRCPsych
Psychopharmacology Unit
School of Medical Sciences
University of Bristol
UK

James C Ballenger, MD
Department of Psychiatry and Behavioral Sciences
Medical University of South Carolina
USA

Jean-Pierre Lépine, MD
Hôpital Fernand Widal, AP–HP
Service de Psychiatrie
Paris
FRANCE

MARTIN DUNITZ

© Martin Dunitz Ltd 1999

First published in the United Kingdom in 1999 by

Martin Dunitz Ltd
The Livery House
7–9 Pratt Street
London NW1 0AE

A CIP record for this book is available from the
British Library.

ISBN 1-85317-518-8

Distributed in the United States by:
Blackwell Science Inc.
Commerce Place, 350 Main Street
Malden, MA 02148, USA
Tel: 1–800–215–1000

Distributed in Canada by:
Login Brothers Book Company
324 Salteaux Crescent
Winnipeg, Manitoba, R3J 3T2
Canada
Tel: 204–224–4068

Distributed in Brazil by:
Ernesto Reichmann Distribuidora de Livros, Ltda
Rua Coronel Marques 335, Tatuape 03440–000
Sao Paulo,
Brazil

Composition by Wearset, Boldon, Tyne and Wear
Printed and bound in Spain by Grafos, S.A. Arte
Sobre papel

CONTENTS

List of Contributors

Sandra L Baker
Clinical Training Programs
Boston University
Center for Anxiety & Related Disorders
648 Beacon St, 6th Floor
Boston, MA 02215
USA

James C Ballenger
Department of Psychiatry and Behavioral
Sciences
Medical University of South Carolina
171 Ashley Avenue
Charleston, SC 29425
USA

David H Barlow
Clinical Training Programs
Boston University
Center for Anxiety & Related Disorders
648 Beacon St, 6th Floor
Boston, MA 02215
USA

C Barr Taylor
Department of Psychiatry and Behavioral
Sciences
Stanford University Medical Center
Stanford, CA 94305
USA

Graham D Burrows
Department of Psychiatry
University of Melbourne
Austin & Repatriation Hospital
Heidelberg, Vic 3084
AUSTRALIA

Anne Chosak
Clinical Training Programs
Boston University
Center for Anxiety & Related Disorders
648 Beacon St, 6th Floor
Boston, MA 02215
USA

Carlo Faravelli
Istituto delle Malattie Nervose e Mentali
Policlinico Careggi
Viale Morgagni 35
50134 Firenze
ITALY

Eric Griez
Department of Psychiatry & Neuropsychology
State University of Limburg
PO Box 616
6200 MD Maastricht
THE NETHERLANDS

David France Jakubec
Department of Psychiatry and Behavioral
Sciences
Stanford University Medical Center
Stanford, CA 94305
USA

Heinz Katschnig
Psychiatr Universitätsklinik
Währinger Gürtel 18–20
1090 Vienna
AUSTRIA

Neil Laufer
Geha Psychiatric Hospital
PO Box 102
28100 Petach Tikva
ISRAEL

Jean-Pierre Lépine
Hôpital Fernand Widal
Assistance Publique Hôpitaux de Paris
Service de Psychiatrie
200, Rue du Faubourg Saint-Denis
75475 Paris Cedex 10
FRANCE

Andrea L Malizia
MRC Cyclotron Unit
Hammersmith Hospital
Du Cane Rd
London W12 0NN
UK

Trevor R Norman
Department of Psychiatry
University of Melbourne
Austin & Repatriation Hospital
Heidelberg, Vic 3084
AUSTRALIA

David J Nutt
Psychopharmacology Unit
School of Medical Sciences
University of Bristol
University Walk
Bristol BS8 ITD
UK

Mark A Oakley-Browne
Department of Psychological Medicine
Christchurch School of Medicine
PO Box 4345
Christchurch
NEW ZEALAND

Alessandra Paionni
Istituto delle Malattie Nervose e Mentali
Policlinico Careggi
Viale Morgagni 35
50134 Firenze
ITALY

Antoine Pélissolo
Hôpital Fernand Widal
Assistance Publique Hôpitaux de Paris
Service de Psychiatrie
200, Rue du Faubourg Saint-Denis
75475 Paris Cedex 10
FRANCE

Raben Rosenberg
Institute for Basic Research in Psychiatry
Department of Biological Psychiatry
Psychiatric Hospital in Aarhus
8240 Risskov
DENMARK

David A Spiegel
Clinical Training Programs
Boston University
Center for Anxiety & Related Disorders
648 Beacon St, 6th Floor
Boston, MA 02215
USA

George R Thorn
Clinical Training Programs
Boston University
Center for Anxiety & Related Disorders
648 Beacon St, 6th Floor
Boston, MA 02215
USA

Kees Verburg
Department of Psychiatry & Neuropsychology
State University of Limburg
PO Box 616
6200 MD Maastricht
THE NETHERLANDS

Abraham Weizman
Director of Research
Geha Psychiatric Hospital
PO Box 102
28100 Petach Tikva
ISRAEL

Preface

Panic disorder is an important clinical diagnosis for many reasons. Firstly, panic disorder is the first psychiatric syndrome to have been defined by a biological response, in that panic attacks were observed to be particularly responsive to treatment with the tricyclic antidepressant imipramine. Thus it stands as an example of what many would see as a new and important branch of psychiatric nosology, namely that based on a biological understanding of a disorder. Panic disorder is also important because of the growing evidence of its prevalence, severity and the consequent personal and economic costs.

It is also a fascinating area for research, in biological and social psychiatry and in psychology. Indeed, the interchange (both positive and negative) between psychiatrists and psychologists involved in the treatment and understanding of panic disorder is one of the most vibrant and active growth areas in the respective disciplines. Many of the concepts, both biological and psychological, that have emerged from research in the field of panic disorder have produced conceptual shifts in their respective disciplines.

It was on the basis of these understandings of the importance and future role of panic disorder as a clinical and research area that the Editors decided to put together this current volume. What we have done is to approach experts in panic disorder from around the world and asked them to contribute chapters targeting what we consider to be the key areas.

The book is designed for everyone interested in the field of panic disorder. It contains rich amounts of clinical diagnostic and treatment information for the practising clinician. There are state-of-the-art reviews of research findings in the field, including the presentation of some novel and important new discoveries for biological research. It also contains several chapters from world leaders in the field of psychological theory and treatment.

With the end of this century upon us, we hope that this volume will provide a strong and effective foundation for the development of research and treatment of panic disorder well into the next millennium.

Acknowledgements
We wish to thank Nancy Pickett for her sterling work in coordinating the production of this book, correcting manuscripts, organizing contributors and liaising with the publishers. We are also grateful to the individual authors for their efforts in producing such a fine collection of chapters.

David J Nutt
Jean-Pierre Lépine
James C Ballenger

1

Anxiety neurosis, panic disorder or what?

Heinz Katschnig

CONTENTS • Panic: what's in a word? • Panic disorder: the development of the disease concept • The modern era • Is panic disorder another American disease? • Conclusions

Panic: what's in a word?

At the beginning of this century, Danish travellers to Greenland used to report a strange syndrome among Eskimo hunters. When, on a sunny day, with completely calm water, they were out in the sea and waiting in their kayak for seals to show up, they suddenly had difficulties in breathing, felt their heart racing and experienced fear of dying. Usually they were able to reach safe land, but did not dare to go out again for hunting. Some could not even leave the igloo any more. The condition was later called 'kayak angst', but has obviously disappeared today with changes in hunting habits. If the descriptions by the travellers are closely analysed, the Eskimo hunters affected have suffered from what we today call panic disorder with agoraphobia.[1,2]

What is interesting in the descriptions of kayak angst is that it tended to occur in a kind of sensory-deprivation situation, when the hunter had been waiting for hours in his kayak, without any breeze disturbing the mirror-like surface of the sea.[3] Kayak angst literally came,

'out of the blue' – as is typical of the first panic attack of panic disorder patients.

The word 'panic', as it is used in modern languages, is derived from Pan, the Greek god of flocks and herds. He used to create turmoil out of the blue – when, for instance, in Arcadia at noon everyone was resting. The story goes that, on one occasion, when everyone was sleeping on the pasture in the heat of early afternoon, he suddenly made a loud noise, frightening animals, shepherds and the nymphs. The nymphs fled, and one of them, Syrinx, froze out of terror, and became a reed (actually the word 'syrinx' means 'tube' in both Greek and Latin). Pan reportedly cut it and made the Pan pipes out of it – rather a symbol of tranquillity and 'bucolic' calm than of terror.

As a rule, the first panic attack indeed occurs out of the blue: usually in a calm situation, when someone is, for instance, out for a walk on a sunny Sunday afternoon. Panic attacks are a sudden and frightening experience, but they are an inner event, with the person experiencing inner terror, trying to hide it outwardly – nothing of a hysterical outbreak, as lay persons might think, when they hear that someone suffers from a panic attack. One other interesting observation fits into this contradiction between tranquillity and sudden fear: it is not rare that panic attacks occur during sleep.

Panic disorder: the development of the disease concept

Consider the following doctor/patient dialogue:

'Well, what is it you suffer from?'
'I get so out of breath. Not always. But sometimes it catches me so that I think I shall suffocate.'
'Sit down here. What is it like when you get "out of breath"?'
'It comes over me all at once. First of all it's like something pressing on my eyes. My head gets so heavy, there's a dreadful buzzing, and I feel so giddy that I almost fall over. Then there's something crushing my chest so that I can't get my breath.'
'And you don't notice anything in your throat?'
'My throat is squeezed together as though I were going to choke.'
'Does anything else happen in your head?'
'Yes, there's a hammering – enough to burst it.'
'And don't you feel at all frightened while this is going on?'
'I always think I'm going to die . . .'

There are enough indications in this dialogue that this patient fulfils diagnostic criteria for a panic attack according to modern diagnostic systems, like DSM or ICD. Yet this conversation is more than one hundred years old. It can be found in case 4 (Katharina) of Freud and Breuer's *Studies on Hysteria*, published in 1895.[4]

It is not widely known that Sigmund Freud – besides presenting this clear clinical description of a panic attack – laid the foundations for the modern classification of anxiety disorders by separating out 'anxiety neurosis' from the then-fashionable concept of neurasthenia. As Berrios[5] (quoting Laplanche and Pontalis[6]) notes, this is surprising, since Freud had 'adduced hardly any examples and quoted no statistics' in his seminal paper on 'The justification for detaching from neurasthenia a particular syndrome: the anxiety neurosis'.[7]

Already before Freud, anxiety states had been clinically recognized, and specific cases of panic attacks (without using the word) had been described in the psychiatric literature as early as 1866.[8] Also, soon after Freud's paper had appeared, clear conceptualizations of separate 'paroxysmal anxiety states' were published.[9,10] Nevertheless, only Freud's all-embracing concept of 'anxiety neurosis' was accepted by his fellow psychiatrists at the time (although few followed his ideas of sexual aetiology), and it survived for nearly a century (for a more detailed account of these developments see Berrios[5]). See Figure 1.1.

In 1978 the Research Diagnostic Criteria (RDC)[11] were the first to split 'anxiety neurosis' into two distinct diagnostic groups. Only when DSM-III[12] was published, and later also in ICD-10,[13] was the separation into two distinct entities, 'panic disorder', characterized by short intensive episodes of anxiety ('paroxysmal anxiety'), and 'generalized anxiety disorder', without such episodes, definitively introduced into official classifications. A fine distinction, though, is kept up between the latest version of the American Diagnostic and Statistical Manual (DSM-IV)[14] and the World Health Organization's ICD-10: in the case of coexistence of panic and agoraphobia, the former gives precedence to panic disorder (calling the condition 'panic disorder with agoraphobia'),

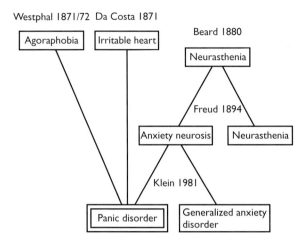

Figure 1.1 Some roots of the modern concept of panic disorder.

open spaces, but should refer more broadly to fear of public places. In this broad meaning, the term was introduced in DSM-III.[12]

Completely separated from these developments within psychiatry, internists have repeatedly described paroxysmal cardiac conditions without any actual cardiac pathology. In 1871, during the American Civil War, Da Costa[19] had already described a condition among soldiers as 'irritable heart', and Oppenheimer et al[20] made similar observations during the First World War, and used the term 'neurocirculatory asthenia'. Today these conditions are clearly recognized as panic attacks. However, medical aspects of panic disorder are still relevant and discussed (see Chapter 8 in this volume).

while the latter sees agoraphobia as dominant and consequently names the same condition 'agoraphobia with panic attacks', which is subsumed under the broader category of 'phobias'. In ICD-9, which is still in use in a number of countries around the world, Freud's definition of 'anxiety neurosis' is still present. It still comprises both today's 'general anxiety disorder' and 'panic disorder'.

In a parallel development, Westphal[15] described three cases of men who could not cross places unaccompanied, and coined the term agoraphobia. He described it as '...impossibility of walking through certain streets or squares, or possibility of so doing only with resultant dread of anxiety'. In 1870, Benedikt[16] in Vienna had already reported on a case of 'Platzschwindel' ('place dizziness'), which he related to otological problems. At that time, obsessions and phobias had not been clearly distinguished, and it was again Freud[17] who succeeded in separating phobia from obsession.[5] Marks[18] stressed that the term 'agoraphobia' should not be restricted to fear of

The modern era

The credit for having started the process of dissecting panic disorder out from 'anxiety neurosis' has to be given to Donald F Klein,[21] who showed that panic attacks responded to imipramine but not to benzodiazepines; for free-floating anxiety without paroxysmal attacks the inverse was true. Consequently, this was later called the 'pharmacological dissection' of 'anxiety neurosis'. While the observation of strict pharmacological separation is no longer valid today (benzodiazepines are also efficacious in panic disorder – though in higher dosages than were originally employed; see Chapter 10 in this volume), antidepressants have become the first-line treatment of panic disorder (see Chapters 9 and 11 in this volume).

In 1981 Klein[22] put forward his new conceptualization of the anxiety disorders. Panic attacks were no longer regarded as 'occasional eruptions from a volcanic sea of anxiousness', as Freud saw them, but as a disease entity of their own. In this new concept, anticipatory anxiety is regarded as the consequence of panic attacks and not as their predecessor, and agoraphobia follows both panic attacks and anticipatory anxiety. Thus Klein[22] brought panic attacks and agoraphobia into one diagnostic concept. However, DSM-III[12] still kept agoraphobia as a separate category, and only some years later was Klein's suggestion taken up by DSM-III-R[23] and DSM-IV,[14] with the diagnosis of panic disorder taking the lead, and being divided into panic disorder with and without agoraphobia.

In addition to these developments, observations in the late 1960s that panic attacks could be challenged by lactate in anxiety patients with panic attacks but not in patients without panic attacks[24] nurtured the idea of separating 'anxiety neurosis' into two distinct disorders. Today's state-of-the-art knowledge of the pharmacological provocation of panic attacks and the evidence from studying brain mechanisms (Chapter 5 in this volume) support the concept of panic disorder as a separate entity, by identifying specific biological mechanisms. Also, respiratory dysregulation seems to play an important specific role in at least a subgroup of panic disorder patients (Chapter 6 in this volume). Furthermore, panic patients tend to have a specific cognitive set, with dominating catastrophizing thoughts, which has led to the development of specific cognitive treatments, emphasizing a vicious circle of catastrophizing thoughts and panic symptoms both in the pathogenesis and in the treatment of panic disorder (Chapter 7 in this volume).

Is panic disorder another American disease?

In 1880 Beard[25] published his most influential book, *A Practical Treatise on Nervous*

Exhaustion (Neurasthenia), and called neurasthenia the 'American disease' of civilization, assuming that its rising frequency could be linked to the pace of civilized life, particularly in urbanized and industrialized countries. As we have noted, Freud[7] had cut out 'anxiety neurosis' from 'neurasthemia', and in 1980, exactly one hundred years after Beard, 'panic disorder' was cut out from 'anxiety neurosis' by the American Psychiatric Association in DSM-III.[12] Suspicion arose that another 'American disease' was being created, and many European psychiatrists kept a reserved stance. However, it is clear today that panic disorder is universal.[1,2] According to the most recent epidemiological surveys (Chapter 2 in this volume), panic disorder is a condition occurring in many different cultures and countries around the world. Also, in clinical studies, panic disorder patients could be identified in sufficiently large numbers to conduct clinical trials in such different countries as Brazil, Norway, Canada, Italy and many others.[26] Finally, an analysis of so-called culture-bound syndromes reveals that conditions like kayak angst among the Eskimos (as it was described above) and koro, anxiety attacks experienced by the Chinese in Southeast Asia and characterized by the sudden fear that the penis would retract into the body and therefore death would ensue,[27,28] are comparable to DSM-III panic disorder. Amering and Katschnig[1,2] have analysed the respective literature, and have found that the case descriptions of both koro and kayak angst corresponded to the diagnostic criteria set out in DSM-III. In Table 1.1 the common features of DSM-III panic attacks, kora and kayak angst are presented, showing the identity of seemingly different conditions.

Table 1.1 Common features of DSM-III panic attacks, koro and kayak angst[1,2]

	DSM-III	Koro	Kayak angst
Speed of onset	'Sudden onset'	'Attack of koro' 'Seized suddenly'	'Attacks' 'Out of the blue' 'Like a fit'
Intensity	'Intense apprehension'	'High intensity' 'Severe'	'Intense state of anxiety'
Symptoms	Dyspnoea Palpitations Chest pain or discomfort Choking or smothering sensations Dizziness, vertigo, or unsteady feelings Feelings of unreality Paresthesias (tingling in hands or feet) Hot and cold flushes Sweatiness Faintness Trembling or shaking Fear of dying, going crazy, or doing something uncontrolled during an attack	Breathlessness Palpitations Precordial discomfort Nausea/abdominal distress Dizziness, nausea Paresthesias Hot and cold sensations Sweating Faintness Trembling and shaking Fear of dying	Palpitations Sweating Dizziness, unsteady feelings, nausea Paresthesias Hot and cold sensations Sweating Faintness Trembling and shaking Fear of dying, fear of losing control
Duration	'Usually minutes, rarely hours'	'20, 30, 60 minutes, terminates spontaneously or by group support or reassurance'	'Terminates on reaching land or with arrival of others'

Conclusions

Both when tracing back the historical developments that led to the definition of panic disorder and when surveying the current evidence for a separate disease entity 'panic disorder' – as opposed to an over-inclusive category of 'anxiety neurosis' – the evidence is overwhelming that panic disorder should be regarded as a separate diagnostic entity. However, a few questions remain open.

American authors tend to characterize panic disorder as a chronic condition,[29] although the evidence points to a heterogeneity in terms of the course of the disorder.[30] The original observations about panic disorder and its course came from the USA, where clinical panic disorder patients usually show the largest proportion of agoraphobia.[1,2] This might be specific for the health-seeking processes at the time when the disorder was defined – not only because doctors were not aware of the diagnosis, but also because the health care system in the USA, with its emphasis on private initiative and responsibility, might have prevented many patients from seeking help at an early stage of the disorder. It might therefore well be that clinical cases in the USA, at least at the time of the first definition of panic disorder, constituted a selected group of the more severely ill with a longer duration of illness.

I should like to suggest that the same heuristic bias might have occurred in panic disorder as it has in schizophrenia. When Kraepelin[31] described dementia praecox, he obviously based his description on those patients who had ended up in the few beds in psychiatric hospitals that existed at that time, and were so severely ill that they could not leave the hospital. A few years later, Bleuler[32] in his famous monograph on *Dementia Praecox or the Group of Schizophrenias*, split schizophrenia into several subgroups. It might well be that this will become a model for dividing panic disorder into several subtypes. Apart from the evidence from longitudinal studies (where about one-third of the patients come into complete remission and 20% show a severely disabling persistent course, with 50% between these two extremes[33,34]), other criteria for subtyping may be important, such as symptoms. Briggs et al[35] have shown that panic attacks with respiratory symptoms tend to respond to antidepressants, whereas panic attacks characterized by palpitations and dizziness respond well to benzodiazepines. It is also interesting that quite a few patients suffer from frequent panic attacks without developing agoraphobia, whereas others develop agoraphobia already after the first panic attack.[36] I conclude that there is no way around a careful description of psychopathological phenomena if progress is to be made. That panic disorder is a distinct diagnostic entity is a good working hypothesis. It might well be that this diagnostic entity is still too large.

References

1. Amering M, Katschnig H, Panic attacks and panic disorder in cross-cultural perspective. *Psychiatric Ann* 1990; **20**: 511–16.
2. Katschnig H, Amering M, Panic attacks and panic disorder in cross-cultural perspective. In: *Clinical Aspects of Panic Disorder* (Ballenger J, ed.). New York: Wiley, 1990: 67–80.
3. Gussow Z, A preliminary report of kayak-angst among the eskimo of West Greenland: a study in sensory deprivation. *Int J Soc Psychiatry* 1963; **9**: 18–26.
4. Breuer J, Freud S, *Studien über Hysterie*. Leipzig: Franz Deuticke, 1895. English translation in: *The Standard Edition of the Complete Works of Sigmund Freud*, Vol 2 (Strachey J, ed.). The Hogarth Press, London, 1961: 125.
5. Berrios GE, History of treatment options for anxiety disorders. In: *Clinical Management of Anxiety* (den Boer JA, ed.). New York: Marcel Dekker, 1997: 1–21.
6. Laplanche J, Pontalis JB, *The Language of Psychoanalysis*. London: The Hogarth Press, 1973: 10–12.
7. Freud S, The justification for detaching from neurasthenia a particular syndrome: the anxiety neurosis. In: *Collected Papers*, Vol 1. London: The Hogarth Press, 1953: 76–106.
8. Morel B, Du délire Emotif. Nervose du systéme nerveux ganglionnaire viscéral. *Arch Gen Med* 1866; **7**: 385–402; 530–51; 700–7.
9. Hartenberg P, *Les Timides et la Timidité*. Paris: Alcan, 1901.
10. Heckel F, *La Névrosa d'Angoisse. Et les Etats d'Emotivité Anxieusé*. Paris: Masson, 1917.
11. Spitzer RL, Endicott J, Robins E, Research diagnostic criteria rationale and reliability. *Arch Gen Psychiatry* 1978; **35**: 773–82.
12. American Psychiatric Association, *Diagnostic and Statistical Manual of Mental Disorders, DSM-III*, ed 3. Washington, DC: American Psychiatric Association, 1980.
13. World Health Organization, *The ICD-10 Classification of Mental and Behavioural Disorders. Clinical Descriptions and Diagnostic Guidelines*. Geneva: WHO, 1992.
14. American Psychiatric Association, *Diagnostic and Statistical Manual of Mental Disorders, DSM-IV*. Washington, DC: American Psychiatric Association, 1994.
15. Westphal C, Die Agoraphobie, eine neuropathische Erscheinung. *Arch Psychiatr Nervenkr* 1871/1872; **34**: 138–61.
16. Benedikt M, Über Platzschwindel. *Allg Wien Med Ztg* 1870; **15**: 488–90.
17. Freud S, L'Hérédité et l'étiologie des névroses. *Rev Neurol* 1896; **4**: 47–62.
18. Marks IM, *Fears and Phobias*. London: Heinemann, 1969.
19. Da Costa JM, On irritable heart. A clinical study of a functional cardiac disorder and its consequences. *Am J Med Sci* 1871; **51**: 17–52.
20. Oppenheimer BS, Levine SA, Morison RA et al, Report on neurocirculatory asthenia and its management. *Military Surgeon* 1918; **42**: 409–26; 711–19.
21. Klein DF, Delineation of two drug-responsive anxiety syndromes. *Psychopharmacology* 1964; **5**: 397–408.
22. Klein DF, Anxiety reconceptualised. In: *New Research and Changing Concepts* (Klein DF, Rabkin JG, eds). New York: Raven Press, 1981.
23. American Psychiatric Association, *Diagnostic and Statistical Manual of Mental Disorders, DSM-III-R*. Washington, DC: American Psychiatric Association, 1987.
24. Pitts FN Jr, McClure JN Jr, Lactate metabolism in anxiety neurosis. *N Engl J Med* 1967; **277**: 1329–36.
25. Beard GW, *A Practical Treatise on Nervous Exhaustion (Neurasthenia)*. New York: William Wood, 1880.
26. Cross-National Collaborative Panic Study Second Phase Investigators, Drug treatment of panic disorder. Comparative efficacy of alprazolam, imipramine and placebo. *Br J Psychiatry* 1992; **160**: 191–202.
27. Gwee AL, Koro – a cultural disease. *Singapore Med J* 1963; **4**: 119–22.
28. Yap PM, Koro – a culture-bound depersonalisation syndrome. *Br J Psychiatry* 1965; **111**: 43–50.
29. Roy-Byrne PP, Cowley DS, Course and outcome in panic disorder. A review of recent follow-up studies. *Anxiety* 1995; **1**: 151–60.

30. Katschnig H, Amering M, Is it possible to predict the long-term course of panic disorder? *J Clin Psychopharm* (in press).
31. Kraepelin E, *Psychiatrie*, 6 Aufl. Leipzig: Barth, 1899.
32. Bleuler E, *Dementia praecox oder die Gruppe der Schizophrenien*. Leipzig: Deuticke, 1911.
33. Katschnig H, Amering M, Stolk JM et al, Long-term follow-up after a drug trial for panic disorder. *Br J Psychiatry* 1995; **167**: 487–94.
34. Katschnig H, Freeman H, Sartorius N (eds), *Quality of Life in Mental Disorders*. Chichester: Wiley, 1997.
35. Briggs AC, Stretch DD, Brandon S, Subtyping of panic disorder by symptom profile. *Br J Psychiatry* 1993; **163**: 201–9.
36. Lelliott P, Marks I, McNamee G, Tobena A, Onset of panic disorder with agoraphobia. Toward an integral model. *Arch Gen Psychiatry* 1989; **46**: 1000–4.

2

Epidemiology, comorbidity and genetics of panic disorder

Jean Pierre Lépine and Antoine Pélissolo

CONTENTS • Introduction • Conceptual and methodological issues • Prevalence of panic in clinical settings • Risk factors • Comorbidity • Suicidality • Family and genetic factors • Conclusions

Introduction

Epidemiological data on prevalence rates, comorbidity, course and risk factors of panic disorder have been provided by a number of community studies conducted during the last 15 years, using operationalized diagnostic criteria. These surveys, based on a diagnostic approach essentially derived from the DSM classification, stressed the wide prevalence of the disorder, with a relatively high agreement in rates and patterns across many countries in the five continents.[1] These findings contrast with previous discrepant data obtained with other methodologies and older classifications. In this chapter, we present community-based data on prevalence rates, comorbidity, risk factors and genetic epidemiology of panic disorder. Clinical course and prognosis issues are considered elsewhere (see Chapter 3).

Conceptual and methodological issues

The definition of a case for epidemiological studies on panic disorder exposes pitfalls associated with the diagnosis of the disorder and with the necessary exclusion of comorbid or confusing conditions. Even if diagnostic criteria for panic disorder are relatively well defined in psychiatric classifications, substantial revisions have been introduced from one version to another, namely between DSM-III, DSM-III-R and DSM-IV versions:[2]

(1) Panic attacks are no longer considered as specific to panic disorder; thus criteria of panic have been placed at the beginning of the anxiety disorder section.

(2) Precise reference to a panic frequency criterion for defining panic disorder has been eliminated and replaced with a more inclusive one.

These types of adjustment may have an impact on the nature or severity of the symptoms required, leading to discrepancies in the findings of epidemiological surveys using different diagnostic criteria. This can also be amplified by the fact that the definitions of the criteria are designed basically to be 'user-friendly' for clinicians, reducing the specificity of the described symptoms.[2]

The second methodological point concerns the assessment procedures used in epidemiological studies. Even if there is now a clear consensus that a structured diagnostic interview is essential to ensure uniformity of the assessment method, the choice of the 'best instrument' remains an unresolved issue. As an example, for the diagnosis of panic disorder, several criteria may require a clinical judgment – for example for the appraisal of the levels of anticipatory anxiety, phobic avoidance or overall impairment. The frequent comorbidity of panic disorder with other anxiety disorders and with affective disorders can also complicate the clinical assessment. Nevertheless, large epidemiological surveys in the community cannot be carried out only by clinicians, mainly because of the cost of such studies.

A recent expert conference report on standardized assessment for panic disorder research listed five structured interviews that were found to be acceptable on the basis of their high inter-rater reliability: three have to be used by clinicians, namely

- the Anxiety Disorders Interview Schedule–Revised (ADIS-R),
- the Schedule for Affective Disorders–Lifetime, Anxiety (SADS-LA),
- the Structured Clinical Interview for DSM-III-R (SCID),

and two can be used by lay, trained interviewers, namely

- the Diagnostic Interview Schedule (DIS),[3]
- the Composite International Diagnostic Interview (CIDI).[4]

These latter two instruments have been employed in several epidemiologic surveys since 1980, improving the comparability of findings in different countries and cultures: the DIS was the key diagnostic instrument used in the Epidemiologic Catchment Area (ECA) program in the USA and in countries involved in the cross-national collaborative group,[1] and the CIDI was used in the recent American National Comorbidity Survey (NCS).[5] The CIDI allows diagnoses to be made according to both the DSM-III (and then the DSM-III-R and DSM-IV) and ICD-10 classification systems.

Prevalence of panic attacks and panic disorder in the general population

Two epidemiologic studies referring to the Research Diagnostic Criteria, before the DSM-III era, found the one-month prevalence rate of panic disorder to be 0.4% and 0.7%.[6,7]

The NCS extensively studied the prevalence of panic symptoms in an 8098-subject sample representative of the entire US population.[8] Table 2.1 shows the prevalences of these symptoms according to the DSM-III-R criteria, and a comparison is made with other rates obtained with similar definitions in previous US studies.

The NCS lifetime prevalence of DSM-III-R panic attacks was 7.3%, and the prevalence in the preceding month was 2.2%. With less specific criteria, in terms of severity and number of associated symptoms, the prevalence of a 'fearful spell' was found to be more than twice as high: 15.6% in the lifetime and 5.8% in the last month.[8] Using the DIS, Von Korff et al[11] and Weissman[12] reported the lifetime prevalence of panic attacks to be around 10%. In other studies, the lifetime rates of panic attacks were more heterogenous: 1.8% in Florence,[13]

Table 2.1 One-month and lifetime prevalence of panic symptoms and panic attacks in the NCS,[8] the ECA study[9] and a household-residing sample in San Antonio, Texas[10]

	Preceding month			Lifetime
	Men	Women	Total	
Fearful spell (NCS)	2.2	5.3	3.8	15.6
Simple panic attack (ECA)				9.7
Limited symptom attack (San Antonio)				11.6
Intense fearful spell[a] (NCS)	1.7	4.4	3.0	11.3
Intense panic attack (ECA)				5.9
Panic attack (San Antonio)				9.4
DSM-III-R panic attack (NCS)	1.1	3.2	2.2	7.3
Recurrent panic attacks[b] (NCS)	0.9	2.5	1.7	4.2

[a]'Intense fearful spell' is defined as a fearful spell with at least four accompanying psychophysiological symptoms.
[b]'Recurrent panic attacks' correspond to four or more attacks within one month or a period of one month with a constant worry about the possibility of an attack.

2.4% in Japan,[14] 1.7% in men and 4.8% in women in Paris,[15] 7.8% in New Zealand,[16] 8.8% in Zurich[17] and 9.3% in Munich.[18]

In summary, the best estimation of lifetime prevalence rates of panic attacks, according to diagnostic criteria, appears to be between 7% and 9% in most countries.

The prevalence rates of panic disorder, explored with diagnostic criteria and structured interviews, has been studied in 15 community epidemiologic surveys (Table 2.2).

Eleven of these studies, conducted in 10 different countries with similar procedures and in a total of more than 40 000 subjects, have been presented together to determine the consistency of findings across various cultures.[1] The lifetime prevalence rates for panic disorder ranged from 0.4% in Taiwan[23] to 3.5% in the NCS.[8] Nevertheless, the majority of studies reported lifetime rates between 1.5% and 2.5%. The prevalence rates of all psychiatric disorders were found to be lower in Taiwan, for reasons which are unclear. Conversely, the NCS obtained high rates for many disorders, for example twice as high as the rate in the ECA for panic disorder, possibly because of the use of the CIDI that includes memory probes potentially improving recollection.[1] The age range of the population included in the NCS was 15–54 years, but convergent data showed that panic disorder is relatively rare in the elderly.[27]

The annual prevalence for panic disorder is

Table 2.2 Prevalence rates of panic disorder per 100 in community-based surveys

Site	n	1-year	Lifetime			Authors and refs
			Women	Men	Total	
USA (ECA)	18 571	1.0	2.3	1.0	1.7	Eaton et al[9]
USA (NCS)	8 098	2.2	5.1	1.9	3.5	Eaton et al[8]
Canada (Edmonton)	3 258	0.9	1.9	0.9	1.4	Bland et al[19]
Puerto Rico	1 551	1.1	1.8	1.4	1.7	Canino et al[20]
France (Savigny)	1 746	0.9	3.0	1.3	2.2	Lépine et al[15]
Germany	481	1.7	3.8	1.4	2.6	Wittchen et al[21]
Italy (Florence)	1 100	1.3	3.9	1.2	2.9	Faravelli et al[13]
Lebanon (Beirut)	234	2.1	3.1	1.1	2.1	Karam[22]
Taiwan	11 004	0.2	0.6	0.2	0.4	Hwu et al[23]
Korea (Seoul)	5 100	1.5	2.9	0.5	1.5	Lee et al[24]
New Zealand (Christchurch)	1 498	1.3	3.3	0.7	2.1	Wells et al[25]
Iceland	862				2.1	Lindal and Stefansson[26]
Japan (Ichikawa)	207				1.0	Aoki et al[14]
USA (San Antonio)	1 306				3.4	Katerndahl and Realini[10]

generally about 1%, ranging from 0.2% in Taiwan to 3.1% in Zurich. There was also a close agreement in the ECA program from one center to another for the one-month prevalence of the disorder, ranging from 0.6% in New Haven to 1.0% in Baltimore.[28]

Prevalence of panic in clinical settings

A recent worldwide survey conducted by the World Health Organization explored the frequency and the nature of psychological problems in primary care or general health settings.[29] Subjects were interviewed with the CIDI in all countries, and the diagnoses were made according to the International Classification of Disease (ICD-10).

The mean prevalence of panic disorder in this population was 1.1% for the current diagnostic, and 3.4% for a lifetime diagnostic.[30,31] The current prevalences of panic attacks and panic disorder in the different countries are presented in Table 2.3. It can be seen that, despite a great discrepancy in the prevalence rates of panic attacks, the prevalence of panic disorder showed a better agreement at about

Table 2.3 Current prevalence rates of panic attacks and panic disorder per 100 in primary care[30,31]		
Site	Panic attacks	Panic disorder
Rio de Janeiro	1.4	0.0
Bangalore	2.0	1.0
Athens	3.0	0.7
Nagasaki	3.3	0.2
Verona	3.3	1.5
Ankara	3.4	0.2
Shanghai	3.8	0.2
Ibadan	4.9	0.7
Santiago	5.5	0.6
Groningen	8.8	1.5
Berlin	10.0	0.9
Mainz	11.2	1.7
Paris	11.3	1.7
Seattle	11.5	1.9
Manchester	16.5	3.5

Risk factors

As previously shown in Table 2.1, the one-month prevalence of panic attacks is consistently higher in women when compared with men in the NCS, with a prevalence more than twice as great among women at each level of severity.[8] The same figures were obtained in the ECA study.[11] The lifetime prevalence rates of panic disorder are also higher in women compared with men in every country (Table 2.2). These differences are statistically significant, except in the Puerto Rico[20] and Taiwan[23] studies.

The age at onset of panic disorder is generally in the early to mid 20s, as was found in the cross-national study and the NCS (Figure 2.1).

By using life-table survey methods, Burke et al[33] found the highest hazard rates in the ECA study to be between 25 and 34 years for women and between 30 and 44 years for men.

The prevalence of panic attacks and panic disorder is usually higher in young subjects, particularly between 15 and 45 years of age.[15]

1%. Low prevalence rates are also reported in Asian sites (Nagasaki, Shanghai).

If prevalence rates of panic disorder in primary care patients seem to have similarities with those observed in the general population, this is not the case for patients referred to specialized consultations. Indeed, 15% of patients attending a clinic for vestibular disorders can be found to be suffering from panic disorder, as well as 16% of cardiac outpatients[32] and up to 35% of general hospital patients with hyperventilation symptoms (see Chapter 8).

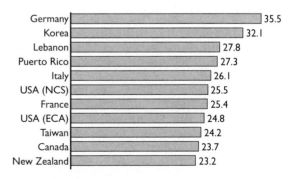

Figure 2.1 Mean age at onset of panic disorder in the cross-national epidemiology study (from Weissman et al[1]).

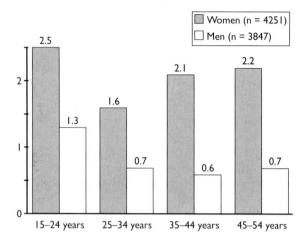

Figure 2.2 One-month prevalence of panic disorder by age group and by sex in the NCS (from Eaton et al[8]).

Another sociodemographic risk factor found to be associated with panic disorder is the fact of living in a city versus rural habitation.[23] Regarding cultural impact, similar prevalence rates were found in Japan, the USA and Canada for example (Table 2.1); the only exception is Taiwan, where very low prevalence rates were observed in both settings.[23]

Lastly, several studies have suggested that life events such as major loss or separation before 15 years of age,[35,36] early separation anxiety[37] or other childhood trauma,[14,38,39] and more specifically parental indifference and physical or sexual abuse[40,41] may enhance the risk of panic attacks and panic disorder in adulthood.

In the NCS study, the gender association of panic disorder seems to differ with age[8] (Figure 2.2).

The age pattern suggests a bimodality, with an early mode in the range 15–24 years, and a later one in the range 45–54 years. In the ECA study, people of 65 years of age or more had very low prevalence rates, of about 0.1%,[34] and panic disorder generally seems to be rare in the elderly.[27]

Marital status constitutes another significant risk factor for panic disorder: the highest lifetime prevalence rates are found in widowed, separated or divorced subjects.[15]

Educational level also produced strong differences in risk for panic disorder in the NCS.[8] People with fewer than 12 years of education were more than 10 times as likely to suffer from this disorder as the comparison sample with 16 or more years of education. However, no association was found between level of income and prevalence of panic disorder.

Comorbidity

The important issue of comorbidity between panic disorder and somatic disorders is discussed elsewhere (see Chapter 8). Our aim is here to consider the association between panic disorder and other psychiatric disorders, especially agoraphobia and affective disorders.

The first epidemiological evidence for comorbidity among anxiety disorders came from ECA data analysis, which showed that almost 50% of all subjects with a lifetime anxiety disorder had at least one other anxiety disorder.[42]

At every cross-national site, panic disorder has been found to be significantly associated with an increased risk for agoraphobia, with the odds ratio ranging from 7.5 in the ECA survey to 21.4 in Puerto Rico (Table 2.4).[1] A comorbidity pattern with agoraphobia is observed in 29.5–58.2% of subjects with panic disorder. In the NCS, where 50% of subjects with panic disorder reported no symptoms of agoraphobia,[8] the lifetime prevalence of panic disorder with agoraphobia was 1.5% and the

Table 2.4 Comorbidity of panic disorder with agoraphobia, with odds ratio adjusted by age and gender within each site (from Weissman et al[1])

	In subjects with panic disorder (%)	In subjects without panic disorder (%)	Odds ratio (95% CI)	
USA (ECA)	33.3	5.5	7.5	(5.6–10.1)
USA (NCS)	38.8	5.1	10.6	(7.3–15.5)
Canada (Edmonton)	31.8	2.7	15.1	(7.6–29.9)
Puerto Rico	58.2	6.0	21.4	(9.2–50.2)
France (Savigny)	48.9	6.5	12.7	(8.0–24.0)
Taiwan	22.5	1.4	17.2	(10.6–27.8)
Korea (Seoul)	34.7	2.1	17.2	(4.2–21.2)
New Zealand (Christchurch)	29.5	3.4	10.6	(7.3–15.5)

one-month prevalence of this association was 0.7%.

Social phobia is another condition frequently associated with panic disorder: 19.2–73.9% of subjects with social phobia reported lifetime symptoms of panic disorder in the cross-national studies. Goisman et al[43] have reported prevalences of 20% for generalized anxiety disorder, 14% for obsessive–compulsive disorder and 6% for post-traumatic stress disorder in patients with panic disorder.

Based on the cross-national sites data (Table 2.5), the lifetime odds ratios for association between panic disorder and major depression ranged from 3.8 in Savigny to 20.1 in Edmonton.[1] In the French study,[15] the odds ratio for lifetime major depressive episode in subjects with agoraphobia were the same for

men (4.33; 95% CI 1.06–17.7) as for women (4.11; 2.10–8.03). In the WHO–ADAMHA CIDI Field Trial study, Lépine et al[44] reported that when studying retrospectively the time sequence of panic disorder and affective disorders in 55 comorbid subjects, both occurred in the same year in 50.9%, 25.5% experienced onset of an affective disorder before panic and 23.6% had the reverse pattern.

In the ECA study, 20.8% of subjects with panic disorder had a comorbid bipolar disorder.[45]

Lastly, Regier et al[34] reported that 36% of subjects with panic disorder had substance or alcohol abuse in the ECA survey. Evidence for this comorbidity has also appeared in clinical studies, where alcoholism is observed in 13–43% of patients with panic disorder.[46]

Table 2.5 Comorbidity of panic disorder with major depression, with odds ratio adjusted by age and gender within each site (from Weissman et al[1])

	In subjects with panic disorder (%)	In subjects without panic disorder (%)	Odds ratio (95% CI)	
USA (ECA)	32.8	4.7	8.7	(6.4–11.7)
USA (NCS)	54.5	16.0	5.7	(4.0–8.1)
Canada (Edmonton)	68.2	9.2	20.1	(10.4–38.8)
Puerto Rico	38.2	3.7	15.3	(6.4–36.6)
France (Savigny)	48.9	17.3	3.8	(2.1–7.1)
Taiwan	22.5	1.3	19.6	(9.1–42.1)
Korea (Seoul)	28.4	2.5	13.2	(8.0–21.6)
New Zealand (Christchurch)	40.8	11.2	4.6	(2.2–9.4)

Suicidality

A significant association between panic disorder and suicide attempts in the general population was originally reported by Weissman et al[47] and Johnson et al.[48] In these reports, the majority of panic disorder subjects had other lifetime psychiatric disorders, but non-comorbid cases also were associated with an increased risk of suicide attempts (7% versus 1% in subjects without psychiatric disorders), as shown in Table 2.6.

In cross-national sites, significant odds ratios for history of suicide attempts in subjects with panic disorder versus those without panic disorder were found, ranging from 11.4 in Christchurch to 78.4 in Edmonton.

Further clinical studies have been conducted

Table 2.6 Lifetime prevalence rate of suicide attempts by diagnosis and comorbidity (from Johnson et al[48])

	Prevalence rate (%)
Panic disorder:	
without lifetime comorbidity	7.0
with lifetime comorbidity	23.6
Major depression:	
without lifetime comorbidity	7.9
with lifetime comorbidity	19.8
Panic disorder plus major depression	19.5
No psychiatric disorder	1.0

Table 2.7 Rate of suicide attempts (%) in patients with panic disorder according to lifetime diagnoses of major depression (MD), alcoholism and other substance abuse (from Lépine et al[49])

	Men (n = 37)	Women (n = 63)	Total (n = 100)
MD with alcoholism and/or substance abuse	57.1	81.8	72.2
MD without alcoholism and/or substance abuse	28.6	55.6	50.0
Alcoholism and/or other substance abuse without MD	42.9	50.0	46.2
No alcoholism, other substance abuse or MD	12.5	21.1	17.1

to examine this issue, and Lépine et al[49] reported that 42% (30% in men and 49% in women) of outpatients with panic disorder had a history of suicide attempts, this proportion being 17.1% in those without lifetime comorbid affective or substance abuse disorder (Table 2.7).

In this study,[49] all suicide attempts were by drug overdose, and 42.9% of cases required hospitalizations of longer than 24 hours. Analysing the time sequencing of disorders, showed the majority (73.8%) of suicide attempts occurred after the first panic attack. Divergent results have been reported by Beck et al,[50] in patients referred to a clinic for cognitive therapy in which no increased association between panic disorder and suicide was found. Methodological and sampling biases have been advanced as explanations of these discrepant results.[51]

Family and genetic factors

Familial and genetic studies are important elements in the validation of a nosologic entity and in enhancing the understanding of its etiopathogenesis.[52] In panic disorder, several familial studies have been conducted, and a few twin and linkage studies have been completed.

Ten studies have examined the prevalence rates of panic disorder, according to the DSM-III and DSM-III-R or Research Diagnostic Criteria (RDC), in first-degree relatives of probands with panic disorder, using direct interview or the family history method (Table 2.8).

When negative results are obtained, these family studies can provide strong evidence against genetic transmission of a disorder. Positive results can only *suggest* the existence of genetic factors, because familial aggregation

Table 2.8 Family studies of panic disorder

Authors and refs	Method[a]	Lifetime prevalence (%) for first-degree relatives		Relative risk
		Probands	Controls	
Crowe et al:[53]				
all relatives	History	31	4	7.8
interviewed only	Direct	41	8	5.1
Crowe et al[54]	Direct	17.3	1.8	9.6
Moran and Andrews[55]	History	12.5	—	—
Noyes et al[56]	Direct	14.9	3.5	4.3
Hopper et al[57]	History	11.6	—	—
Weissman[58]	Direct	14.2	0.8	17.7
Mendlewicz et al[59]	Direct	13.2	0.9	14.6
Maier et al[60]	Direct	7.9	2.3	3.4
Fyer et al[61] (panic disorder with agoraphobia)	Direct	10	3	3.3

[a]'Direct' indicates direct interview of relatives; 'History' indicates the family history method.

may be due to shared environment factors.[62] The lifetime rates of panic disorder in relatives of probands ranged between 7.9% and 41% versus 8% and less in controls. It should be noted that earlier studies, using prior concepts of 'irritable heart' (Da Costa syndrome), 'soldier's heart' or 'anxiety neurosis', also had reported familial aggregation for these conditions usually considered as close to panic disorder.[56,63,64]

Three studies have suggested a specific famil-ial aggregation for panic disorder, with a pattern distinct from that for generalized anxiety disorder (GAD).[54,56,65] Furthermore, Goldstein et al[66] observed specific familial aggregation for panic disorder, not associated with another anxiety or other psychiatric disorders, when proband comorbidity was controlled for. One exception could be for social phobia, with a significantly increased risk in relatives of panic disorder probands (5.7%, versus 1.6% in controls). Maier et al[60,67,68] also found an increased familial risk of major depression and alcoholism in panic patients, but Schuckit et al[69] did not find a high rate of panic disorder (3.4%) in 591 interviewed first-degree relatives of alcohol-dependent subjects. So these family studies suggest that the relative risk for first-degree relatives of panic disorder probands ranges from 2.6- to 20-fold, with a median value of 7.8.[62] These findings are consistent with a genetic transmission of panic disorder, with a relatively high specificity of heritability pattern.

There have been no adoption studies of panic disorder reported, but several twin studies have been conducted in order to compare the concordance rates between monozygotic and dizygotic pairs. Torgersen[70] published the first twin study on panic disorders, in a small Norwegian sample of 13 monozygotic twin pairs and 16 dizygotic twin pairs. This study showed a higher rate of concordance in monozygotic pairs (31%) than in dizygotic pairs (0%) for anxiety disorder with panic, but no significant difference for other psychiatric disorders. Methodological limitations of this study were a small sample size of twin pairs with panic disorder and the absence of blindness for co-twin interviews.

Skre et al[71] also found a more than twice higher concordance for panic disorder in 20 monozygotic twin pairs when compared with 29 dizygotic twin pairs. Nevertheless, Andrews et al[72] found no concordance difference between monozygotic and dizygotic twins for panic disorder, in an Australian registry of 446 twin pairs.

In a large sample of interviewed female twins from a population-based registry, Kendler et al[73] also assessed the genetic epidemiology of panic disorder. In this study, the familial aggregation of panic disorder appeared to be largely due to genetic factors, with moderate heritability of liability (30–40%). This lower heritability, as compared with the Torgensen study, can possibly be explained by the fact that the types of samples were not the same (population-based versus clinical samples, and only females in the Kendler study) and by methodological limitation of the first study as previously noted. Furthermore, Knowles and Weissman[62] underlined discrepancies between family studies and twin studies, since the risk in first-degree relatives of panic disorder probands is between 8% and 50% while concordance rates between dizygotic twins were 15% or less in twin studies.

Several genetic linkage studies have been conducted in pedigrees with panic disorder.

The first linkage study used 29 polymorphic blood antigenes in 26 families.[73] Most of the markers provided evidence against linkage, but a marker for α-haptoglobin, located on chromosome 16q22, gave a suggestive lod score of 2.27, even if the threshold level of 3 was not reached. Nevertheless, when confirmatory investigations were performed in the same sample families and in 10 additional families, these findings were not replicated, the maximum lod score then being 0.67.[74]

Candidate genes of tyrosine hydroxylase, pro-opiomelanocortin, adrenergic receptors and GABA$_A$ β1 receptor subunits have been excluded in such studies.[75-79] A recent study on 495 subjects from 26 pedigrees of probants with panic disorder found negative lod scores for eight GABA$_A$ receptor subunit genes.[80] Locus 20q13.2–13.3 has been proposed as a potent candidate gene in another linkage study conducted in 16 families with at least three subjects with DSM-III-R panic disorder (lod score 2.6), but these findings were not replicated by Crowe and colleagues.[62]

These linkage studies suggest that single-gene transmission is not probable. The findings support either genetic heterogeneity across different families and/or in favour of a polygenic model.[62] Moreover, more recent research in this area suggests genetic methods other than linkage studies (sib pairs, case-control studies and non-parametric analyses), to have improved efficacy for the study of the genetic factors of mental disorders.

Conclusions

During recent years, several epidemiologic studies conducted around the world have determined the relative consistency of the prevalence of panic disorder in the community. The annual prevalence is about 1%, and the lifetime prevalence has been found to range between 1.4% and 3.5%, with lower rates in some Asian countries. Rates are higher in women than in men, in younger, and in widowed, separated and divorced subjects. Comorbidity of panic disorder with other anxiety disorders and affective disorders has also been consistently reported in these studies. These comorbidity patterns have a large impact on the course and outcome of panic disorder (see Chapter 3) and may play a role on suici-dality associated with the disorder. Early-life events and parental attitudes have been stressed in retrospective studies as possible risk factors for panic disorder in adulthood. There is a familial aggregation of the disorder as shown by several studies, but, to date, evidence for genetic factors are still lacking.

Many unresolved issues remain in the epidemiologic field:

- the impact of modification of diagnostic criteria in the different classification systems;
- the role of the age of onset and a comparison of early- versus late-onset panic disorder;
- the risk factors for comorbidity;
- the interplay of developmental, environmental and genetic factors.

Studies addressing these different questions are currently ongoing, and one can expect that, in the near future, fruitful findings from the epidemiologic data, in conjunction with other fields of enquiry, will shed more light on the understanding of the pathophysiology of panic disorder.

References

1. Weissman MM, Bland RC, Canino GJ et al, The cross-national epidemiology of panic disorder. *Arch Gen Psychiatry* 1997; **54**: 305–9.
2. Barlow DH, Brown TA, Craske MG, Definitions of panic attacks and panic disorder in the DSM-IV: implications for research. *J Abnormal Psychol* 1994; **104**: 553–64.
3. Robins LN, Helzer JE, Croughan JL, The NIMH diagnostic interview schedule: its history, characteristics, and validity. *Arch Gen Psychiatry* 1981; **38**: 381–9.
4. Robins LN, Wing J, Wittchen HU et al, The composite international diagnostic interview: an epidemiologic instrument suitable for use in conjunction with different diagnostic systems and in different cultures. *Arch Gen Psychiatry* 1989; **45**: 1069–77.
5. Kessler RC, McGonagle KA, Zhao S et al, Lifetime and 12-month prevalence of DSM-III-R psychiatric disorders in the United States. Results from the National Comorbidity Survey. *Arch Gen Psychiatry* 1994; **51**: 8–19.
6. Weismann MM, Myers JK, Psychiatric disorders in a U.S. community: the application of Research Diagnostic Criteria to a resurveyed

community sample. *Acta Psychiatr Scand* 1980; **62**: 99–111.

7. Dean C, Surtees PG, Sashidharan SP, Comparison of research diagnostic systems in an Edinburgh community sample. *Br J Psychiatry* 1983; **142**: 247–56.

8. Eaton WW, Kessler RC, Wittchen HU, Magee WJ, Panic and panic disorder in the United States. *Am J Psychiatry* 1994; **151**: 413–20.

9. Eaton WW, Drymon A, Weissman MM, Panic and phobias. In: *Psychiatric disorders in America: The Epidemiologic Catchment Area Study* (Robins LN, Regier DA, eds). New York: The Free Press, 1991: 155–79.

10. Katerndahl DA, Realini JP, Lifetime prevalence of panic states. *Am J Psychiatry* 1993; **150**: 246–9.

11. Von Korff MR, Eaton WW, Keyl PM, The epidemiology of panic attacks and panic disorder: results of three community surveys. *Am J Epidemiol* 1985; **122**: 970–81.

12. Weissman MM, The hidden patient: unrecognized panic disorder. *J Clin Psychiatry* 1990; Suppl: 5–8.

13. Faravelli C, Degl'Innocenti BG, Aiazzi L et al, Epidemiology of anxiety disorder in Florence. *J Affect Disord* 1989; **19**: 1–5.

14. Aoki Y, Fujihara S, Kitamura T, Panic attacks and panic disorder in a Japanese nonpatient population: epidemiology and psychosocial correlates. *J Affect Disord* 1994; **32**: 51–9.

15. Lépine JP, Lellouch J, Classification and epidemiology of anxiety disorders. In: *Current Therapeutic Approaches to Panic and Other Anxiety Disorders* (Darcourt G, Mendlewicz J, Racagni G, Brunello N, eds). Int Acad Biomed Drug Res, Vol 8. Basel: Karger, 1994: 1–14.

16. Joyce PR, Bushnell JA, Oakley-Browne MA et al, The epidemiology of panic symptomatology and agoraphobic avoidance. *Comp Psychiatry* 1989; **30**: 303–12.

17. Angst J, Dobler-Mikola A, The Zurich study. V. Anxiety and phobia in young adults. *Eur Arch Psychiatry Clin Neurosci* 1985; **235**: 171–8.

18. Wittchen HU, Natural course and spontaneous remissions of untreated anxiety disorders: results of the Munich Follow-Up Study (MFS). In: (Hand I, Wittchen H-U, eds). *Panics and Phobias*, Vol. 2. Berlin: Springer-Verlag, 1986.

19. Bland RC, Orn H, Newman SC, Lifetime prevalence of psychiatric disorders in Edmonton. *Acta Psychiatr Scand* 1988; **77**(Suppl 338): 24–32.

20. Canino GJ, Bird HR, Shrout PE et al, The prevalence of specific psychiatric disorders in Puerto Rico. *Arch Gen Psychiatry* 1987; **44**: 727–35.

21. Wittchen HU, Essau CA, von Zerssen D et al, Lifetime and six-month prevalence of mental disorders in the Munich follow-up study. *Eur Arch Psychiatry Clin Neurosci* 1992; **241**: 247–58.

22. Karam E, Dépression et guerres du Liban: méthodologie d'une recherche. *Ann Psychol Sci Educ, Univ St Joseph (Beyrouth)* 1992: 99–106.

23. Hwu HG, Yeh EK, Chang LY, Prevalence of psychiatric disorders in Taiwan defined by the Chinese Diagnostic Interview Schedule. *Acta Psychiatr Scand* 1989; **79**: 136–47.

24. Lee CK, Kwak KS, Yamamoto J et al, Psychiatric epidemiology in Korea. Part I: Gender and age differences in Seoul. *J Nerv Ment Dis* 1990; **178**: 242–6.

25. Wells JE, Bushnell JA, Hornblow AR et al, Christchurch psychiatric epidemiology study, I: Methodology and lifetime prevalence for specific psychiatric disorders. *Aust NZ J Psychiatry* 1989; **23**: 315–26.

26. Lindal E, Stefansson JG, The lifetime prevalence of anxiety disorders in Iceland as estimated by the US National Institute of Mental Health Diagnostic Interview Schedule. *Acta Psychiatr Scand* 1993; **88**: 29–34.

27. Flint AJ, Epidemiology and comorbidity of anxiety disorders in the elderly. *Am J Psychiatry* 1994; **151**: 640–9.

28. Weissman MM, Leaf P, Tischler GL et al, Affective disorders in five United States communities. *Psychol Med* 1988; **18**: 141–53.

29. Sartorius N, Üstün B, Costa e Silva JA et al, An international study of psychological problems in primary care. *Arch Gen Psychiatry* 1993; **50**: 819–24.

30. Lecrubier Y, A worldwide primary care perspective. Paper presented at the 6th World Congress of Biological Psychiatry, Nice, France, 22–27 June 1997.

31. Ustun TB, Sartorius N, *Mental Illness in General Health Care: An International Study.* Chichester: Wiley, 1995.

32. Chignon JM, Lépine JP, Adès J, Panic disorder in cardiac outpatients. *Am J Psychiatry* 1993; **150**: 780–5.

33. Burke KC, Burke JD, Regier DA, Rae DS, Age at onset of selected mental disorders in five community populations. *Arch Gen Psychiatry* 1990; **47**: 511–18.

34. Regier DA, Boyd JH, Burk JD Jr et al, One-month prevalence of mental disorders in the United States: based on five Epidemiological Catchment Area sites. *Arch Gen Psychiatry* 1988; **45**: 977–86.

35. Battaglia M, Bertella S, Politi E et al, Age at onset of panic disorder: influence of familial liability to the disease and of childhood. *Am J Psychiatry* 1995; **152**: 1362–4.

36. Servant D, Parquet PJ, Early life events and panic disorder: course of illness and comorbidity. *Prog Neuropsychopharmacol Biol Psychiatry* 1985; **18**: 373–9.

37. Silove D, Harris M, Morgan A et al, Is early separation anxiety a specific precursor of panic disorder–agoraphobia? A community study. *Psychol Med* 1995; **25**: 405–11.

38. Dumas CA, Katerndahl DA, Burge SK, Familial patterns in patients with infrequent panic attacks. *Arch Fam Med* 1995; **4**: 863–7.

39. David D, Giron A, Mellman JA, Panic-phobic patients and developmental trauma. *J Clin Psychiatry* 1995; **56**: 113–17.

40. Brown GW, Harris TO, Aetiology of anxiety and depressive disorders in an inner-city population. 1. Early adversity. *Psychol Med* 1993; **23**: 143–54.

41. Stein MB, Walker JR, Anderson G et al, Childhood physical and sexual abuse in patients with anxiety disorders and in a community sample. *Am J Psychiatry* 1996; **153**: 275–7.

42. Weissman MM, Leaf P, Blazer DG et al, Panic disorder: clinical characteristics, epidemiology, and treatment. *Psychopharmacol Bull* 1986; **22**: 787–91.

43. Goisman RM, Warshaw MG, Peterson LG et al, Panic, agoraphobia and panic disorder with agoraphobia data from a multicenter anxiety disorders study. *J Nerv Ment Dis* 1994; **182**: 72–9.

44. Lépine JP, Wittchen HU, Essau CA and participants of the WHO–ADAMHA CIDI Field Trials, Lifetime and current comorbidity of anxiety and affective disorders: results from the International WHO–ADAMHA CIDI Field Trials. *Int J Meth Psy Res* 1993; **3**: 67–77.

45. Chen YW, Dilsaver SC, Comorbidity of panic disorder in bipolar illness: evidence from the epidemiologic catchment area survey. *Am J Psychiatry* 1995; **152**: 280–2.

46. Wittchen HU, Essau CA, Epidemiology of panic disorders: progress and unresolved issues. *J Psychiat Res* 1993; **27**(Suppl 1): 47–68.

47. Weissman MM, Klerman GL, Markowitz JS, Ouelette R, Suicidal ideation and suicide attempts in panic disorder and attacks. *N Engl J Med* 1989; **321**: 1209–41.

48. Johnson J, Weissman MM, Klerman GL, Panic disorder, comorbidity, and suicide attempts. *Arch Gen Psychiatry* 1990; **47**: 805–8.

49. Lépine JP, Chignon JM, Téhérani M, Suicide attempts in patients with panic disorder. *Arch Gen Psychiatry* 1993; **50**: 144–9.

50. Beck AT, Steer RA, Sanderson WC, Skeie TM, Panic disorder and suicidal ideation and behavior: discrepant findings in psychiatric outpatients. *Am J Psychiatry* 1991; **148**: 1195–9.

51. Weismann MM, Panic disorder: epidemiology and genetics. In: *Treatment of Panic Disorder. A Consensus Development Conference* (Wolfe BE, Maser JD, eds). Washington, DC: American Psychiatric Press, 1994: 31–9.

52. Weissman MM, Merikangas KR, John K et al, Family-genetic studies of psychiatric disorders. Developing techniques. *Arch Gen Psychiatry* 1986; **43**: 1104–16.

53. Crowe RR, Pauls DL, Slymen DJ, Noyes R, A family study of anxiety neurosis. Morbidity risk in families of patients with and without mitral valve prolapse. *Arch Gen Psychiatry* 1980; **37**: 77–9.

54. Crowe RR, Noyes R, Pauls DL, Slymen D, A family study of panic disorder. *Arch Gen Psychiatry* 1983; **40**: 1065–9.

55. Moran C, Andrews G, A familial occurrence of agoraphobia. *Br J Psychiatry* 1985; **146**: 262–7.

56. Noyes R Jr, Crowe RR, Harris EL, Relationship between panic disorder and agoraphobia. *Arch Gen Psychiatry* 1986; **43**: 227–32.

57. Hopper JL, Judd FK, Derrick PL, Burrows GD, A family study of panic disorder. *Genet Epidemiol* 1986; **4**: 33–41.

58. Weissman MM, Family genetic studies of panic disorder. *J Psychiat Res* 1993; **27**(Suppl 1): 69–78.

59. Mendlewicz J, Papadimitriou G, Wilmotte J, Family study of panic disorder: comparison with generalized anxiety disorder, major depression, and normal subjects. *Psychiatric Genet* 1993; **3**: 73–8.

60. Maier W, Lichtermann D, Minges J et al, A controlled family study in panic disorder. *J Psychiatr Res* 1993 27(Suppl 1): 79–87.

61. Fyer AJ, Mannuzza S, Chapman TF et al, Specificity in familial aggregation of phobic disorders. *Arch Gen Psychiatry* 1995; **52**: 564–73.

62. Knowles JA, Weissman MM, Panic disorder and agoraphobia. In: *Review of Psychiatry*, Vol. 14 (Oldham JM, Riba MB, eds). Washington, DC: American Psychiatric Press, 1995: 383–404.

63. Brown FW, Aetiology of Da Costa's syndrome. *Br Med J* 1941; i: 845–51.

64. Oppenheimer BS, Rotschild MA, The psychoneurotic factor in the irritable heart of soldiers. *J Am Med Assoc* 1918; **70**: 1919–22.

65. Harris EL, Noyes R Jr, Crowe RR, Chaudhry DR, Family study of agoraphobia: report of a pilot study. *Arch Gen Psychiatry* 1983; **40**: 1061–4.

66. Goldstein RB, Weissman MM, Adams PB et al, Psychiatric disorders in relatives of probands with panic disorder and/or major depression. *Arch Gen Psychiatry* 1994; **51**: 383–94.

67. Maier W, Minges J, Lichtermann D, Alcoholism and panic disorder: co-occurrence and co-transmission in families. *Eur Arch Psychiatry Clin Neurosci* 1993; **243**: 205–11.

68. Maier W, Minges J, Lichtermann D, The familial relationship between panic disorder and unipolar depression. *J Psychiatr Res* 1995; **29**: 375–88.

69. Schuckit MA, Hesselbrock VM, Tipp J et al, The prevalence of major anxiety disorders in relatives of alcohol dependent men and women. *J Stud Alcohol* 1995; **56**: 309–17.

70. Torgersen S, Genetic factors in anxiety disorders. *Arch Gen Psychiatry* 1983; **40**: 1085–9.

71. Skre I, Onstad S, Torgersen S et al, A twin study of DSM-III-R anxiety disorders. *Acta Psychiatr Scand* 1993; **88**: 85–92.

72. Andrews G, Stewart G, Allen R, Henderson AS, The genetics of six neurotic disorders: a twin study. *J Affect Disord* 1990; **19**: 23–9.

73. Kendler KS, Neale MC, Kessler RC et al, Panic disorder in women: a population-based twin study. *Psychol Med* 1993; **49**: 109–16.

74. Crowe RR, Noyes R, Wilson AF et al, A linkage study of panic disorder. *Arch Gen Psychiatry* 1987; **44**: 933–7.

75. Crowe RR, Noyes R, Samuelson S et al, Close linkage between panic disorder and α-haptoglobin excluded in 10 families. *Arch Gen Psychiatry* 1990; **47**: 377–80.

76. Mutchler K, Crowe RR, Noyes R Jr et al, Exclusion of tyrosine hydroxylase gene in 14 panic disorder pedigrees. *Am J Psychiatry* 1990; **147**: 1367–9.

77. Crowe RR, Noyes R, Persico AM, Pro-opiomelanocortin (POMC) gene excluded as a cause of panic disorder in a large family. *J Affect Disord* 1987; **12**: 23–7.

78. Wang ZW, Crowe RR, Noyes RJ, Adrenergic receptor genes as candidate genes for panic disorder: a linkage study. *Am J Psychiatry* 1992; **149**: 470–4.

79. Schmidt SM, Zoega T, Crowe RR, Excluding linkage between panic disorder and the γ-aminobutyric acid β1 receptor locus in five Icelandic pedigrees. *Acta Psychiatr Scand* 1993; **88**: 225–8.

80. Crowe RR, Wang Z, Noyes R Jr et al, Candidate gene study of eight $GABA_A$ receptor subunits in panic disorder. *Am J Psychiatry* 1997; **154**: 1096–100.

3

Panic disorder: clinical course, etiology and prognosis

Carlo Faravelli and Alessandra Paionni

CONTENTS • **Introduction** • **Panic disorder** • **Clinical course** • **Interpretations**

Introduction

Panic is the acute, sudden and intense form of anxiety. A panic attack is defined as a discrete period of intense fear or discomfort accompanied by somatic and cognitive symptoms. The anxiety that is characteristic of a panic attack can be differentiated from generalized anxiety by its intermittent, almost paroxysmal nature and its typically greater severity. The attack has a sudden onset and rapidly builds to a peak (usually in 10 minutes or less), and is often accompanied by a sense of imminent danger or impending doom and an urge to escape. A panic attack is also accompanied by clear and marked bodily symptoms: cardiocirculatory (palpitations, pounding heart, accelerated heart rate), respiratory (dyspnea, chest pain or discomfort, sensations of shortness of breath or smothering), neurological-like (dizziness, trembling or shaking, paresthesias), sweating, nausea or abdominal distress, and chills or hot flushes. The concomitant psychic symptoms are feelings of dizziness, unsteadiness, lightheaded-

ness or fainting, derealization or depersonalization, fear of losing control or going crazy, and fear of dying.

DSM IV[6] lists 13 symptoms, 4 of which are necessary in order to satisfy the criteria for a panic attack. Attacks where less than four symptoms are present are usually referred to as limited-symptom attacks. ICD-10[7] considers approximately the same set of symptoms. Individuals seeking help for panic attacks will usually describe the fear as intense and report that they thought they were about to die, lose control, have a heart attack or stroke, or 'go crazy'. They also usually report an urgent desire to flee from wherever the attack is occurring.

Often, the somatic symptoms mask anxiety, and such patients are primarily referred to non-psychiatric physicians.

Almost all physical symptoms are due to the activation of the sympathetic system: elevated plasma and urinary concentrations of adrenaline, noradrenaline and their metabolites (mainly 3-methoxy-4-hydroxyphenylethylene glycol, MHPG) have been reported.[1,2] Increased activity of platelet monoamine oxidase and reductions in the numbers of beta and alpha receptors have also been observed in patients with panic disorder.[3] The increased plasma levels of MHPG shown by panic patients exposed to phobic stimuli that previously elicited panic attacks give indirect support to the concept of the over-functioning of the noradrenergic system in panic disorder.[2,4] However, other studies have produced conflicting results: Woods et al[5] found that CO_2 inhalation that induced panic attacks had no effect on plasma free-MHPG levels.

The symptoms of panic may be present in a variety of situations: physical effort, use of or withdrawal from drugs, and medical conditions, including hyperthyroidism, pulmonary embolism, hypoglycemia, hyperparathyroidism, pheochromocytoma, vestibular dysfunctions, seizure disorders and cardiac conditions (arrhythmias, supraventricolar tachycardia), are commonly associated with the same set of symptoms. Generally, all the acute cardiopulmonary diseases may produce the same symptoms as panic. For this reason, the DSM IV[6] criteria for a panic attack require the explicit exclusion of organic causes – Criterion C states that 'the panic attacks are not due to the direct physiological effects of a substances (e.g. a drug of abuse, a medication) or a general medical condition (e.g. hyperthyroidism)'.

Even in the field of mental disorders, the panic attack can be part of several other conditions, including all the phobic states. In determining the differential diagnostic significance of a panic attack, it is important to consider the context in which the attack occurs.

Basically, there are two types of panic, depending on the presence or absence of situational triggers: unexpected panic attacks, in which the onset of the attack is not associated with a situational trigger (i.e. occurring spontaneously, 'out of the blue'), and situationally bound panic attacks, in which the attack almost invariably occurs immediately on exposure to, or in anticipation of, the situational cue. A third variation is that of situationally predisposed panic attacks, which are more likely to occur on exposure to the situational cue or trigger, but are not invariably associated with the cue and do not necessarily occur immediately after the exposure (for example, attacks are more likely to occur while driving, but there are times when the individual drives and does not have a panic attack or times when the attack occurs after driving for half an hour).

Unexpected panics and cued panics do not differ in terms of severity, although the relative frequency of symptoms differs according to the kind of panic. Subjects with unpredictable panic more often report symptoms such as dizziness, paresthesia, shaking, chest pain, and fear of going crazy or losing control. More than 90% of patients with unpredictable panic report feelings of loss of control and dizziness, which are less common among people suffering from situationally bound panic.[8] The kind of phobic stimuli may also be associated with a different somatic symptom pattern: shortness of breath is a common symptom in panic attacks associated with agoraphobia, whereas blushing is common in panics related to social or performance anxiety.[6]

Apart from phobic states, where panic is a basic aspect of the disorder, panic attacks may also be observed during the course of several other psychiatric conditions, including major depression, obsessive–compulsive disorder, borderline personality disorder, brief psychosis and others. In these cases it is controversial whether the panic attack should be considered as part of the original symptomatology or rather as an independently occurring phenomenon. Classifications that use an hierarchical approach tend to consider panic as secondary to the original state, whereas nosological systems that allow comorbidity enforce a double diagnosis.

Panic attacks may occasionally occur in otherwise healthy people without any particular pathological consequence (so-called sporadic or infrequent panic attacks). Between 2% and 30% of the adult population have panic attacks without ever meeting the criteria for panic disorder.

Panic disorder

Because panic attacks may be observed during the course of many psychiatric conditions and in healthy people, the DSM IV criteria[6] for panic disorder (PD) require that the presence of unexpected panic attack(s) is followed by at least one month of persistent concern about having another attack, worry about the possible implications or consequences of the attacks, or a significant behavioral change (Criterion A).

An unexpected panic attack is defined as one that is not associated with a situational trigger. At least two unexpected panic attacks are required for the diagnosis, but most individuals have considerably more. Individuals with PD frequently also have situationally predisposed panic attacks (i.e. those more likely to occur on, but not invariably associated with, exposure to a situational trigger). Situationally bound attacks (i.e. those that occur almost invariably and immediately on exposure to a situational trigger) can also occur, but are less common.

Panic disorder is therefore characterized by:

- recurrent panic attacks;
- anticipatory anxiety;
- agoraphobia;
- hypochondriasis;
- demoralization/secondary depression.

Recurrent panic attacks
The frequency and severity of the panic attacks vary widely: some individuals have moderately frequent attacks (e.g. once a week) that occur regularly for months at a time; others report short bursts of more frequent attacks (e.g. daily for a week) separated by weeks or months without any attacks, or with less frequent attacks (e.g. one attack per month) over many years. Limited-symptom attacks are also very common in individuals with panic. Although the distinction between full panic attacks and limited-symptom attacks is somewhat arbitrary, full-blown attacks are generally associated with a greater morbidity. Most individuals who have limited-symptom attacks have also had full panic attacks at some time during the course of the disorder. It is quite common to observe that the frequency of full-blown attacks tends to decrease during the course of the illness, whereas the limited-symptom attacks may persist for longer periods.

Anticipatory anxiety
After the first attack(s), most patients develop the fear that another attack may occur. During the intervals between attacks, therefore, the level of nonpanic (diffuse) anxiety increases. Anticipatory anxiety has many characteristics of the generalized anxiety: increase of attention, apprehension and hyperactivity. This condition can be so intrusive as to obscure the difference between a panic attack and generalized anxiety. It is speculated that such a higher level of diffuse anxiety may lower the threshold for panic, thus increasing the risk of new attacks.

Agoraphobia
'The essential feature of agoraphobia is anxiety about being in places or situations from which escape might be difficult (or embarrassing) or in which help may not be available in the event

of having a panic attack or panic-like symptoms (e.g. fear of having a sudden attack of dizziness or a sudden attack of diarrhea)'.[6] Other defining characteristics are physiological changes associated with accompanying panic attacks. These can include palpitations, lightness in the head, weakness, atypical chest pain, and dyspnea. Most agoraphobics also express fear of losing control, going insane, embarrassing themselves and others, dying, and fainting. The anxiety typically leads to a pervasive avoidance of a variety of situations, which may include being alone outside the home or being home alone, being in a crowd of people, traveling in a car, bus or airplane, or being on a bridge or in an elevator. The level of discomfort may range from mild uneasiness (with no avoidance) to severe distress with marked avoidance. Some individuals are able to expose themselves to the feared situations so endure these experiences but with considerable dread. Often an individual is better able to confront a feared situation when accompanied by a companion; other forms of support such as pushchairs and walking sticks can be helpful. In other cases, agoraphobia may become chronic, and individuals' avoidance of situations may impair their ability to travel to work or to carry out homemaking responsibility; therefore agoraphobia is a severely disabling illness.

The onset of agoraphobia usually follows the first panic attack (at least in clinical samples), with a time lag varying from a few days to several years. The course of agoraphobia and its relationship to the course of panic attacks is variable. In some cases, a decrease or remission of panic attacks is followed closely by a corresponding decrease in agoraphobic avoidance and anxiety. In other cases, the agoraphobia may become chronic regardless of the presence of panic attacks.

Approximately one-third to one-half of individuals diagnosed with PD in community samples also have agoraphobia, although the rate of agoraphobics is higher in clinical samples (around 75% of PD patients are agoraphobic).

Panic attacks, anticipatory anxiety and agoraphobia constitute the core system components of the panic/agoraphobia syndrome.[9–11] As Klein[10] points out, this disorder starts with the initial panic attack, which is followed by the fear of subsequent attacks (anticipatory anxiety) and then by the avoidance of situations that are believed to trigger panic attacks or result in embarrassment and/or danger in case of a new attack.

Cognitive factors related to panic anxiety have been described as contributing to the development of agoraphobia.[12,13] It has been hypothesized that the perception of the panic attack as a catastrophic medical problem, rather than a manifestation of anxiety, results in an exaggerated fear of having subsequent panic attacks. This unrealistic and exaggerated fear results in elevated anticipatory anxiety and in a stronger tendency to avoid situations that are believed to precipitate additional panic attacks.

Hypochondriasis

Most patients develop a particular attention towards their bodily sensations, with an exaggerated sensitivity to minor and normal changes. This sort of 'cenestophobia' makes some subjects avoid activities that provoke physical sensations that can be interpreted as anxiety-like (e.g. physical effort or drinking coffee). Many patients (around 20%) develop a true hypochondriacal elaboration, during which they are seriously afraid of being ill or even convinced that they have a medical problem. The hypochondriacal worries concern mainly the fear of cardiac illness or of epilepsy/other psychoneurological illness.

Demoralization

Some patients with PD or PD/agoraphobia (about 30%) develop feelings of sadness, guilt and anhedonie. Generally this state may be considered as psychological demoralization because patients' ability to live normally and to achieve social goals is seriously compromised by the disorder. In other cases, the possibility of a true depressive episode must be taken into account. This has major implications for treatment – see later chapters.

Sex ratio

The preponderance of women among patients with anxiety disorders is a consistent epidemiological and clinical finding. For PD without agoraphobia, the ratio of females to males is around one. The ratio of total numbers of patients is more like 3:1. The Epidemiologic Catchment Area (ECA) study in the USA suggested that the ratio in epidemiologic samples is approximately 3:2.[25] Women mainly predominate in agoraphobia cases: over three-quarters of PD patients manifesting extensive avoidance are women.[26–29] Women are also more likely to develop phobic complications, to present with generalized anxiety[30] and to have more depression.[31,32] (see also Chapter 2)

Male patients have a significantly longer duration of illness compared with females.[33] Women suffer significantly more frequently from anticipatory anxiety and from current or past depressive mood. In spite of the longer duration of illness in male patients, the less frequent occurrence of concomitant phobic avoidance and depressive disorders in males indicates that men might be less severely impaired than female patients. Males also display less frequent search for help;[32–34] the economic imperative for males to work may help reduce agoraphobia.

Early-life events

It has been suggested that there may be a link between the experience of traumatic life events during childhood and adolescence and the development of anxiety disorder in adults: Raskin et al,[35] examining developmental antecedents in a variety of types of anxiety disorder, found that 53% of the panic disorder group had some record of parental separation in childhood.

Faravelli et al[36] and Tweed et al[37] found that agoraphobics with panic attacks experience more traumatic life events (such as death of parents, prolonged separation from parents and divorce of parents) during childhood and adolescence compared with normal subjects.

Although part of the excess of these events is the result of a greater prevalence of psychiatric disorders in their families,[15] this does not entirely account for the bulk of the difference, and a cause-and-effect relationship between traumatic early-life events and anxiety disorders should be considered.

The occurrence of separation events during childhood/adolescence seems to be specifically associated with later development of agoraphobia. In fact, two-thirds of patients with panic and agoraphobia showed at least one traumatic event in the first 16 years of life, compared with 22% of panic patients without agoraphobia.[38]

Recently there has been increasing interest in child sexual abuse as a risk factor for the development of mental disorders. Saunders et al[39] report that in children physically and sexually abused before the age of five, the most common adult psychiatric disorder is agoraphobia, which occurs in 44%.

Maternal overprotection

It is a common clinical impression that the parents of patients with PD appear to be overprotective, stern and rigid.[40,41] On empirical grounds, Terhune,[42] Webster[43] and Tucker[44] all described a background of parental overprotection (especially maternal) in their agoraphobic patients.

Some support for this view comes from controlled studies, using the Maternal Overprotection Questionnaire, Solyom et al[45] found that the mothers of agoraphobics were more protective than those of normal controls.

Parker,[46] using the Parental Bonding Instrument (PBI), reported that patients suffering from anxiety neurosis scored both their parents as significantly less caring and more overprotective than did matched normal controls, whereas another study by Parker[47] found that agoraphobics differed from controls only on the scale measuring maternal care, which was reduced among patients.

Using the PBI in operationally defined PD, it was found that patients affected by PD reported childhood interactions with significantly less caring and more controlling parents.[48,49] No differences emerged between agoraphobic and non-agoraphobic patients, nor was there any correlation with the level of phobic avoidance. However, although the PBI has been shown to be an acceptable measure of actual, and not merely perceived parental characteristics, it is possible that subjects with emotional pathology might search in the past for the causes of their problems. They might attribute a more negative value to their earlier interactions with parents than these in fact warrant. On the other hand, as a family concentration of anxiety does exist, it is reasonable to conceive that parents with an anxious or phobic condition might have a reduced capacity to care for children and might overprotect the child as they protect themselves from the feared situations. Conversely, phobic-type behaviors of children, such as those frequently reported in the past personal history of patients with PD, could induce reactions of overprotection in their parents.

Separation anxiety

Increasing evidence points to an association between childhood anxiety and PD during adult life,[14,35,50–58] though some reports have failed to confirm this association.[59–62]

Silove et al[63–65] found that early separation anxiety was associated with risk of adult PD and that subjects with a lifetime history of PD/agoraphobia had more separation anxiety symptoms than those with generalized anxiety disorders (GAD) or other phobic disorders without a history of PD.

Pollack et al[56] reported that 55% of adult patients with PD met the criteria for childhood anxiety disorder, and found that those cases where a childhood history of anxiety was retraceable had a higher rate of comorbid anxiety disorder. Patients with a childhood history of anxiety disorders were also characterized by greater avoidance and greater fear of anxiety symptoms, even though they did not demonstrate a greater overall severity of PD.

Only one prospective study of well-diagnosed children with separation anxiety has been conducted:[55] PD was infrequent in these cases, but was significantly more elevated than in the controls. This supports the earlier work of Kagan et al[66] reported that behavioral inhibition in childhood may be a risk factor for the later development of anxiety disorders. Similarly Rosenbaum et al[67] reported a high rate of behavioral inhibition in young children of parents with PD and agoraphobia. To investigate further the link between behavioral inhibition and anxiety disorders, Biederman et al[68] examined the psychiatric correlates of behavioral inhibition by evaluating a sample of offspring of parents with PD and agoraphobia and an existing epidemiologically derived sample of children, followed during a seven-year period by Reznick et al.[69] They found that inhibited children had increased risk of multiple anxiety, overanxiety and phobic disorders, especially social phobia.

Further evidence for the link between childhood and adult anxiety psychopathology comes from family studies reporting high rates of childhood anxiety difficulties in the offspring of adult patients with PD;[17,51,70] whether childhood anxiety predisposes the individual to adult PD by influencing cognitive or behavioral reactions to symptoms, or is an early manifestation of the same disorder, is still unclear.

Personality

Anecdotal reports contend that PD subjects had a normal or even sociable and outgoing nature, before the onset of the disorder. Even though this is true as a superficial observation, clinicians have long suspected that patients with agoraphobia have more dependent personality traits than the average person. Andrews[71] hypothesized that dependence on others was a major coping style of agoraphobic patients. To some extent this was reported by Shafar,[72] who, using undefined ratings, concluded that dependence problems were present in 38% of her agoraphobic patients, and Buglass et al,[73] although reporting an overall negative study, found that 27% of their patients and none of their control subjects were aware of dependence about which they were resentful. Finally, Torgersen,[74] in his study of monozygotic twins, found that the agoraphobic twin was most likely to be dependent.

Faravelli et al[75] investigated the personality of subjects affected by PD during a phase of remission. Personality scales revealed pessimism, excessive preoccupation for physical functions, insecurity, egocentrism, immaturity, excessive ruminations, indecisiveness and

excessively high standards of morality. The Maudsley Personality Inventory revealed high levels of neuroticism, and the Sensation Seeking Scale showed the wish of agoraphobic subjects to cope with those situations they do not dare confront in reality.

Since all these studies are retrospective, it is not clear whether the dependent personality traits observed are primary or secondary to the occurrence of the symptoms. On the one hand, the possibility that this disorder might be a predisposing condition for the development of PD is supported by the findings of Nystrom and Lyndergard:[76] in a prospective study of more than 3000 subjects, these authors found dependent premorbid personality traits in persons who later developed anxiety disorders. Consequently, it is not unreasonable to believe that personality traits or disorders contribute to the development of an illness. On the other hand, it may be that personality disturbances are secondary to panic disorder, especially when complicated by phobic avoidance. Some patients claim that before the onset of their phobic disorder they had been independent and self-confident, in contrast to the fearful clinging to a companion that later accompanied their illness. Their avoidant behavior and phobic cognitive style may well have contributed to an unwelcome dependence.

Age of onset

The age of onset for PD varies considerably, but most typically is situated between late adolescence and the mid-30s. In clinical samples, the mean age of onset is around 25 years. There may be a bimodal distribution, with one peak in late adolescence and a second smaller peak in the mid-30s.[28] A small number of cases begin during childhood. In about 15% of the patients, onset is after age 40.[33,77] Whereas PD without agoraphobia prevailed during the late 20s, PD with agoraphobia most frequently developed during the early 20s.

Prodromal experiences

Klein[10] suggested that patients are often feeling quite well when they suddenly are struck by a panic attack. After the first panic attacks, they develop persistent anticipatory anxiety and hypochondriacal fears. These lead to avoidant behavior, so that agoraphobia ensues. Several papers report that, in psychiatric samples, panic precedes agoraphobia.[10,50,78] However, Roth[79] first observed that, even though the first attack of panic often develops abruptly, 'more detailed investigation will usually reveal that the disorder has not emerged out of an entirely clear sky and that the complex repertoire of avoidance behaviors and helpless dependence on others were not entirely without premorbid antecedents'. Fava et al[80] confirm Roth's remarks: the large majority of patients (90%) suffered from mild phobic or hypochondriacal symptoms before the onset of panic attacks. Anxiety and hypochondriacal fears and beliefs were also exceedingly common.

Lelliott et al[81] found that, at least in Britain, the first panic attack occurred more often in late spring–summer and during warm weather than in winter and cold weather.

Situations of onset

Following a study on the context in which the first panic attack occurs, Lelliott et al[81] reported that 92% of their agoraphobic patients with panic experienced their first panic attack in a phobogenic situation rather than at home. These sites are usually a loosely knit agoraphobic cluster of public places, such as streets, stores, public transportation, auditoria and crowds, and, less centrally, elevators, tunnels, bridges, open spaces and heights.

The findings of Lelliott et al are consistent with those reported by Faravelli et al,[82] who found that most agoraphobic patients experienced their first panic attack in a phobogenic situation. In addition, they found that such an onset was significantly less common among patients with panic disorder who did not develop agoraphobia.

The association between public onset and agoraphobia merits special interest. A possible interpretation is that a sort of subclinical agoraphobia precedes clinical panic, thus supporting the previously mentioned view that some predisposition predates the acute onset of PD. Lelliott et al[81] suggest a role for an ethological factor (an evolutionary vulnerability to extraterritoriality), in addition to the biological and learning components of the disorder. While such a model is fascinating, it does not explain satisfactorily why such an onset is rare among patients with PD without agoraphobia. Another simpler interpretation could be taken into account. The different psychological meaning of the context in which panic occurs might explain the evolution of the disorder. Experiencing the drama of an unexpected panic attack in a setting in which, objectively, help is not available has a different psychological impact than experiencing the same symptoms in protected settings (e.g. at home). It is possible that undergoing such a stressful experience as having an attack in contexts in which one is helpless might affect the later course of the disorder. In this case, the basic core of PD would be the pathological evolution of panic, rather than panic itself.

Precipitants

Panic attacks could be artificially provoked in predisposed subjects by a series of chemical challenges: sodium lactate, bicarbonate, caffeine, cholecystokinin or hypercapnia (see Chapter 5). Outside such experimental challenging procedures, the occasional use of these substances may induce the first attack in predisposed people (e.g. caffeine contained in tablets for migraine, or adrenergic agonists prescribed therapeutically).

Some patients report that panic attacks may be triggered by physical exercise (through accumulation of lactate?), sexual intercourse and sudden temperature changes.[83–85]

Stressful life events

Uncontrolled clinical descriptions have reported that often the first panic attack is preceded by some stressful life event.[35,86,87] Controlled studies generally confirm the excess of life stress prior to the onset of PD.[88–90] Faravelli and Pallanti[88,89] found that panic patients experience more life events in the year before the onset of the illness than do healthy control subjects, and that the highest concentration of life stress occurs in the last few months before the initial symptoms. However, they did not confirm the findings of Finlay-Jones and Brown,[87] who reported that danger events were significantly overrepresented among patients with 'anxiety', whereas loss events were more frequent among patients with 'depression'. Roy-Byrne et al[91] examined the subsequent course of illness in patients with PD as a function of whether or not the onset of illness had been preceded by major loss or separation. Their results suggest that the occurrence of severe loss before the onset is not related to the severity of subsequent anxiety symptoms, but does appear to be related to the subsequent occurrence of a major depression.

Since events preceding the onset of the disorder are generally assigned a causative–precipitating role, it is plausible to suggest that the same types of events would have a role in maintaining or exacerbating the disorder. This would be consistent with a recent study showing that agoraphobic patients who continued to experience adverse life events after behavioral treatment had a poorer outcome.[92]

Clinical course

Clinical course, short- and long-term outcome

Anxiety neurosis, a forerunner of panic disorder, was generally thought to be a mild condition, not severely disabling and with a favorable outcome. However, even the earliest follow-up studies revealed that the long-term recovery rates for this disorder were low.[93] After the DSM III reclassification of anxiety disorders,[94] several reports focused on the long-term outcome of PD. Retrospective descriptions by individuals seen in clinical settings suggest that the usual course of the illness is generally chronic, with waxing and waning. Some individuals may have episodic outbreaks with years of remission in between, and others may have continuous severe symptomatology.

Specific follow-up studies confirm the general chronicity of PD, although through an ample variety of possible outcomes. Although the earliest studies, which included relatively brief follow-up periods, showed a relatively good prognosis, with recovery rates ranging from 25% to 72% after one or two years,[95–97] further studies reported less-favorable outcomes.[98–101] After five years of prospective follow-up, only 10–12% of patients had fully recovered (i.e. with no symptoms and no treatment).

Moreover, higher risks of suicide, major depressive episodes and cardiovascular diseases, as well as increased general morbidity and mortality, have been reported in these patients.[19,102,103] However, since PD is frequently comorbid with other axis I and II disorders, the long-term consequences could be attributed to the comorbid condition rather than to PD itself. Recent studies seem to confirm this position: the worst consequences in terms of fatality, morbidity and substance abuse seem to be related to the associated conditions.[103–105]

Noyes et al[100] found that patients with extensive phobic avoidance or agoraphobia have a more severe form of panic disorder, with a longer duration of illness, more severe symptoms and greater social maladjustment than subjects with limited or no phobic avoidance. Breier et al,[34] Lesser et al[106] and Noyes et al[100] found that subjects with panic disorder plus secondary depression (current or past) were part of a more severely ill group. They had been ill longer and had more severe anxiety symptoms, more frequent panic attacks and more extensive phobic avoidance, and they more frequently had personality disorders. There is some evidence that concomitant personality disorders influence the outcome of patients with PD: the presence of a personality disturbance in fact predicts a less favorable treatment response.[100,107,108]

Faravelli et al,[101] in a naturalistic follow-up study, in which only patients with PD as the primary psychopathologic condition were studied, found that the rate of recovery is relatively low (12%) and that PD tends to be a chronic disturbance. The long-term outcome shows a wide variability, with the intermediate outcome of being neither ill nor well being the most common. Among the predictors taken into consideration, only duration of the disorder before treatment showed a close relationship to outcome: patients with a shorter duration of illness more frequently experienced complete recovery or remission and reported fewer relapses. In this sample, the number of patients exhibiting suicidal type behavior was small.

Comorbidity

Panic disorder is often associated with other anxiety disorders and with depression. There are reports that 35–91% of patients with panic disorder also suffer from major depressive episodes during their life.[109–111] In many cases, both disorders occur at the same time.[112] In others, PD occurs before the onset of depressive disorder as well as before the onset of substance abuse.[113] (See Chapter 2)

Breier et al[34] found that patients with PD and/or agoraphobia who had a current or past major depressive episode had more severe symptoms of both anxiety and depression than those who had never been depressed. In a naturalistic study, Van Valkenburg et al[114] reported that patients with secondary depression had an earlier age at onset of their PD, but did not differ from nondepressed patients with panic disorder in their treatment response or psychosocial outcome. While it might be reasonable to expect that patients with depression would have suffered from PD longer than those without depression, patients with and without histories of depression have had PD for similar periods of time.[115] Also, while it is conceivable that patients with more severe agoraphobic avoidance would be more likely to experience depression than patients with less severe avoidance, such a pattern was not supported by empirical evidence. Thus there is little support for the hypothesis that the depression that frequently complicates PD is etiologically secondary to the long-term demoralizing effects of chronic agoraphobic avoidance.

The coexistence of social phobia and PD is far from rare. While neither duration of PD nor agoraphobic severity was related to a history of major depression, the concomitant diagnosis of social phobia was associated with significantly greater lifetime risk of depression. The data, however, should not be used to support a casual relationship. It is possible that, in making concomitant diagnoses of social phobia, we are identifying a subgroup of PD patients with a constellation of personality traits that includes low self-esteem, extreme self-consciousness and a tendency toward negative self-appraisal. Such a subgroup could be at considerable risk of depression on the basis of psychological – particularly cognitive – factors. Additionally, the social isolation experienced as a result of social avoidance could contribute to a propensity to become depressed. Alternatively, concomitant social phobia may merely be a marker for a more severe illness.

Since the co-occurrence of significant obsessive–compulsive symptoms has also been noted to increase the lifetime risk of depression in patients with PD, it is possible that PD complicated by the presence of any other disorder, rather than social phobia specifically, may increase the risk of depression.

Another risk factor in PD is the development of alcohol abuse, which some view as 'self-medication'.[23] Unquestionably, intake of alcohol initially decreases anticipatory anxiety in patients with panic disorder, but alcoholism later becomes a complication.[116] Several studies[16,20] suggest that PD has a higher than expected prevalence among alcoholics compared with the general population. The question concerning primacy and any causal relationship between the two disorders, i.e. whether alcoholism leads to the development of anxiety disorders or vice versa, is less clear. George et al[117] suggest that a possible mechanism for the link between alcoholism and anxiety is a kindling process: the hyperresponsive CNS state that results from repeated alcohol withdrawal may, in susceptible individuals, give rise to a heightened state of anxiety and panic attacks, even during sobriety.

A model based on a kindling process has been proposed for alcohol dependence by Ballenger and Post.[118] They demonstrate that the alcohol withdrawal syndrome becomes progressively more severe with increasing years of heavy daily alcohol abuse, irrespective of age. They propose that repeated episodes of withdrawal in chronic alcoholics serve as stimuli for kindling of subcortical structures, primarily limbic, hypothalamic and thalamic nuclei. They hypothesize that the spectrum of withdrawal symptoms from mild withdrawal with tremor and autonomic symptoms to the more severe withdrawal symptoms of hallucinations, psychic symptoms, epileptic seizures and delirium tremens are secondary to cumulative physiological changes that accompany a kindling-like process. Malcolm et al,[119] in a double-blind controlled study, found that carbamazepine, because of its ability to both retard the development of kindling and suppress established kindled foci, is as effective and safe as benzodiazepine treatment for alcohol withdrawal.

Apart from the above-mentioned affective disorders, there are relatively few other psychiatric conditions appearing after the onset of PD. Thus PD appears to be more likely to be preceded by another psychiatric disorder than to be a chronologically primary condition. This finding implies that some primary disorders (e.g. simple phobia, social phobia or substance abuse) may represent a specific predisposition for the development of PD, and has treatment implications (see later chapters).

Suicide and quality of life

Using data from the Epidemiologic Catchment Area (ECA) study, Markowitz et al[120] reported that PD (with or without agoraphobia) was associated with a greater risk of poor physical and emotional health, alcohol and other drug abuse, suicide attempts, poorer marital functioning and greater financial dependence. The risk of PD was even greater than for major depression for many measures, including alcohol abuse and financial dependence. ECA suicide rates for the separate diagnoses of PD or major depression alone were similar, and were higher than rates for the general population. Coryell[121] reviewed earlier studies from 1936 to 1986, and concluded that patients with anxiety states appeared as likely as patients with primary depression to commit suicide. Weissman et al[102] found a very high rate of suicide attempt and suicidal ideation in subjects suffering from PD, even when controlling for lifetime major depressive episode and alcoholism. Lepine et al[103] found that 42% of outpatients with PD had attempted suicide at some time during their lives. In patients with PD, they found demographic determinants for suicide attempts to be similar to those of other clinical populations, such as depressed patients: the suicide attempts occur most frequently in single, divorced or widowed women. In this study, the authors found a significantly longer duration of PD at the time of referral in suicide attempters. Otherwise, the severity of the worst episode of PD did not differ between suicide attempters and non-attempters. They found that suicide attempts in patients with PD were often associated with a lifetime diagnosis of major depressive episodes and alcohol and/or other substance abuse. Warshaw et al[122] found that suicidal behavior in subjects with PD seems to be better related to factors not inherent in the PD. The presence of depression, post-traumatic stress disorder, eating disorders, substance abuse/dependence or personality disorders (in particular, borderline and antisocial personality disorders) increased the risk. Factors related to quality of life (in fact, being married or having a child, and working

full-time reduced the risk of suicide attempts protective factors).

Areas of controversy and debate

Since the introduction of the DSM III,[94] the nosological position of panic disorder has been controversial. Two positions have arisen and given rise to a long-lasting debate.

On the one hand, most North American psychiatrists consider the panic attack as the central feature of the disorder. Panic is seen as an inherently pathological, primary phenomenon, central to the origin of the disorder. Its association with agoraphobia is interpreted as the avoidance behavior being a secondary or a derived phenomenon, from both etiopathogenetic and chronological points of view.[10,78] This position considers the panic attack as a predominantly biological event, qualitatively distinct from the other forms of anxiety. Moreover, the American view of panic disorder is that repeated, sudden and spontaneous panic attacks are only seen in panic disorder. Panic attacks seen in other conditions are not spontaneous.

Since agoraphobia is considered solely as a consequence of panic, this position denies its existence without panic. Several studies support this view. First, there is Klein's observation[86] of a specific response of panic attacks to tricyclic antidepressants, which were considered not effective on other anxiety disorders.[123,124] The fact that panic attacks could be artificially provoked in predisposed subjects by a series of chemical challenges reinforced the hypothesis of a biological origin of this disorder. The possibility of provoking anxiety in normal subjects and of increasing the frequency of panic attacks in panic patients by the use of yohimbine or isoproterenol point to an important role for the noradrenergic system in this disorder. These studies suggest a possible subsensitivity of post-synaptic α_2 inhibitory adrenoceptors in panic patients, with an increasing firing rate of the locus ceruleus.[4] Consistent with this hypothesis is the observation that drugs that prevent spontaneous panic attacks appear to reduce the locus ceruleus firing rate,[125] whereas the panicogenic stimuli usually increase this firing. The increased plasma levels of 3-methoxy-4-hydroxy-phenylethylene glycol shown by panic patients exposed to phobic stimuli give indirect support to the noradrenergic hypothesis,[2,4] although other studies have produced conflicting results.[5]

In favor of the American view are also electroencephalographic data, which show that night panics occur outside rapid eye movement phases of sleep.[126–128] Alterations of EEG[129–131] and cerebral blood flow,[132–134] anatomical abnormalities in the mesiotemporal region on magnetic resonance imaging,[135] hyposensitivity to benzodiazepines[136] and neurological soft signs have all been reported in PD. As a confirmation of some biological abnormality, Nutt et al[137,138] have demonstrated that flumazenil is anxiogenic in patients with PD: possible explanations of this finding are that in PD there is a relative deficiency of an anxiolytic ligand, or that the setpoint of the benzodiazepine receptor is shifted in the inverse agonist direction. (For a detailed analysis of the brain mechanism and circuits of PD see Chapter 5).

Not all these findings may be unequivocally interpreted as in favor of the biological view. The response to a chemical challenge, for instance, can be seen as the intrapsychic dramatization of bodily sensations, rather than as a specific substance response. The fact that the various chemical challenges do not share any common mechanism could be explained on this basis. Also, the broad range of drugs effec-

tive for panic could suggest a low biological specificity. Moreover, the specificity of the response of panic anxiety to tricyclic antidepressants has not been confirmed in other trials, where other forms of anxiety e.g. GAD proved to respond to these drugs.[139,140]

Two main categories of clinicians disagree with this so-called biological theory: many European psychiatrists and cognitive–behavioral psychologists. They contend that the single panic attack is an aspecific phenomenon, which can be found in many other conditions: somatic illnesses, depression, alcohol abuse, anorexia nervosa, borderline states, acute psychosis, etc.[34,100,106,117,141,142] Isolated panic attacks are also frequent in normal subjects.[143,144] This position therefore contends that panic per se is neither specific nor pathological. Panic becomes pathological when its occurrence is combined with specific premorbid vulnerability factors. Preconstitutive aspects of panic must exist either as a peculiar cognitive pattern or as a vulnerability to environmental events. The European position maintains that a phobic attitude precedes the development of panic and that specific temperamental features are necessary in order for PD to occur. There are findings that seem to support this position. All community epidemiological studies report the presence of a consistent rate of subjects affected by agoraphobia without panic attacks.[28,145–147] Patients affected by PD were reported to show prodromal symptoms before the onset of the disorder.[80,81,148,149] The presence of personological–temperamental traits predisposing to agoraphobia is also supported by studies of the premorbid personality of these patients. The importance of early environmental factors was confirmed by empirical verification. As often happens with biological data, however, all of these findings may lend themselves to different interpretations. For instance, the abnormal response to life events could be due to impairment of the cerebral neuroendocrine systems that should cope with stress. Recent findings report that patients with PD show a blunted adrenocorticotropic hormone response to corticotropin-releasing hormone in association with basal hypercortisolism.[150–152]

The above-mentioned positions represent extreme views of the problem, and many authors admit the possibility of an intermediate view. In an integrated model, in which biological and environmental factors should necessarily be interconnected, the autonomic nervous system (ANS) could have a basic role in the pathogenesis of PD. This involvement may be inferred on the basis of several considerations:

(a) most of the somatic symptoms of the panic attack are mediated by the ANS;
(b) increased values of autonomic functions are common observations in patients with PD even outside the panic attacks;
(c) several papers have reported dys- (over-) functioning of the noradrenergic system in PD at both the central and peripheral levels;[1,2]
(d) some theoretical models, of which the learning theory[153] is probably the best known, propose that hyperactivity of the ANS, interacting with conditioning, is at the basis of neuroses.

Given that personal autonomic reactivity may vary from birth, we can hypothesize that childhood development of cognition may be influenced by different degrees of bodily sensations. We can imagine that one child will react with severe palpitations, shortness of breath and excessive sweating when exposed to a moderately fearful stimulus, while another will experience only mild sensations. It is possible to speculate that the development of the personal cognitive pattern will be different in the two children, leading to an insecure temperament in one case and to self-confidence in the other. A tendentially insecure child will limit his or her exposure to new situations and thus reinforce his or her tendency to avoid and escape. In turn, insecurity on the part of the child is likely to induce protective behavior in his or her parents.

On the other hand, the same factors, acting on the parents' side, are likely to influence their upbringing patterns. Anxious and insecure mothers will protect their children from situations they fear. The child will grow up in a context characterized by an increased level of anxiety, overprotection and low quality of care. This environment might provoke phobic behavior in the child, which in turn increases parental overprotection, in a vicious circle. Children with such a background will be more prone to developing peculiar personality traits. They may reasonably tend to dramatize any circumstance that may challenge the stability they have achieved. The 'catastrophizing' pattern described by cognitive psychologists[154,155] could well be consistent with this.

Further anxiety-inducing events (stressful events, chemicals, primarily somatic sensations) will cause a pathological level of anxiety in these subjects, because of both the persisting biological predisposition and the psychic dramatization of the bodily symptoms.

References

1. Charney DS, Heninger GR, Noradrenergic dysfunction in panic anxiety. Aetiology and treatment studies. *Clin Neuropharmacol* 1984; 7(Suppl): S99.
2. Ko GN, Elsworth JD, Roth RH et al, Panic induced elevation of plasma MHPG levels in phobic-anxious patients. *Arch Gen Psychiatry* 1983; 40: 425–30.
3. Cameron OG, Smith CB, Platelet alpha 2 adrenergic receptor binding and plasma catecholamines before and during imipramine treatment in patients with panic anxiety. *Arch Gen Psychiatry* 1984; 41: 114–48.
4. Charney DS, Heninger GR, Breier A, Noradrenergic function and panic anxiety effects of yohimbine in healthy subjects and patients with agoraphobia and panic disorder. *Arch Gen Psychiatry* 1984; 41: 751–63.
5. Woods SW, Charney DS, Goodman WK et al, Carbon dioxide-induced anxiety: behavioural physiologic and biochemical effects of carbon dioxide in patients with panic disorder and healthy subjects. *Arch Gen Psychiatry* 1988; 45: 43–52.
6. American Psychiatric Association, *Diagnostic and Statistical Manual of Mental Disorders*, 4th edn draft. Washington: APA, 1993.
7. World Health Organization, *The ICD-10 Classification of Mental and Behavioural Disorders: Clinical Descriptions and Diagnostic Guidelines*. WHO: Geneve, 1992.
8. Barlow DH, Vermileyea J, Blanchard EB et al, The phenomenon of panic. *Abnormal Psychol* 1985; 94: 320–8.
9. Marks IM, Agoraphobic syndrome (phobic anxiety state). *Arch Gen Psychiatry* 1970; 23: 538–53.
10. Klein DF, Anxiety reconceptualized. In: *Anxiety: New Research and Changing Concepts* (Klein DF, Raskin J, eds). New York: Raven Press, 1981: 235–63.
11. Sheehan DV, Panic attacks and phobias. *N Engl J Med* 1982; 3: 235–63.
12. Goldstein AJ, Chambless DL, A reanalysis of agoraphobia. *Behavior Ther* 1978; 9: 47–59.
13. Thorpe GL, Burns LE, *The Agoraphobic Syndrome*. New York: Wiley, 1983.
14. Crowe RR, Noyes R, Pauls DL, Slymen D, A family study of panic disorder. *Arch Gen Psychiatry* 1983; 40: 1065–9.
15. Harris EL, Noyes R, Crowe RR et al, Family study of agoraphobia. *Arch Gen Psychiatry* 1983; 40: 1061–4.
16. Leckman JF, Weissman MM, Merikangas KR et al, Panic disorder and major depression: increased risk of depression, alcoholism, panic, and phobic disorders in families of depressed probands with panic disorder. *Arch Gen Psychiatry* 1983; 40: 1055–60.
17. Weissman MM, Leckman JF, Merikangas KR et al, Depression and anxiety disorders in parents and children: results from the Yale Family Study. *Arch Gen Psychiatry* 1984; 41: 845–52.
18. Goldstein RB, Weissman MM, Adams PB et al, Psychiatric disorders in relatives of probands with panic disorder and/or major depression. *Arch Gen Psychiatry* 1994; 51: 383–94.
19. Coryell WH, Endicott J, Andreasen NC et al, Depression and panic attacks: the significance of overlap as reflected in follow-up and family study data. *Am J Psychiatry* 1988; 145: 293–300.
20. Noyes R, Crowe RR, Harris EL et al, Relationship between panic disorder and agoraphobia: a family study. *Arch Gen Psychiatry* 1986; 43: 227–32.
21. Mendlewicz J, Papadimitriou G, Wilmotte J, Family study of panic disorder: comparison with generalized anxiety disorders, major depression, and normal subjects. *Psychiatr Genet* 1993; 3: 73–8.
22. Bowen RC, Kohut J, The relationship between agoraphobia and primary affective disorders. *Can J Psychiatry* 1979; 24: 317–21.
23. Munjack M, Moss HB, Affective disorder and alcoholism in family of agoraphobics. *Arch Gen Psychiatry* 1981; 38: 869–71.
24. Torgersen S, Genetic factors in anxiety disorders. *Arch Gen Psychiatry* 1983; 40: 1085–9.
25. Von Korff MR, Eaton WW, Keyel PM, The epidemiology of panic attacks and panic disorder. *Am J Epidemiol* 1985; 122: 970–81.

26. Myers JK, Weissman MM, Tischler CE et al, Six-month prevalence of psychiatric disorders in three communities. *Arch Gen Psychiatry* 1984; **41**: 959–67.

27. Thyer BA, Parrish RT, Curtis GC et al, Ages of onset of DSM-III anxiety disorders. *Compr Psychiatry* 1985; **26**: 113–22.

28. Wittchen HU, Epidemiology of panic attacks and panic disorders. In: *Panic and Phobias: Empirical Evidence of Theoretical Models and Longterm Effects of Behavioral Treatments* (Hand I, Wittchen HU, eds). Berlin: Springer-Verlag, 1986: 18–28.

29. Barlow DH, *Anxiety and Its Disorders*. New York: The Guildford Press, 1988.

30. Aronson TA, Logue CM, On the longitudinal course of panic disorder. Developmental history and predictors of phobic complications. *Compr Psychiatry* 1987; **28**: 344–55.

31. Dealy RS, Ishiki DM, Avery DM, Secondary depression in anxiety disorders. *Compr Psychiatry* 1981; **22**: 612–18.

32. Buller R, Maier W, Benkert O, Clinical subtypes in panic disorder: Their descriptive and prospective validity. *J Affective Disord* 1986; **11**: 105–14.

33. Scheibe G, Albus M, Age at onset, precipitating events, sex distribution, and co-occurrence of anxiety disorders. *Psychopathology* 1992; **25**: 11–18.

34. Breier A, Charney DS, Heninger GR, Major depression in patients with agoraphobia and panic disorder. *Arch Gen Psychiatry* 1984; **41**: 1129–35.

35. Raskin M, Peeke HVS, Dickman W et al, Panic and generalized anxiety disorders: developmental antecedents and precipitants. *Arch Gen Psychiatry* 1982; **39**: 587–9.

36. Faravelli C, Webb T, Ambonetti A et al, Prevalence of traumatic early life events in 31 agoraphobic patients with panic attacks. *Am J Psychiatry* 1985; **142**: 1493–4.

37. Tweed JL, Schoenbach VJ, George LK et al, The effects of childhood parental death and divorce on six-month history of anxiety disorders. *Br J Psychiatry* 1989; **154**: 823–8.

38. Faravelli C, Pallanti S, Frassine R et al, Panic attacks with and without agoraphobia: a comparison. *Psychopathology* 1988; **21**: 51–6.

39. Saunders BE, Villeponteaux LA, Lipovsky JA et al, Child sexual assault as a risk factor for mental disorders among women. *Interpersonal Violence* 1992; **7**: 189–204.

40. Errera P, Some historical aspects of the concept, phobia. *Psychiatr Q* 1962; **36**: 325–36.

41. Marks IM, *Fears and Phobias*. London: Heinemann, 1969.

42. Terhune WB, The phobic syndrome. *Arch Neurol Psychiatr* 1949; **62**: 162–72.

43. Webster AS, The development of phobias in married women. *Psychol Monographs* 1953; **67**(367).

44. Tucker WI, Diagnosis and treatment of the phobic reaction. *Am J Psychiatry* 1956; **112**: 825–30.

45. Solyom L, Silberfeld M, Solyom C, Maternal overprotection in the etiology of agoraphobia. *Can Psychiatr Assoc J* 1976; **21**: 109–13.

46. Parker G, Parental representations of patients with anxiety neurosis. *Acta Psychiatr Scand* 1981; **63**: 33–6.

47. Parker G, Reported parental characteristic of agoraphobics and social phobics. *Br J Psychiatry* 1979; **135**: 555–60.

48. Faravelli C, Panichi C, Pallanti S et al, Perception of early parenting in panic and agoraphobia. *Acta Psychiatr Scand* 1991; **84**: 6–8.

49. Silove D, Parker G, Hadzi-Pavlovic D, Parental representations of patients with panic disorder and generalised anxiety disorder. *Br J Psychiatry* 1991; **159**: 835–41.

50. Breier A, Charney D, Heninger G, Agoraphobia with panic attacks. *Arch Gen Psychiatry* 1986; **43**: 1029–36.

51. Turner SM, Beidel DC, Costello A, Psychopathology in the offspring of anxiety disorders patients. *J Consult Clin Psychol* 1987; **55**: 229–35.

52. Zitrin C, Ross D, Early separation anxiety and adult agoraphobia. *J Nerv Ment Dis* 1988; **176**: 621–5.

53. Klein RG, Klein DF, Adult anxiety disorders and childhood separation anxiety. In: *Handbook of Anxiety*. Vol I. *Biological, Clinical and Cultural Perspectives* (Roth M, Noyes R, Burrows GD, eds). Amsterdam: Elsevier Science, 1988: 213–29.

54. Klein RG, Adult consequences of childhood separation anxiety disorder. In: *New Prospects*

in Psychiatry/The Bioclinical Interface I (Macher JP, Crocq MA, eds). Amsterdam: Elsevier Science, 1992: 233–44.

55. Klein RG, Is panic disorder associated with childhood separation anxiety disorder? *Clin Neuropharmacol* 1995; **18**(Suppl): 7–14.

56. Pollack MH, Otto MW, Rosenbaum JF et al, Longitudinal course of panic disorder: findings from the Massachussetts General Hospital Naturalistic Study. *J Clin Psychiatry* 1990; **51**: 12–16.

57. Rosenbaum JF, Biederman J, Bolduc-Murphy EA et al, Behavioral inhibition in childhood: a risk factor for anxiety disorders. *Harvard Rev Psychiatry* 1993; **1**: 2–16.

58. Laraia MT, Stuart GW, Frye LH et al, Childhood environment of women having panic disorder with agoraphobia. *J Anxiety Disord* 1994; **8**: 1–17.

59. Thyer B, Nesse R, Cameron O, Curtis G, Agoraphobia: a test of the separation anxiety hypothesis. *Behav Res Ther* 1985; **23**: 75–8.

60. Thyer B, Nesse R, Curtis G, Cameron O, Panic disorder: a test of the separation anxiety hypothesis. *Behav Res Ther* 1986; **24**: 209–11.

61. van der Molen G, van den Hout M, van Dieren A, Griez E, Childhood separation anxiety and adult-onset panic disorders. *J Anxiety Disord* 1989; **3**: 97–106.

62. Lipsitz JD, Martin LY, Mannuzza S et al, Childhood separation anxiety disorder in patients with adult anxiety disorders. *Am J Psychiatry* 1994; **151**: 927–9.

63. Silove D, Manicavasagar V, Adults who feared school: is early separation anxiety specific to the pathogenesis of panic disorder? *Acta Psychiatr Scand* 1993; **88**: 385–90.

64. Silove D, Manicavasagar Y, O'Connell D et al, Reported early separation anxiety symptoms in patients with panic and generalized anxiety disorders. *Aust NZ J Psychiatry* 1993; **27**: 487–94.

65. Silove D, Harris M, Morgan A et al, Is early separation anxiety a specific precursor of panic disorder–agoraphobia? A community study. *Psychol Med* 1995; **25**: 405–11.

66. Kagan J, Reznick JS, Clarke C et al, Behavioral inhibition to the unfamiliar. *Child Dev* 1984; **55**: 2212–25.

67. Rosenbaum JF, Biederman J, Gersten M et al, Behavioral inhibition in children of parents with panic disorder and agoraphobia: a controlled study. *Arch Gen Psychiatry* 1988; **45**: 463–70.

68. Biederman J, Rosenbaum JF, Hirshfeld MA et al, Psychiatric correlates of behavorial inhibition in young children of parents with and without psychiatric disorders. *Arch Gen Psychiatry* 1990; **47**: 21–6.

69. Reznick JS, Kagan J, Snidman N et al, Inhibited and uninhibited children: a follow-up study. *Child Dev* 1986; **51**: 660–80.

70. Last CG, Hersen M, Kazdin A et al, A family study of childhood anxiety disorders. *Arch Gen Psychiatry* 1991; **48**: 928–34.

71. Andrews JDW, Psychotherapy of phobias. *Psychol Bull* 1966; **66**: 455–80.

72. Shafar S, Aspects of phobic illness – a study of 90 personal cases. *Br J Med Psychol* 1970; **49**: 211–36.

73. Buglass D, Clarke J, Hendersen AS et al, A study of agoraphobic housewives. *Psychol Med* 1977; **7**: 73–86.

74. Torgersen S, The nature and origin of common phobic fears. *Br J Psychiatry* 1979; **134**: 343–51.

75. Faravelli C, Guerrini Degl'Innocenti B, Sessarego A et al, Personality features of patients with panic anxiety. *New Trends Exper Clin Psychiatry* 1987; **3**: 13–23.

76. Nystrom S, Lyndegard B, Predisposition for mental syndromes: a study comparing predisposition for depression, neurasthenia, and anxiety state. *Acta Psychiatr Scand* 1975; **51**: 69–76.

77. Buller R, Maien W, Goldenberg IM, Lavori PW, Benkert O, Chronology of panic and avoidance, age of onset in panic disorder, and prediction of treatment response. A report from the Cross-National Collaborative Panic Study. *Eur Arch Psychiatry Clin Neurosci* 1991; 163–8.

78. Klein DF, Anxiety reconceptualized. In: *Anxiety* (Klein DF, ed). Basel: Karger, 1987, pp. 253–65.

79. Roth M, Agoraphobia, panic disorder and generalized anxiety disorder. *Psychiatr Dev* 1984; **2**: 31–52.

80. Fava GA, Grandi S, Canestrari R, Prodromal

symptoms in panic disorder with agoraphobia. *Am J Psychiatry* 1988; **145**: 1564–7.

81. Lelliott P, Marks I, McNamee G, Tobena A, Onset of panic disorder with agoraphobia. *Arch Gen Psychiatry* 1989; **46**: 1000–4.

82. Faravelli C, Pallanti S, Biondi F et al, Onset of panic disorder. *Am J Psychiatry* 1992; **149**: 827–8.

83. Cohen AS, Barlow DH, Blanchard EB, Psychophysiology of relaxation-associated panic attacks. *J Abnormal Psychology* 1985; **9**: 96–101.

84. Heide FJ, Borkovec TD, Relaxation-induced anxiety: paradoxical anxiety enhancement due to relaxation training. *J Consult Clin Psychology* 1983; **51**: 171–82.

85. Heide FJ, Borkovec TD, Relaxation-induced anxiety: mechanisms and theoretical implications. *Behaviour Res Ther* 1984; **22**: 1–12.

86. Klein DF, Delineation of two drug-responsive anxiety syndromes. *Psychopharmacologia* 1964; **5**: 397–408.

87. Finlay-Jones R, Brown GW, Types of stressful life events and the onset of anxiety and depressive disorders. *Psychol Med* 1981; **11**: 803–15.

88. Faravelli C, Life events preceding the onset of panic disorder. *J Affective Disord* 1985; **9**: 103–5.

89. Faravelli C, Pallanti S, Recent life events and panic disorder. *Am J Psychiatry* 1989; **146**: 622–6.

90. Roy-Byrne P, Geraci M, Uhde T, Life events and the onset of panic disorder. *Am J Psychiatry* 1986; **143**: 1424–7.

91. Roy-Byrne P, Geraci M, Uhde T, Life events and course of illness in patients with panic disorder. *Am J Psychiatry* 1986; **143**: 1033–5.

92. Wade S, Monroe S, Michelson L, Chronic life stress and treatment outcome in agoraphobia with panic attacks. *Am J Psychiatry* 1993; **150**: 1491–5.

93. Wheeler EO, White PD, Reed EW, Cohen ME, Neurocirculatory asthenia (anxiety neurosis, effort syndrome, neurasthenia). *J Am Med Assoc* 1950; **142**: 878–88.

94. American Psychiatric Association, *Diagnostic and Statistical Manual of Mental Disorders*, 3rd edn. Washington, DC: APA, 1980.

95. Gloger S, Grunhaus L, Birmacher B, Troudert T, Treatment of spontaneous panic attacks with clomipramine. *Am J Psychiatry* 1981; **138**: 1215–17.

96. Faravelli C, Albanesi G, Agoraphobia with panic attacks: 1-year prospective follow-up. *Compr Psychiatry* 1987; **28**: 481–7.

97. Maier W, Buller R, The course of panic attacks and agoraphobia (letter). *Arch Gen Psychiatry* 1988; **45**: 501.

98. Coryell W, Noyes R, Clancy J, Panic disorder and primary unipolar depression. A comparison of background and outcome. *J Affective Disord* 1983; **5**: 311–17.

99. Nagy LM, Krystal JH, Woods SW, Clinical and medication outcome after short-term alprazolam in behavioral group treatment of panic disorder. *Arch Gen Psychiatry* 1989; **46**: 993–9.

100. Noyes R, Reich J, Christiansen J et al, Outcome of panic disorder. Relationship to diagnostic subtypes and comorbidity. *Arch Gen Psychiatry* 1990; **47**: 809–18.

101. Faravelli C, Paterniti S, Scarpato MA, 5-year prospective, naturalistic follow-up study of panic disorder. *Compr Psychiatry* 1995; **36**: 271–7.

102. Weissman MM, Klerman GL, Markowitz JS, Suicidal ideation and suicide attempts in panic disorder and attacks. *N Engl J Med* 1989; **321**: 1209–14.

103. Lepine JP, Chignon JM, Teherani M, Suicide attempts in patients with panic disorder. *Arch Gen Psychiatry* 1993; **50**: 144–9.

104. Wittchen HU, Essau CA, Comorbidity of anxiety disorders and depression: does it affect course and outcome? *Psychiatr Psychobiol* 1989; **4**: 315–23.

105. Johnson J, Weissman MM, Klerman GL, Panic disorder, comorbidity, and suicide attempts. *Arch Gen Psychiatry* 1990; **47**: 805–8.

106. Lesser IM, Rubin RT, Pecknold JC et al, Secondary depression in panic disorder and agoraphobia, I: Frequency, severity, and response to treatment. *Arch Gen Psychiatry* 1988; **45**: 437–43.

107. Reich J, Noyes R Jr, Troughton E, Dependent personality disorder associated with phobic avoidance in patients with panic disorder. *Am J Psychiatry* 1987; **144**: 323–6.

108. Roy-Byrne P, Ashleigh EA, Carr J, Personality and the anxiety disorder: a review of clinical findings. In: *Handbook of Anxiety* (Noyes R, Roth M, Burrows GD, eds). New York: Elsevier Science, 1988: 175–88.

109. Cloninger CR, Martin RL, Clayton P, Guze SB, A blind follow-up and family study of anxiety neurosis: preliminary results of the St. Louis 500. In: *Anxiety: New Research and Changing Concepts* (Klein DF, Rabtkin J, eds). New York: Raven Press, 1981, pp. 137–48.

110. Breier A, Charney DS, Heninger GR, The diagnostic validity of anxiety disorder and their relationship to depressive illness. *Am J Psychiatry* 1985; **142**: 787–97.

111. Stein MB, Tancer ME, Uhde TW, Major depression in patients with panic disorder: factors associated with course and recurrence *J Affect Disord* 1990; **19**: 287–96.

112. Vollrath M, Koch R, Angst J, The Zurich Study, IX: Panic disorder and sporadic panic: symptoms, diagnosis, prevalence, and overlap with depression. *Eur Arch Psychiatry Neurol Sci* 1990; **239**: 221–30.

113. Wittchen HU, Natural history and spontaneous remissions of untreated anxiety disorders: results of the Munich Follow-up Study (MFS). In: *Panic and Phobias 2. Treatment and Variables Affecting Course and Outcome* (Hand I, Wittchen HU, eds). New York: Springer-Verlag, 1988, pp. 3–17.

114. Van Valkenburg C, Akiskal HS, Puzantian V, Rosenthal T, Anxious depressions: clinical, family history and naturalistic outcome: comparisons with panic and major depressive episode. *J Affect Disord* 1984; **6**: 67–82.

115. Starcevic V, Uhlenhuth EH, Kellner R, Pathak D, Comparison of primary and secondary panic disorder: a preliminary report. *J Affect Disord* 1993; **27**: 81–6.

116. Cox BJ, Norton R, Dorward J, Fergusson PA, The relationship between panic attacks and chemical dependencies. *Addict Behav* 1989; **14**: 53–60.

117. George DT, Nutt DJ, Dwyer BA, Linnoila M, Alcoholism and panic disorder: is the comorbidity more than coincidence? *Acta Psychiatr Scand* 1990; **81**: 97–107.

118. Ballenger JC, Post RM, Kindling as a model for alcohol withdrawal syndromes. *Br J Psychiatry* 1978; **133**: 1–14.

119. Malcolm R, Ballenger JC, Sturgis ET, Anton R, Double-blind controlled trial comparing carbamazepine to oxazepam treatment of alcohol withdrawal. *Am J Psychiatry* 1989; **146**: 617–21.

120. Markowitz JS, Weissman MM, Ouellette R et al, Quality of life in panic disorder. *Arch Gen Psychiatry* 1989; **46**: 984–92.

121. Coryell W, Panic disorder and mortality. *Psychiatr Clin North Am* 1988; **11**: 433–40.

122. Warshaw MG, Massion AO, Peterson LG et al, Suicidal behavior in patients with panic disorder: retrospective and prospective data. *J Affect Disord* 1995; **34**: 235–47.

123. Zitrin CM, Klein DF, Woerner MG, Behaviour therapy, supportive psychotherapy, imipramine and phobias. *Arch Gen Psychiatry* 1978; **37**: 63–72.

124. Zitrin CM, Klein DF, Woerner MG et al, Treatment of phobias: I. Comparison of imipramine hydrochloride and placebo. *Arch Gen Psychiatry* 1983; **40**: 125–38.

125. Svenson TH, Usdin T, Feedback inhibition of brain noradrenaline neurons by tricyclic antidepressant alpha-receptor mediation. *Science* 1978; **202**: 1089–91.

126. Akiskal HS, Lemmi H, Dickson H, Chronic depression: Part 2. Sleep EEG differentiation of primary dysthymic disorders from anxious depression. *J Affect Dis* 1984; **6**: 287–95.

127. Hauri P, Friedman M, Ravaris CL, Sleep in patients with spontaneous panic attacks. *Sleep* 1989; **12**: 323–37.

128. Mellman TA, Uhde TW, Electroencephalographic sleep in panic disorder. *Arch Gen Psychiatry* 1989; **46**: 178–84.

129. Beauclaire L, Fontaine R, Epileptiform abnormalities in panic disorders. Presented at the Society of Biological Psychiatry Annual Convention, 1986.

130. Edlund JM, Swann AC, Clothier J, Patients with panic attacks and abnormal EEG results. *Am J Psychiatry* 1987; **144**: 508–9.

131. Lepola U, Nou siainen U, EEG and CT findings in patients with panic disorder. *Biol Psychiatry* 1990; **28**: 721–7.

132. Reiman EM, Raichle ME, Butler FK, A focal

brain abnormality in panic disorder, a severe form of anxiety. *Nature* 1984; **310:** 683–5.

133. Reiman EM, Raichle ME, Robins E, Application of positron emission tomography to the study of panic disorder. *Am J Psychiatry* 1986; **143:** 469–77.

134. Reiman EM, Raichle ME, Robins E, Involvement of temporal poles in pathological and normal forms of anxiety. *J Blood Flow Metab* 1989; **9**(Suppl 1): S589.

135. Fontaine R, Breton G, Dery R et al, Temporal lobe abnormalities in panic disorders: a MRI study. *Arch Gen Psychiatry* 1990; **27:** 304–10.

136. Roy-Byrne PP, Cowley DS, Greenblatt DJ et al, Reduced benzodiazepine sensitivity in panic disorder. *Arch Gen Psychiatry* 1990; **47:** 534–8.

137. Nutt DJ, Glue P, Lawson C, Wilson S, Flumazenil provocation of panic attacks. *Arch Gen Psychiatry* 1990; **47:** 917–25.

138. Nutt DJ, Lawson C, Panic attacks. A neurochemical overview of models and mechanisms. *Br J Psychiatry* 1992;, **160:** 165–78.

139. Kahn RS, McNair DM, Lipman RS et al, Imipramine and clordiazepoxide in depressive and anxiety disorders. *Arch Gen Psychiatry* 1986; **43:** 79–85.

140. Klein DF, Rabkin G, Gorman JM, Etiological and pathophysiological inferences from the pharmacological treatment of anxiety. In: *Anxiety and the Anxiety Disorders* (Tuma AH, Maser JD, eds). Hillsdale: Lawrence Erlbaum, 1985: 41–50.

141. Himle JA, Hill EM, Alcohol abuse and the anxiety disorders: evidence from the Epidemiological Catchment Area Survey. *J Anxiety Disord* 1991; **5:** 237–45.

142. Krystal JH, Leaf PS, Bruce ML et al, Effects of age and alcoholism on the prevalence of panic disorder. *Acta Psychiatr Scand* 1992; **85:** 77–82.

143. Joyer PR, Bushnell JA, Oakley-Browne HA, The epidemiology of panic symptomatology and agoraphobic avoidance. *Compr Psychiatry* 1989; **30:** 303.

144. Klerman GL, Weissman GL, Weissman MM et al, Panic attacks in the community. Social morbidity and health care utilization. *J Am Med Assoc* 1991; **265:** 742–6.

145. Angst J, Dobler-Mikola A, The Zurich Study: anxiety and phobia in young adults. *Eur Arch Psychiatr Neurol Sci* 1985; **235:** 171–8.

146. Weissman MM, Loof PJ, Holzer CE, The epidemiology of anxiety disorder: a highlight of recent evidence. *Psychopharmacol Bull* 1985; **21:** 538–41.

147. Faravelli C, Guerrini Degl'Innocenti B, Giardinelli L, Epidemiology of anxiety disorders in Florence. *Acta Psychiatr Scand* 1989; **79:** 308–12.

148. Garvey MJ, Cook B, Noyes R, The occurrence of a prodrome generalized anxiety in panic disorder. *Compr Psychiatry* 1988; **29:** 445–9.

149. Fava GA, Grandi S, Rafanelli C et al, Prodromal symptoms in panic disorder with agoraphobia. A replication study. *J Affect Disord* 1992; **26:** 85–8.

150. Roy-Byrne PP, Uhde TW, Post RM et al, The corticotropin-releasing hormone stimulation test in patients with panic disorder. *Am J Psychiatry* 1986; **143:** 896–9.

151. Gold PW, Pigott TA, Kling MA, Basic and clinical studies with corticotropin-releasing hormone. Implications for a possible role in panic disorder. *Psychiatry Clin North Am* 1988; **11:** 327–34.

152. Holsboer F, Staiger A, v Bardeleben U et al, Role of CRH and other neuropeptides in panic disorder. Presented at 5th World Congress of Biological Psychiatry, Florence, 1991.

153. Eysenck HJ, Learning theory and behavior therapy. *J Ment Sci* 1959; **105:** 61–75.

154. Clark DM, A cognitive approach to panic. *Behav Res Ther* 1986; **24:** 461–70.

155. Clark DM, Anxiety states. Panic and generalized anxiety. In: *Cognitive Behavior Therapy for Psychiatric Problems* (Hawton K, Salkovskis PM, Kirk J et al, eds). Oxford: Oxford Medical Publications: 1989.

4

Health economic aspects of panic disorder

Mark A Oakley-Browne

Introduction

Anxiety and depressive disorders are a major public health problem,[1] and impose substantial burdens on individuals, their families, the wider community and the health system. As clinicians, we know well that illness imposes a significant burden on our patients and their families. We tend to be less aware of the wider societal costs. In this chapter an attempt is made to describe the economic aspects of panic disorders. Only a very brief overview of the economic analyses will be provided, and for a fuller discussion the reader is referred to two excellent texts by experts in the area.[2,3] For reviews of the principles of economic analyses applied to mental health, the reader is referred to the paper by Knapp and Beecham[4] and the chapter by Wilkinson and Pelosi.[5] In this chapter an epidemiological perspective is taken, since a population-based perspective is necessary to understand the efficacy and efficiency of health care interventions. If optimum results are to be obtained from spending on health, then '... we must finally be able to express the results in the form of the benefit and cost to the population of a particular type of activity, and the increased benefit that could be obtained if more money were made available'.[6]

Prevalence, risk factors and morbidity of panic disorder

Community epidemiological studies have shown panic disorder and panic attacks to be common, with lifetime prevalence rates of approximately 2.0% and 15.0% respectively.[7,8] The disorder tends to have onset in late teenage years and early adulthood, and follows a chronic or episodic course.[7,9] Females have twice the rate of disorder, and it is more common amongst persons who are separated, widowed or divorced.[7] Markowitz et al[10] used data from the Epidemiologic Catchment Area (ECA) program, and found that a diagnosis of panic disorder was associated with pervasive social and health consequences similar to or greater than those associated with depression. The negative consequences included subjective feelings of poor physical and emotional health, substance abuse, impaired social and marital functioning, financial dependency, increased use of psychoactive medications and health services, and increased frequency of suicide attempts. These findings were not explained by comorbidity with major depression, agoraphobia and substance use. Leon et al[11] also used ECA program data to examine the societal costs of all anxiety disorders. Amongst persons with panic disorder, they found increased financial dependency, increased rates of chronic unemployment and increased use of health services. Other authors have also noted the high rate of health service utilization amongst persons with panic disorder.[9,12] In a study of a clinical population, Sherbourne et al[13] compared the health-related quality of life of patients with panic disorder to that of patients with other major chronic medical and psychiatric conditions. They found that patients with panic disorder had lower levels of mental health and role functioning compared with patients with other major chronic medical illnesses, but higher levels compared with patients with major depression.

Treatment of panic disorder

Panic disorder is a common disorder with significant associated morbidity, but it is a treatable disorder and there are a number of treatment options. A number of systematic reviews, which used meta-analytic methods to aggregate and summarize the results of treatment, are available.[14–17] Both psychological (cognitive–behavioural therapy) and pharmacological treatments (imipramine, clomipramine, SSRIs, alprazolam and clonazepam) have been shown to be effective in the short-term. However, there is a high relapse rate associated with cessation of pharmacological treatments,

while the gains of cognitive–behavioural therapy tend to persist.[18,19] Unfortunately, many persons with panic disorder are not diagnosed, and do not receive appropriate treatment for the condition.[20]

Why consider the economics of panic disorder?

Given the good evidence base about the prevalence, risk factors, health service use patterns, associated morbidity and treatments, why should we need to consider the economic aspects of panic disorder? Surely, our responsibility as mental health care providers is to advocate that our patients have access to the best care possible, regardless of cost? Drummond[3] provides the answer to this question: 'To put it simply, resources – people, time, facilities, equipment, and knowledge – are scarce. Choices must and will be made concerning their deployment...'. The treatments and other services that we may wish to provide to our patients need to be considered in balance with treatments and services that might be provided to others. Economic evaluation provides us with a set of tools to identify the options and attempt to measure the benefits and costs associated with the different options. 'Economics, at its best, is a logical way of analysing the costs and benefits of alternative ways of achieving competing objectives: it is the science of deciding how to allocate scarce means among competing ends.'[21]

Over the last 30 years in the developed economies, health care costs have increased substantially. Approximately two-thirds of the excess increase (the proportion of the increase that is more than the general inflation rate and population growth) is attributable to increases in the volume and intensity of services.[22] Even in the strongest of economies, it is not possible to sustain this rate of increase, and rationing is inevitable.[23] Increased awareness of panic disorder and treatment options for panic disorder will inevitably lead to increased demand for treatment. Increased recognition and improved diagnosis will lead to increased treatment provision. New treatment options (e.g. the SSRIs) are likely to be more expensive than older treatment options (e.g. imipramine). There will also be an expectation of increased intensity of service: for instance, an expectation that expertly delivered cognitive–behavioural therapy be more freely available at the primary care level. Finally, since panic disorder is a chronic and episodic condition with considerable comorbidity with major depression,[24] it may become more prevalent as the population ages and if cohort trends for increasing rates of major depression continue.[25] If we are to provide increased access to effective treatments for patients with panic disorder, we shall need to provide 'more for less'. To accomplish this, we shall need to identify and eliminate inefficiencies in the diagnosis and treatment of panic disorder. Economic evaluation will help us to identify and eliminate these inefficiencies.

Types of economic evaluation

To understand how economic evaluation may be used to identify and eliminate inefficiencies related to panic disorder, it is necessary to consider the types of analyses that are most commonly used. The main methods of economic evaluation are cost-of-illness studies, cost-minimization analysis, cost–effectiveness analysis, cost–utility analysis and cost–benefit analysis. Each of these methods will be briefly described, and, if possible, examples of their application in panic disorder (or related disorders) will be presented.

Cost-of-illness studies

Cost-of-illness studies are descriptive studies that aim to identify and estimate all direct and indirect costs related to a particular disorder so as to give a measure of its economic burden to a community. This information may be used, along with estimates of prevalence, incidence and severity of disorder, to 'weigh up' the relative importance of different health problems.

There have been a number of studies that have attempted to estimate direct and indirect costs of mental disorders to the health system and the wider community. Unfortunately, these studies do not allow for extraction of the costs related to panic disorder alone, but they do provide information about total costs. In the USA there have been a number of studies that have used models to estimate the total direct and indirect costs of mental illness. In these studies, anxiety disorders, including panic disorder, have been aggregated with other mental disorders and substance abuse/dependence disorders. Rice et al[26] estimated that in 1985 the total economic costs of mental illness were US$103.7 billion. This comprised 41% direct treatment and support costs (11.5% of total personal health care spending for all illnesses) 46% for reduced or lost productivity, 9% for lost value of productivity because of premature death, and 4% for other related costs, including care-giver services. In a report of the National Advisory Mental Health Council[27] it is estimated that the 1990 total cost (direct, indirect and related costs) for all mental disorders was US$148 billion, and for severe mental disorders (schizophrenia, manic-depressive illness, major depression, panic disorder and obsessive–compulsive disorder) US$74 billion. The direct treatment costs for all mental illness represented 10%, and severe mental illness represented 4%, of the total US direct health care costs.

Evidence that the contribution of anxiety disorders to direct costs may be significant may be obtained from an Australian model in which the costs of an ideal mental health system for a catchment area were estimated. Andrews[28] used data on the treated prevalence and costs of treatment to estimate the mental health service costs for a catchment area of 200 000. It was found that the costs of services for schizophrenia (380 cases) were A$3.65 million, for affective psychosis (280 cases) A$1.28 million, and for neuroses (2840 cases, 50% anxiety disorders, 50% depressive neuroses) A$7.32 million. In this model, although the cases of schizophrenia cost four times as much as anxiety disorders to treat (A$9700 per schizophrenia case versus A$2600 per anxiety disorder case), the total direct treatment costs of all the anxiety disorder cases was approximately the same as that for all the schizophrenia cases, because the treated prevalence of anxiety disorders is much greater than that of schizophrenia.

Croft-Jeffreys and Wilkinson[29] have estimated the cost of 'neurotic' disorder to UK general practice and the UK economy. The ICD-9 system was used to define the neuroses. The total direct and indirect cost of all neuroses in UK general practice was estimated to be £373 million, or just over 9% of the total spent on family practitioner services in 1984–85. The costs to the economy due to lost production of sufferers were estimated at £5.6 billion, or approximately one-third of the total cost of the National Health System. Croft-Jeffreys and Wilkinson present data that indicate that anxiety disorder accounted for approximately 38% of consultations in general practice per 1000 at risk, and 32% of home visits and surgery consultations. The authors emphasized that the greatest effects and hence costs for neurotic disorder were in the areas of lost production and impaired economic functioning of sufferers rather than the cost of treatment.

Simon et al[30] examined the health care costs associated with depressive and anxiety disorders in primary care. They found that primary care patients with anxiety or depressive disorders had markedly higher baseline costs ($2390) than patients with subthreshold disorders ($1098) or no anxiety/depressive disorders ($1397). These large cost differences persisted after adjustment for medical morbidity, and were a consequence of higher use of general medical services rather than mental health treatment.

Edlund and Swann[31] studied 30 patients with panic disorder over a four-month period. They computed the indirect costs of work loss due to disability for the period (a total of 79.5 years). The total loss of work disability alone came to $1 010 207 in 1984 dollars or $33 674 per patient. Although this sample was small and not representative, the findings do confirm those of the community and primary care studies previously described. The indirect costs associated with anxiety disorders are high and mostly the consequence of work disability.

These studies all suggest that the direct and indirect costs of anxiety disorders are substantial. Although the costs of treatment per individual patient for anxiety disorders are probably less than that for schizophrenic disorders, the high treated prevalence of anxiety disorders results in total treatment costs to a community of the same order as that for schizophrenia. The indirect costs of anxiety disorder are far greater than the direct costs, and are mainly the result of work disability. It might be assumed that panic disorder makes a large contribution to the indirect and direct costs of all anxiety disorders. In the community epidemiological studies described previously, panic disorder was found to be the mental disorder most likely to lead to persons seeking health care, and, compared with other anxiety disorders, persons with panic disorder were more likely to be unemployed or financially disadvantaged. Further studies that disentangle the economic burden to the community of the different mental disorders are needed.

Cost-minimization analysis

The aim of cost-minimization studies is to compare the costs of two or more interventions that are known to have equivalent effect. The intention is to determine which intervention is the cheapest. For instance, two pharmacological treatments known to be of equal effectiveness might be compared in terms of their respective costs. Although it usual to compare pharmacological treatments in randomized controlled trials (RCTs), until recently it has been rare for such trials to include an economic evaluation. A literature search failed to locate any such published studies related to the treatment of panic disorder. It is essential that such studies be undertaken, if resources are to be used efficiently.

Cost–effectiveness analysis

The term 'cost–effectiveness analysis' is often used to mean any form of economic evaluation. Within health economics, the term has a more specific meaning. Cost–effectiveness analysis is undertaken when two or more interventions may differ in terms of their effects but the effects can be measured in the same units, and it is possible to measure the costs of the interventions. It is then possible to compare the interventions in terms of the cost per unit of effect. Cost–effectiveness analysis is probably the most widely used form of economic evaluation in medicine. However, no published studies of cost–effectiveness analysis

of interventions for panic disorder were located in the literature search.

Two published RCTs that included cost–effectiveness analysis of alternative interventions for 'neuroses' (which includes panic disorder) were located. These studies are discussed here since they provide useful models of how such studies may be conducted and challenge some assumptions about methods of delivery of care. The two studies are RCTs that demonstrate the cost–effectiveness of nurse-administered therapy for neurotic patients compared with routine outpatient psychiatrist follow-up[32] or general-practitioner care.[33] The first study is a prospective RCT of chronic psychiatric patients, the majority of whom had neurotic disorders. The patients were randomly allocated either to community psychiatric nurse care or to routine outpatient psychiatrist follow-up. The clinical and social outcomes were comparable in both groups at follow-up. Consumer satisfaction was significantly greater among the community psychiatric nurse care patients. Over the total 18-month study period, the nursing care group had lower direct costs. These direct costs of psychiatric care comprised a small proportion of the total public expenditure, which was not significantly different between the two groups. In the second study, neurotic patients were randomly assigned to behavioural psychotherapy from a nurse therapist or to routine care from their general practitioner. At the end of one year, the nurse therapist group fared significantly better for clinical outcome. The economic outcome to one year, compared with the year before the patients entered the trial, showed a slight decrease in the health service use by the nurse therapist group, and an increase in health service use by the GP-treated group. The increased costs in the GP-treated group were mainly due to increased absence from work and more hospital treatment and medications compared with the nurse therapist group. These two studies suggest that in the population of persons suffering from neurotic disorders, care by nursing staff, who are more likely to use non-pharmacological treatments such as behavioural therapy, is as efficacious and more cost-effective than care provided by psychiatrists, who are more likely to use pharmacological interventions. Clearly, more studies need to be done to define more specifically the subgroups of persons with neurotic disorders, such as panic disorder, who might have differing treatment needs.

Cost–utility analysis

Cost–utility analysis is undertaken when two or more interventions produce different effects in terms of both quality and quantity of life. In this situation, the comparison is undertaken with 'utilities'. Utilities are units that comprise both measures of time and quality of life. An example of a utility is the QALY (quality-adjusted life-years).

No cost–utility analyses with a focus on panic disorder were located in the literature search. One study was found that compared the interventions for schizophrenia, affective and neurotic disorders. This study was an economic evaluation of the Buckingham Mental Health Service in which cost–utility analysis was used to evaluate the service and cost per QALY was used as an outcome measure.[34] The cost per QALY provided was lowest in people with schizophrenia (approximately £6000), higher in those with affective disorders (£10 000) and higher in those with neurotic disorders (£25 000). Apparently, patients with chronic and severe obsessive-compulsive disorder made a large contribution to the high cost per QALY for the neurotic disorders (I Falloon, personal communication).

Cost–benefit analysis

Cost–benefit analysis is used when both the inputs and outputs (effects) of an intervention can be expressed in monetary terms and the aim is to determine whether the benefits of the intervention justify the costs. With cost–benefit analysis, it is also possible to compare the inputs and outputs of different interventions in terms of monetary units.

An example of cost–benefit analysis is provided by the study of Salvador-Carulla et al,[35] who examined the costs before and after the diagnosis and provision of effective treatment for panic disorder. A 24-month pre–post design was used to collect data on clinical status and health care services use in a natural environment. Sixty-one patients with panic disorder were assessed, and the assessment included measurements on general functioning, improvement, severity of symptoms, level of disability, health care services used and workdays lost. It was found that the total direct costs of health care use were US$29 158 during the year prior to diagnosis and US$46 256 during the year after the diagnosis. The indirect costs of lost productivity were US$65 643 in the year prior to diagnosis and US$13 883 in the year after diagnosis. Thus the costs of increased health service use as a consequence of diagnosis and effective treatment were offset by the reduced costs due to increased productivity. The authors commented that this strong 'offset effect' was greater than that usually described for psychiatric disorders as a whole.

Summary

This limited, non-systematic review suggests that there are very few economic evaluations of interventions for panic disorder. The limited data available suggest the following:

(1) The anxiety disorders, including panic disorder, are common, and are associated with significant morbidity and, most notably from an economic perspective, decreased productivity and increased financial dependency.

(2) The anxiety disorders, including panic disorder, are associated with substantial direct and indirect costs to the health care system and community. The indirect costs outweigh the direct costs, and are mainly attributable to lost productivity. These direct and indirect costs may be equal to or greater than those associated with severe disorders such as schizophrenia.

(3) The increased costs associated with the diagnosis and effective treatment of panic disorder may be offset by savings due to increased productivity amongst treated persons.

(4) Treatment for 'neuroses' (including panic disorder) by nurse practitioners in primary care or mental health outpatient settings is as effective as treatment by general practitioners or psychiatrists, and costs are less. In the studies discussed, the treatments provided by nurse practitioners were non-pharmacological, and mainly consisted of support, education and cognitive-behavioural interventions.

(5) Despite the large number of trials comparing different pharmacological treatments for panic disorder, there appears to be an information vacuum about their comparative costs and benefits. There is also a lack of comparative information about the costs and benefits of pharmacological and psychological treatments. The latter is a major concern, since the present evidence suggests a high relapse rate on cessation of pharmaceutical treatments while the gains of cognitive–behavioural treatment tend to be maintained over time. This suggests that the costs of pharmacological interventions may be ongoing, while those associated with psychological intervention may be time-limited and consequently less than those of pharmacological treatments in the medium to long term.

If we are to deliver effective and efficient care to persons with panic disorder, further economic evaluations must be undertaken. It is essential that cost-minimization and cost–effectiveness studies comparing different interventions for panic disorder be undertaken. When considering this further work, three of the principles proposed by Eddy[36] should be kept in mind.

(1) Because financial resources are limited, when deciding about appropriate use of treatments, it is both valid and important to consider the financial costs.

(2) Because financial resources are limited, it is necessary to set priorities.

(3) A consequence of priority setting is that it will not be possible to cover from shared resources every treatment that might have some benefit.

References

1. Üstün TB, Sartorius N, Public health aspects of anxiety and depressive disorders. *Int Clin Psychopharmacol* 1993; 8(Suppl 1): 15–20.
2. Jefferson T, Demicheli V, Mugford M, *Elementary Economic Evaluation in Health Care*. London: BMJ Publishing Group, 1996.
3. Drummond MF, Stoddart GL, Torrance GW, *Methods for the Economic Evaluation of*

   Health Care Programmes. Oxford: Oxford University Press, 1997.

4. Knapp M, Beecham J, Costing mental health services. *Psychol Med* 1990; **20:** 893–908.

5. Wilkinson G, Pelosi A, *Economic appraisal.* In: *The Scope of Epidemiological Psychiatry: Essays in Honour of Michael Shepherd.* London: Routledge, 1989, pp. 63–73.

6. Cochrane AL, *Effectiveness and Efficiency. Random Reflections on Health Services.* Cambridge: Cambridge University Press, 1986.

7. Oakley-Browne MA, The epidemiology of Anxiety Disorders. *Int Rev Psychiatry* 1991; **3:** 243–52.

8. Eaton WW, Kessler RC, Wittchen HU, Magee WJ, Panic and panic disorder in the United States. *Am J Psychiatry* 1994; **151:** 413–20.

9. Eaton WW, Dryman A, Weissman MM, *Panic and Phobia. Psychiatric Disorders in America: The Epidemiologic Catchment Area Study,* 1st edn. New York: The Free Press, 1991.

10. Markowitz JS, Weissman MM, Ouellette R et al, Quality of life in panic disorder. *Arch Gen Psychiatry* 1989; **46:** 984–92.

11. Leon AC, Portera L, Weissman MM, The social costs of anxiety disorders. *Br J Psychiatry Suppl* 1995; **27:** 19–22.

12. Boyd JH, Use of mental health services for the treatment of panic disorder. *Am J Psychiatry* 1986; **143:** 1569–74.

13. Sherbourne CD, Wells KB, Judd LL, Functioning and well-being of patients with panic disorder. *Am J Psychiatry* 1996; **153:** 213–8.

14. Mattick RP, Andrews G, Hadzi-Pavlocic D, Christensen H, Treatment of panic and agoraphobia. An integrative review. *J Nerv Ment Dis* 1990; **178:** 567–76.

15. Wilkinson G, Balestrieri M, Ruggeri M, Bellantuono C, Meta-analysis of double-blind placebo-controlled trials of antidepressants and benzodiazepines for patients with panic disorders. *Psychol Med* 1991; **21:** 991–8.

16. Jonas JM, Cohon MS, A comparison of the safety and efficacy of alprazolam versus other agents in the treatment of anxiety, panic, and depression: a review of the literature. *J Clin Psychiatry* 1993; **54**(10 Suppl): 25–48.

17. Boyer W, Serotonin uptake inhibitors are supe-rior to imipramine and alprazolam in alleviating panic attacks: a meta-analysis. *Clin Psychopharmacol* 1995; **10:** 45–9.

18. Pollack MH, Smoller JW, The longitudinal course and outcome of panic disorder. *Psychiatr Clin North Am* 1995; **18:** 785–801.

19. Otto MW, Whittal ML, Cognitive–behavior therapy and the longitudinal course of panic disorder. *Psychiatr Clin North Am* 1995; **18:** 803–20.

20. Weissman MM, The hidden patient: unrecognized panic disorder. *J Clin Psychiatry* 1990; **51**(Suppl): 5–8.

21. Maynard A, Logic in medicine: an economic perspective. *Br Med J* 1987; **295:** 1537–41.

22. Eddy DM, Rationing resources while improving quality. How to get more for less. *J Am Med Assoc* 1994; **272:** 817–24.

23. Eddy DM, Health system reform: Will controlling costs require rationing services? *J Am Med Assoc* 1994; **272:** 324–8.

24. Robins LN, Locke BZ, Regier DA, *Psychiatric Disorders in America: The Epidemiologic Catchment Area Study. An Overview of Psychiatric Disorders in America,* 1st edn. New York: The Free Press, 1991.

25. The Cross-National Collaborative Group, The changing rate of major depression. Cross-national comparisons. *J Am Med Assoc* 1992; **268:** 3098–105.

26. Rice DP, Kelman S, Miller LS, The economic burden of mental illness. *Hosp Community Psychiatry* 1992; **43:** 1227–32.

27. The National Advisory Mental Health Council, Health care reform for Americans with severe mental illnesses: report of the National Advisory Mental Health Council. *Am J Psychiatry* 1993; **150:** 1447–65.

28. Andrews G, *The Tolkien Report: A Description of a Model Mental Health Service.* Sydney: Clinical Research Unit for Anxiety Disorders, 1991.

29. Croft-Jeffreys C, Wilkinson G, Estimated costs of neurotic disorder in UK general practice 1985 [editorial]. *Psychol Med* 1989; **19:** 549–58.

30. Simon G, Ormel J, VonKorff M, Barlow W, Health care costs associated with depressive and anxiety disorders in primary care. *Am J Psychiatry* 1995; **152:** 352–7.

31. Edlund MJ, Swann AC, The economic and social costs of panic disorder. *Hosp Community Psychiatry* 1987; **38**: 1277–9, 1288.
32. Mangen SP, Paykel ES, Griffith JH et al, Cost-effectiveness of community psychiatric nurse or out-patient psychiatrist care of neurotic patients. *Psychol Med* 1983; **13**: 407–16.
33. Ginsberg G, Marks I, Waters H, Cost–benefit analysis of a controlled trial of nurse therapy for neuroses in primary care. *Psychol Med* 1984; **14**: 683–90.
34. Wilkinson G, Croft-Jeffreys C, Krekorian H et al, QALYs in psychiatric care? *Psychiatric Bull* 1990; **14**: 582–5.
35. Salvador-Carulla L, Segui J, Fernandez-Cano P, Canet J, Costs and offset effect in panic disorders. *Br J Psychiatry Suppl* 1995; **27**: 23–8.
36. Eddy DM, Principles for making difficult decisions in difficult times. *J Am Med Assoc* 1994; **271**: 1792–8.

5

Brain mechanisms and circuits in panic disorder

Andrea L Malizia and David J Nutt

Introduction

Animal experimentation can produce fundamental leads in medical research. However, for psychiatric conditions there is no satisfactory substitute for human research, despite the constraints that this entails. In anxiety disorders the human neurobiology of panic disorder (PD) has received much attention in the last 20 years. Thus far, the most informative experimental strategy has recorded behavioural, physiological and cognitive responses to pharmacological probes where the aim has been to characterize the central neurochemical processes underlying panic.[1] It is easiest to interpret these challenges when they provoke panic symptoms in patients (Table 5.1) than when they reduce general symptoms of anxiety, since these may be non-specific. These pharmacological challenges have produced findings that are important for generating hypotheses about the biology of this disorder and that will be reviewed in the first part of this chapter.

However, human pharmacological challenges are limited by their intrinsic inability to

Table 5.1 Panicogenic challenges	
Metabolic	
Lactate, biocarbonate	
Respiratory	
Hypercapnia, hypocapnia	
Pharmacological	
GABA	Flumazenil, FG7142
5-HT	mCPP, fenfluramine
Noradrenaline	Yohimbine, isoproterenol
CCK-B	CCK4, pentagastrin
Adenosine	Caffeine

characterize neural networks in detail. Even when the pharmacological effects of the probes are very specific for a receptor at a particular anatomical site (for example, serotonergic neuroendocrine effects are due to post-synaptic occupancy in the hypothalamus/pituitary, while serotonergic body temperature regulation is thought to be due to presynaptic action in the brain stem), it is not possible to achieve a descriptive power that is at all comparable to what can be done in animal pharmacology. Thus, with pharmacological challenge techniques, complex and distributed brain processes are summated and then reduced to the same state as a Skinnerian 'black box' with little neuroanatomical information and limited explanatory power. The solution to this problem is the use of the emerging brain imaging techniques, which can describe the functional anatomy, pharmacology and functional neurochemistry of the human brain with macroanatomical (about 1 cm) resolution. In the second part of this chapter we review the evidence thus far produced in panic disorder by these methods and outline future research strategies.

Pharmacological investigations of panic disorder

Lactate challenge

The development of the concept of panic attacks is historically linked to lactate. Following the observation that anxious people have a reduced exercise tolerance, Pitts and McClure conducted experiments that showed that lactate infusions provoked the sudden appearance of severe anxiety symptoms in man. Lactate infusion (usually 0.5 M sodium DL-lactate given i.v. over 20 minutes) produces anxiety increases in up to 85% of patients with PD and up to 25% of controls.[2] In addition, provocation of disorder congruent psychopathology is also seen in post-traumatic stress

disorder[3] but not in many patients with social phobia.[4] The panicogenic effects of lactate challenge in PD are blocked by antipanic treatments such as benzodiazepines, clonidine and antidepressants.[5–7] The panicogenic effects are probably a state rather than a trait marker, since they do not seem to indicate genetic vulnerability to the disorder.[8] The mechanism by which lactate provokes symptoms is still unknown. A number of theories involving CO_2, hypocalcaemia, alkalosis or direct transport into the brain have been falsified experimentally.[7,9–12] However, out of these, the lack of cisternal increase in lactate following lactate infusion in primates has to be viewed with extreme caution, since many studies have demonstrated lactate transport in sheep, guinea pig,[13] rat[14,15] and man.[16] It is of interest to note that co-administration of 5% dextrose reduces the proportion of patients experiencing panic attacks[11] and that lactate infusion induces cerebrovascular[17] and vagal cardiovascular[18–21] changes, which also occur while patients are asleep[22] and which may underlie its mode of action.

CO_2 challenge

Another 'non-specific' pharmacological challenge is the administration of CO_2. This is fully reviewed in Chapter 6, but will be briefly discussed here since it may be related to specific neurotransmitter systems. The administration of CO_2 provokes panic attacks in PD patients and to a lesser extent in volunteers. The proportion of subjects experiencing symptoms has a dose-dependent relationship, and a single breath of 35% CO_2 produces a panic attack in up to 70% of patients and up to 10% of volunteers;[23] these panicogenic effects of CO_2 may be related to a history of panic attacks,[24] but are not strongly predictive of the occurrence of panic attacks on follow-up in the year subsequent to the challenge.[25] CO_2-provoked panic attacks do not occur in obsessive–compulsive disorder or social phobia more frequently than in controls,[23,24,26] are blocked by antipanic medication,[27] are enhanced in the early follicular phase of the menstrual cycle,[28] and may be a marker for increased genetic vulnerability to PD.[29,30] The mechanism by which CO_2 causes the symptoms is not understood, and has led to the hypothesis that PD is the expression of an abnormally sensitive suffocation alarm. However, there has been little supporting evidence for this unifying concept, and many other explanations are possible, including the profound effects that small variations of CO_2 plasma concentrations have on cerebral blood flow, on locus coeruleus firing[31,32] and on benzodiazepine–$GABA_A$ function.[33,34] In this context, the observation that yohimbine administration does not increase the number of anxiety symptoms following the administration of 35% CO_2 to healthy volunteers[35] is of interest, but does not necessarily exclude locus coeruleus noradrenergic involvement, because of possible ceiling effects.

Noradrenergic system

Preclinical studies have indicated that locus coeruleus activation corresponds to orienting and alerting responses and that the net computational effect of noradrenergic stimulation is an increase in signal-to-noise ratio in the target neuronal fields. As such, it would be expected that noradrenergic modulation would have large effects on anxiety and anxiety disorders. In PD, α_2 probes that increase noradrenergic function (e.g. yohimbine (20 mg p.o. or 0.4 mg/kg i.v.) – an antagonist that blocks noradrenergic autoreceptors) have the effect of precipitating panic attacks in about 60% of PD patients and about 5% of controls.[36–39] The panic attacks thus precipitated have a different phenomenology than naturally occurring panic

attacks, and their frequency in target populations is not always reduced by effective PD treatments.[40] However, since increased noradrenergic function produces an increase in anxiety symptoms in other anxiety disorders, these effects cannot be considered as specific to PD.

Further, studies with clonidine (an α_2 agonist) have produced data that are difficult to synthesize in a unifying theory of altered adrenergic function. These experiments demonstrate that in PD patients' presynaptic α_2 receptors are supersensitive while hypothalamic postsynaptic α_2 receptors are subsensitive.[39,41–47] The subsensitivity is not specific to PD,[48] and may thus indicate a mechanism associated with pathological anxiety. Presynaptic supersensitivity (i.e. a greater fall in 3-methoxy-4-hydroxyphenylethylene glycol clonidine) is reversed by treatment with imipramine. Successful selective serotonin reuptake inhibitor (SSRI) treatment also modifies the responses to noradrenergic probes in PD patients.[49]

Peripheral β receptor function has also been investigated by using the non-selective β agonist isoproterenol. One group has repeatedly demonstrated that isoproterenol induces panic attacks in PD patients, which they interpreted as suggesting receptor hypersensitivity.[50] However, this has not been replicated by others,[51] who have suggested that peripheral β receptors are actually downregulated as part of an adaptive response to increased sympathetic activity during panic attacks. However, these provocation data are difficult to interpret, since isoproterenol induces marked palpitations, which can lead to secondary cognitive effects and may also have central effects. Spectral analysis of heart-rate variability, which represents the balance between vagal and sympathetic efferent output, has revealed that PD patients have abnormal sympathovagal responses after isoproterenol infusion and that therefore this paradigm may be a good method to investigate cardiac autonomic physiology, which is abnormal in these patients at rest[52] and recovers with treatment.[53]

In the clinic, antidepressants with predominant noradrenaline reuptake blocking properties may not be as effective in PD as agents which have serotonin reuptake blocking properties.[54,55]

Serotonergic system

The role of the serotonergic system in the treatment of PD is reviewed in detail in Chapter 11. As a whole, manipulations of serotonergic transmission have produced seemingly contradictory results. These may have been due to the poor receptor subtype specificity of some of the probes and to the uncertain balance between effects at cortical postsynaptic receptors and at somatic presynaptic raphe receptors. A further complication may be due to the differential effects of specific ascending projections from dorsal (DRN) and median raphe nuclei (MRN) proposed by Graeff et al.[56] In their model, DRN efferents to frontal cortex and amygdala increase conditioned fear, DRN efferents to periaqueductal grey matter inhibit innate responses to danger pain and asphyxia, and MRN efferents to the hippocampus facilitate the process of adaptation to stress.

Notwithstanding these limitations, it appears that increases in net serotonin (5-hydroxytryptamine, 5-HT) transmission decrease panic, while they may facilitate anticipatory anxiety. Serotonergic pharmacological challenges have demonstrated that the precursors 5-HT and 5-HTP (which result in an immediate but moderate increase in serotonin synthesis) are either neutral or panicolytic,[57–60] while tryptophan depletion causes anxiety in remitted PD patients.[61] In contrast, acute SSRI, acute tricyclic antidepressant (TCA) and fenfluramine[62] administration induce anxiety (possibly by

suppressing net 5-HT transmission via the stimulation of presynaptic 5-HT_{1A} receptors). m-Chlorophenylpiperazine (mCPP) is a serotonergic agent that has considerable anxiogenic properties in PD patients and controls;[63–66] however, it has a very complex neuropharmacology, being an agonist at 5-HT_{2C}, 5-HT_{1A} and α_2 adrenergic receptors and an antagonist at 5-HT_{2A} and 5-HT_3 receptors, and therefore the interpretation of its actions is very complex. Further characterization of the dynamic changes in the serotonergic system may result from two specific leads. First, PD patients are subsensitive to the neuroendocrine and thermoregulatory effects of 5-HT_{1A} agonists.[67] In addition, PD patients do not respond clinically to 5-HT_2 antagonists such as ritanserin, which may actually exacerbate some of the symptoms.[68] Ritanserin challenges in healthy volunteers seem to support the Graeff–Deakin serotonergic anxiety model, since this compound facilitates anxiety in simulated public speaking (unconditioned anxiety),[69] but it decreases some aspects of the anxiety response in a human conditioned-anxiety model.[70]

In the clinic, drugs that block serotonergic reuptake are very effective antipanic agents, although they may cause transient initial increases in anxiety; no consistent beneficial effects have been demonstrated for 5-HT_{1A} partial agonists.

Dopaminergic system

Anxiety can produce an increase in dopaminergic tone in the prefrontal cortex in experimental animals;[71,72] however, there is no evidence of dopaminergic tone alteration in PD. The suggestion that there may be increased dopamine function in PD patients, as evidenced by an increased endocrine response to apomorphine,[73] has not been confirmed when an appropriate control group has been selected.[74]

GABAergic system

γ-Aminobutyric acid (GABA) is the most common neurotransmitter in the brain. Its effects are mediated by action at two types of receptor: $GABA_A$ and $GABA_B$. $GABA_A$ receptors are on chloride ionophores, and their stimulation increases chloride conductance as well as channel opening, thus inhibiting the postsynaptic neurones. These receptors are pentamers, and have a number of binding sites where other molecules such as barbiturates, alcohol and benzodiazepines bind. Benzodiazepine sites are allosteric modulators of GABA function, and the ligands binding to these sites can be divided into agonists (e.g. diazepam), which increase GABA effects, antagonists (e.g. flumazenil), which bind to the site but have no net effects, and inverse agonists (e.g. FG 7142), which decrease GABA effects. There is strong evidence that benzodiazepine site inverse agonists are specifically panicogenic in man,[75] and this observation seems to be mirrored in simian studies.[76,77] In addition, agonists at this site (which reduce anxiety and panic symptoms) are less effective in PD patients than in controls,[78] and antagonists (which are usually neutral in control subjects) provoke panic attacks in PD patients[79,80] in a dose-dependent manner but do not have this effect in post-traumatic stress disorder.[81] These observations have led to theories that there may either be a 'shift' in benzodiazepine–$GABA_A$ receptor function in PD (Figure 5.1) or that putative endogenous agonists are released in PD in an attempt to block the symptoms.[79] The panicogenic effects of flumazenil would then be due to removing this compensatory effect.

Evidence from direct agonists and antagonists at the $GABA_A$ receptor is in keeping with the above observations in that antagonists are panicogenic[82] and agonists anxiolytic.[83] However, although the same picture emerges from animal studies,[84,85] the patient data are mainly anecdotal and limited by the other effects that such compounds have (e.g. seizures). The later section of this chapter discusses new PET scanning data that confirm GABA-A receptor involvement in PD.

Adenosinergic system

Caffeine is anxiogenic in patients and controls, and PD patients[86] may have supersensitive adenosine receptors,[87] but it is not clear whether the mechanism through which it operates is indeed adenosine$_2$ (A_2) antagonism. Until more selective ligands become available, the involvement of this system in anxiety and PD will have to remain an open question.

CCK/pentagastrin

CCK-4 is a tetrapeptide that has been demonstrated to precipitate panic attacks in PD patients in a dose-dependent manner and to

Possible alteration in benzodiazepine receptor set-point

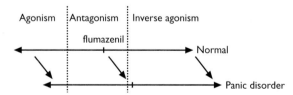

Figure 5.1 Change in benzodiazepine–$GABA_A$ spectrum of activity – the 'receptor shift'. This theory postulates that the set point of the receptor is altered in panic disorder so that antagonists become partial inverse agonists and agonists are less effective. This would explain the panicogenic properties of flumazenil and the reduced sensitivity to benzodiazepine agonists.

increase anxiety symptoms in healthy volunteers.[88–91] Pentagastrin, which shares 4 out of 5 amino acids with CCK-4, has similar properties.[92–94] In addition, although early clinical reports of the efficacy of CCK-4 antagonists in the treatment of PD have been disappointing, both L-365,260 and CI988 attenuate the CCK-4-induced anxiety response, which speaks to the effect being at least partially mediated via these receptors.[95,96] The mechanism by which CCK induces anxiety is unclear, but does not involve inverse agonism at the $BZ–GABA_A$ site, since it is not prevented by flumazenil administration.[97] It is possible that the main site of action for all these probes is outside the brain, since doubts still exist whether they cross the blood–brain barrier, and their onset is very fast.

Cholinergic system

The administration of physostigmine,[98] given with propantheline to block peripheral effects, did not provoke anxiety or endocrine responses that were different between nine PD patients and nine controls, and thus did not support the notion that increased cholinergic transmission is associated with increased anxiety.

Opiates

Naloxone, an antagonist at all opiate receptor subtypes (μ, κ, δ) does not precipitate panic attacks in PD patients, nor does it modify the response to lactate, indicating that it is unlikely that endogenous opiates alone are involved in panic anxiety.[99] However, Charney and Heninger have demonstrated that naloxone and yohimbine are anxiogenic when given together, and this result may speak to the regulation of locus ceruleus activity by opiate receptors and may indicate that ligands acting at opiate receptors may yet be useful in the regulation of anxiety.[100]

Cognitive modulation of pharmacologically induced panic attacks

Some studies have demonstrated that cognitive manipulation of expectation affects the proportion of patients who experience a panic attack with particular probes. Given the nature of reporting, it is difficult to know whether this applies to all the probes or just to those with published results. The finding of effective modulation by cognitive means is often viewed as a limitation of the challenge paradigms. We view this interpretation as unnecessarily dualistic: expectation modulates many experiences that are consciously mediated (pain, visual processing, witness reports) but this does not deny the underlying brain biology. In addition, the statement that the anxiety symptoms are always and only precipitated by a cognitive misinterpretation of bodily symptoms caused by the administered drug is misleading, since not all probes that produce bodily symptoms produce increased anxiety and panic attacks (cf TRH).

Conclusions

Pharmacological challenges have demonstrated that panic symptoms can be precipitated by lactate and CO_2 and by altering monoaminergic, GABAergic and possibly CCK transmission. Many of these effects are not specific to panic disorder, and can be interpreted as altering the modulation of anxiety states in general. However, findings at benzodiazepine sites and possibly serotonergic and CCK-B receptors seem to be specific to PD, implying that anomalies in these systems may be specific to its underlying neurochemical pathology. Further, with all the other probes, PD patients seem to be more easily provoked than patients with other anxiety disorders, perhaps indicating that systems such as the noradrenergic one are involved in more general aspects of the anxiety response. These important leads should be followed up by more specific psychopharmacological, genetic and imaging experiments. It is likely that, even in the improbable event that only one fundamental biochemical abnormality is found to underlie PD, multiple changes in brain biochemistry will be found in people with the established condition, as compensatory and downstream changes take place.

Principles of human imaging

In order to make sense of imaging studies, the principles underlying data acquisition and analysis have to be understood. This section introduces the ideas that we regard as salient for such an interpretation. EEG, MEG, evoked potentials and their computed averaging maps are not discussed, because there are very few data from such neurophysiological experiments in panic disorder. These techniques are, however, likely to be of importance in the future, since they allow accurate temporal resolution of cerebral events that can be investigated following the spatial identification of areas employed for particular tasks by using the imaging techniques discussed below. This section of the chapter can be omitted without loss of continuity.

Anatomical imaging

Anatomical images of the human brain can be produced by the use of X-ray computed tomography (CT) or magnetic resonance imaging (MRI). MRI provides better resolution of soft tissues, and, by varying the parameters of acquisition, can reveal white-matter lesions and areas of altered signal intensity that reflect non-specific pathology. Since MRI does not employ ionizing radiation its use is not restricted by radiation-dose considerations. Magnetic resonance spectroscopy can also be used to produce spectra associated with particular compounds in the brain. In this sense, it is a form of functional imaging, and it produces information on the regional presence and concentration of chemicals of interest (e.g. lactate). While some interesting data have emerged from anatomical and spectroscopy studies, it is unlikely that these techniques will make further significant contributions to the understanding of PD.

Functional imaging

Functional images (physiological and neurochemical) of brain processing can be obtained by the use of nuclear medicine techniques such as positron emission tomography (PET) and single-photon-emission computed tomography (SPECT). These involve the recording of signals emitted by a radiolabelled compound that has been administered to the subject. The observed tomographic signal represents the total radioactive counts from a particular region, and thus is the sum of radioactivity from parent compound and metabolites (if present), both in blood and the various tissue compartments. PET and SPECT are used either to generate maps of brain activity associated with particular tasks or conditions or to measure neurochemical parameters such as receptor or transporter density.

When neuronal populations are engaged in a mental process, they use energy. This can be imaged directly by administering radiolabelled glucose or glucose analogues, or indirectly by imaging the increased blood flow, which is tightly coupled to increased local oxygen requirements in the brain. Regional metabolism or blood flow maps thus produced represent changes in energy requirements at synaptic sites, since synapses are the neuronal elements that consume the most energy. Blood flow maps can, however, also be influenced globally by CO_2 concentrations and regionally by neurotransmitter nerves (noradrenaline, acetylcholine, serotonin and a number of peptides) acting on cerebrovascular adventitia. It is essential to realize that these maps represent the summation of synaptic activity over hundreds of thousands of neurons and that this can therefore lead to seemingly paradoxical effects. For instance, increasing GABAergic activity in 'activated' cortex results in a decrease in local cerebral blood flow, despite the increased synaptic work at inhibitory synapses, because this signal is overwhelmed by the decreased metabolism in excitatory neuron synapses.[101] However, the same result may not apply to resting cortex or to other areas of the brain, where the balance between excitatory and inhibitory cells may be different.[102,103]

[18]F-labelled deoxyglucose ([18]FDG) and ^{11}C-labelled glucose have been used for direct measure of glucose metabolism. [18]FDG is preferable, since it is accumulated in the cells proportionally to the glucose transport rates, and is not further metabolized (unlike [^{11}C]glucose), thus requiring less complex mathematical modelling to interpret the tomographic data. [18]FDG produces a map of integrated glucose transport into the cells dominated by activity over a period of approximately 20 minutes, 20 minutes after injection. Therefore it provides a static picture of brain function in any particular state, which can be maintained for tens of minutes.

[15]O-labelled injected water or inhaled CO_2 (converted to water in the lung capillaries) have been used to delineate blood flow with PET, while ^{133}Xe and ^{99}Tc-HMPAO (a ligand that is freely diffusible across the blood–brain barrier but gets trapped intracellularly by the change in pH) have been used with SPECT. Oxygen PET has been used to map blood flow over a period of up to 2 minutes post injection, with most of the information being acquired in the first 30 seconds. The amounts of radioactivity administered to produce good images with contemporary PET cameras allow up to 12 scans to be performed in a single individual at 8- to 10-minute intervals without exceeding the yearly recommended radiation dose limit for healthy volunteers in the UK. Thus repeated 'activation' experiments can be performed where statistically significant changes in regional activity are interpreted as mapping the cerebral regions associated with particular tasks. This technique has been very successful in delineating areas of the brain involved in particular sensory, motor, affective, language and memory tasks.

[133]Xe is a breathed-in, freely diffusible inert gas used in the original non-tomographic studies that measured brain metabolism. It has been employed tomographically by some laboratories to quantify cerebral blood flow with SPECT. ^{99}Tc-HMPAO produces a 'frozen' picture of cerebral blood flow over a period of 2–3 minutes after injection, which, because of the slow decay of ^{99}Tc, can be imaged for some hours after injection. This has been particularly useful when it has been advantageous to inject patients at sites (e.g. a ward) away from the camera in order to record a particular transient event such as hallucinations. However, slow decay also means an increased amount of absorbed radiation per radioactive dose administered, and most HMPAO 'activation' studies can only perform two scans to keep subjects' exposure to a level of radioactivity that is within acceptable limits; this is a severe limitation, since it greatly reduces the statistical power of the technique.

Much of the activation work, pioneered with nuclear medicine techniques, is going to be continued using functional MRI (fMRI) in the future. fMRI images changes in deoxyhaemoglobin associated with neuronal activation. Although some technical issues have not been fully resolved, the advantages of the absence of ionizing radiation and better spatial and temporal resolution are so great that many research centres have enthusiastically embarked on research protocols with this technique. Much of these initial data are going to be difficult to interpret because of unreliable motion artefact-correction methods. Anxiety research, however, may be one of the areas that is going to benefit least from this new technology, since the environment of MRI scanners generates considerable anxiety, which some patient populations find difficult to tolerate and which adds a further uncontrollable dimension to the experimental procedure.

PET and SPECT have also been used to image pharmacokinetic parameters related to receptors, transporters, enzymes and transmitters. Ligands appropriate for the system under study are labelled with a radiation-emitting nucleus to produce maps of their brain distribution after injection. PET is far more versatile than SPECT for this purpose, since it usually labels nuclei such as carbon that are universal in molecules with biological activity. However, finding compounds that have the ideal characteristics (e.g. very selective receptor/transporter binding, low non-specific binding, easily cross the blood–brain barrier, no lipophillic metabolites, rapid brain–blood equilibration, no physiological action) and that can be radiolabelled is extremely expensive in terms of time and resources. In addition, with single-scan protocols, B_{max} and K_d cannot be separated, and the pharmacokinetic parameters may also include tissue delivery effects and non-specific binding. When semiquantitative methods are applied (as most often in SPECT), errors may also arise by scanning too early after injection, which results in the data being heavily influenced by delivery to the brain rather than binding to the receptors. These methodological problems, accompanied by unsophisticated experimental design, characteristic of new technology, are reflected by the small number of adequate radioligand studies in the current brain research literature. Indeed, very few centres worldwide are able to meet the methodological challenges. However, an additional exciting development is that these imaging techniques may also be used to detect the endogenous release of neurotransmitters, thus allowing the study of functional neurochemistry in vivo in man, which would parallel in vivo microdialysis in animals.

Findings: structural imaging

Structural imaging has been used to investigate the notion that panic disorder may be associated with temporal lobe abnormalities. The results thus far indicate that this may indeed be the case. In a study of 30 consecutive patients from their clinic with PD, Ontiveros et al[104] compared them with 20 healthy volunteers using structural MRI. Eleven patients and one control were thought to have significant abnormalities on their MRI scans, particularly in the right temporal lobe (mainly areas of increased signal intensity, which indicate white matter abnormalities in the medial portion of the lobe), while five patients and one control showed dilatation of the temporal horn of the lateral ventricle. Patients with the temporal lobe abnormalities were younger at onset of PD, had longer duration of illness and had more panic attacks. Applying different criteria to a similar sample of patients, the same group found that 40% of patients with PD and 10% of healthy volunteers had medial temporal structural abnormalities.[105] The strength of these studies is that they investigated consecutive PD patients who were referred to a psychiatric clinic, thus avoiding some of the possible selection biases; however, the sample may not be representative, since many patients with PD do not get referred to secondary care. These findings are echoed in a preliminary report of a large study of 120 PD patients and 28 controls by Dantendorfer et al,[106] which also suggests that temporal lobe abnormalities as detected with MRI are much more common in PD patients than in controls (29% versus 4%). The prevalence of these abnormalities increased to 61% if only PD patients with 'non-epileptic' EEG abnormalities were selected for comparison.

Functional anatomy of panic disorder

Panic disorder received some early attention in imaging research because of the clear definition of the disorder and because of the relative ease with which panic attacks could be induced to study the activated state. In general, however, the early scanners did not have the necessary sensitivity to detect significant changes in metabolism at rest, and investigators focused the experiments by separating out the PD patients who were sensitive to lactate. This strategy produced results that seem to strengthen the case for a biology of PD, since the activated areas were congruous with theories of brain function in anxiety.[107] However, it later became apparent that the most significant activations were due to extracerebral signal secondary to teeth clenching.[108] This reinterpretation of the data has produced a backlash in anxiety disorder research, with many laboratories shunning it and others forsaking statistical power by the introduction of teeth clenching paradigms that are probably not necessary when modern scanners are used. The situation at present is that there have been relatively few studies in anxiety disorders and in PD in partic-

ular when compared with schizophrenia, depression or obsessive–compulsive disorder. While a pattern is starting to emerge, the data are still scarce, and a synthesis is difficult because of the variety of techniques and analyses used, with a particular paucity of pixel-based analyses, which report both increases and decreases. On the other hand, PD patients are amongst the most difficult people to study in the confines of a scanner, since the occurrence of a panic attack almost invariably precludes volunteers from wanting to carry on with the experiment.

In the original studies, Reiman et al[107] demonstrated that patients with PD (some being on medication) had a decreased left-to-right ratio of parahippocampal cerebral blood flow at rest. This was particularly significant in patients who were sensitive to lactate challenge. Other areas (hippocampus, amygdala, inferior parietal lobule, anterior cingulate, hypothalamus, orbito-insular gyri) had no significant left-to-right differences. Two years later, another study was published, which included many of the subjects from the first[109] and which compared eight lactate-sensitive PD patients with eight lactate-insensitive PD patients and 25 controls at rest. The lactate-sensitive patients had lower left-to-right parahippocampal blood flow, volume and metabolic rate for oxygen, which the authors interpreted as an increase in metabolism in the right hippocampus. In a subsequent study,[110] 17 patients and 15 controls were compared before and during lactate infusion. Lactate infusion seemed to produce small increases in blood flow in the superior colliculi bilaterally and the left anterior cerebellar vermis. Only patients who had a panic attack showed bilateral increases in the temporal poles, in the claustrum/pallidum/insula bilaterally, in the superior colliculi bilaterally and in the left anterior cerebellar vermis.

At the same time, Stewart et al[111] studied ten patients with PD and five healthy controls with ^{133}Xe-SPECT scans before after either a lactate or a saline infusion. Six patients had a panic attack, and were compared with non-panickers and controls. Hemispheric blood flow was increased post lactate infusion in non-panickers and controls. This change was greatest on the right, but it did not reach statistical significance. People who experienced a panic attack did not, however, show such a change – possibly because of overbreathing, which would in itself decrease blood flow. In addition, panickers showed a significant increase in the occipital lobe blood flow normalized to hemispheric blood flow bilaterally, as well as a trend for a decrease in left prefrontal blood flow with panic attacks.

Three studies have since examined basal blood flow in PD. Nordahl et al[112] reported the results of comparing ^{18}FDG-PET resting scans between 12 medication-free patients with PD and 30 healthy volunteers. Ten patients had a history of lifetime co-morbidity, but none had other diagnoses at the time of examination. All subjects were scanned during an auditory continuous performance task (CPT) in order to control the environmental conditions. The investigators found a significantly lower metabolic rate in the left interior parietal lobule, trends towards significant increases in the right hippocampal region, medial orbito-frontal cortex, and towards significant decreases in the anterior cingulate. Anxiety measures did not correlate with metabolism in any particular area, while depressed mood ratings and CPT performance correlated positively with medial orbito-frontal metabolism. In a SPECT study, De Cristofaro et al[113] examined nine patients with PD and five controls at rest with ^{99}Tc-HMPAO. They then reported the results for the seven patients who were lactate-sensitive. This population had significantly increased asymmetry (interpreted as increased right-sided flow) in the inferior (orbito-) frontal cortex, increased flow in the left occipital cortex and decreased flow in the hippocampal/amygdala bilaterally. These PD patients were treatment-niaive (although some of them had occasionally taken benzodiazepines) and young, and had a mean duration of illness of 11 months. More recently, Malizia et al[114] compared resting PET ligand delivery (a measure indicative of regional cerebral blood flow) between 11 patients with PD on no medication and 7 healthy controls who were being scanned for the first time, and found that patients had significantly lower delivery in posterior temporal, inferior parietal and cerebellar cortex bilaterally. In patients, but not controls, the Spielberger State Anxiety Inventory administered 1 hour prior to scanning covaried positively with anterior cingulate and negatively with middle temporal and cerebellar delivery. This indicates that the experience of anxiety in this group correlates with increases in blood flow in the cingulate and with decreases in flow in posterior structures.

Only one study has been conducted using a pharmacological challenge.[115] In this study, yohimbine provocation of panic resulted in large decreases in HMPAO-SPECT signal in the frontal cortex. The study has not, however, been described in more detail elsewhere, so that a detailed comment is not possible.

Altogether, these data have to be interpreted in the light of comparative findings in studies other anxiety disorders.[116,117] In general, two sets of areas seem to be activated in anxiety and anxiety disorders, whether at rest or after a challenge. The first set comprises the supragenual anterior cingulate, medial temporal structures (amygdala, parahippocampal gyrus) especially on the left, the orbito-frontal cortex, the insulae, the cerebellum, and a pontine locus variously described as superior colliculi or PAG

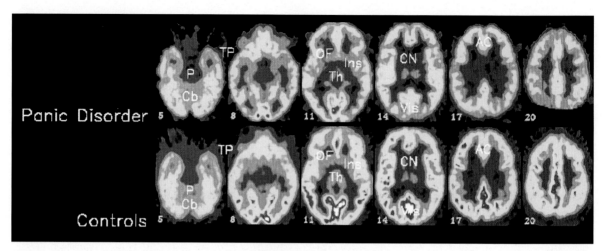

Figure 5.2 Areas of significant increased blood flow in the brain during increased anticipatory anxiety demonstrated by [^{15}O]water PET. The colour coded (see bar) Z values for a group of 16 healthy volunteers are superimposed on transverse slices of an average T_1-weighted MRI to demonstrate the anatomical location. Slices are at 4 mm intervals from 40 mm below to 40 mm above the anterior commissure–posterior commissure plane. The brain is viewed from the feet.

(Figure 5.2). All of these (except the cerebellum) are areas that are directly involved with the evaluation of noxious stimuli and that produce autonomic responses when stimulated. In essence, they may represent the essential circuits of the anxiety responses. The surprising element here is the activation of the cerebellum, which speaks to its hitherto unsuspected involvement in processes that do not have a primary motor component. This finding is not specific to anxiety.[118]

The second set of activations represents areas of sensory or polymodal association cortices, which may represent the processing of relevant anxiogenic stimuli or their imagery.

In conclusion, these data have to be regarded as preliminary, but are tantalizing in that they demonstrate that constructs derived from lesion and animal studies can be valid in the intact human brain and also because they have generated unsuspected new leads, such as the potential involvement of the cerebellum in anxiety. Future developments will come from repeated studies using standardized protocols, contrasting in vivo versus in imagination anxiety provocation, maps of functional connectivity between areas (e.g. amygdala and orbito-frontal), the effects of pharmacological manipulations on loci of activation, and the dissection of fundamental processes such as conditioning and startle.

In vivo neurochemistry of panic disorder

Receptor binding

The only system that has been investigated has been the benzodiazepine–GABA$_A$ one. Following the lead from the psychopharmaco-

logy challenge findings,[79] three lomazenil SPECT studies of PD thus far published have attempted to address the question of whether benzodiazepine-site binding is decreased in particular cortical areas.[119–121] Regrettably, all have significant methodological problems (inappropriate control groups, relative quantitation only, presence of medication, and, most impor-

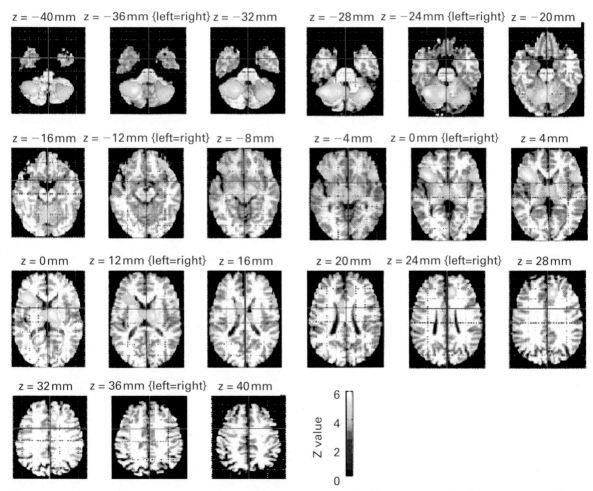

Figure 5.3 Median benzodiazepine binding values for control subjects and panic disorder patients. The binding measure used here is the volume of distribution (VD) and the colour scale corresponds to VD values (red/white high, yellow/green middle, blue/black low). There is a global decrease in benzodiazepine binding in panic disorder patients. Slices are about 1 cm apart from bottom (left) to top (right) of brain. P, Pons; Cb, cerebellum; TP, temporal pole; OF, orbito-frontal cortex; Ins, insula; Th, thalamus; CN, caudate nucleus; AC, anterior cingulate.

tantly, too short an interval between injection and scanning to separate delivery effects from binding[122]), which result in considerable difficulty in interpreting the data. At best, these can only be regarded as pilot data.

Schlegel et al[119] were the first to report decreased benzodiazepine receptor binding in PD using lomazenil SPECT, comparing, at 90–110 minutes post injection, 10 patients with PD with 10 patients with epilepsy on carbamazepine. The decreases were significant in the occipital and frontal lobes and maximal in the temporal lobes. Kaschka et al[121] studied 9 medicated patients with PD *and* depression with a matched group of medicated patients with dysthymia using lomazenil SPECT (2 hours). Decreases in binding were seen in the inferior temporal lobes both medially and laterally and in the inferior frontal lobes. These changes were already detectable at 10 minutes post injection, reflecting changes dominated by delivery effects. All participants were on antidepressants. On the other hand, Kuikka et al,[120] using two different SPECT cameras (at 90 minutes post injection), studied 17 unmedicated patients with PD and 17 healthy age- and sex-matched controls using lomazenil, and found an increase in lomazenil signal bilaterally in the temporal cortex and in the right middle/inferior lateral frontal gyrus.

In the only fully quantitative study so far attempted, Malizia et al[123] employed [^{11}C]flumazenil PET and found a global decrease in binding in benzodiazepine-naïve, drug-free patients with PD who had no comorbid conditions and did not abuse alcohol (Figure 5.3). These changes were maximal in ventral basal ganglia, orbito-frontal and temporal cortex. After correction for the global decrease in binding, PD patients showed a further statistically significant regional decrease in binding in the inferior parietal temporo-occipital areas, which was maximal in the lat-

eral posterior temporal lobes, as well as decreases in orbito-frontal cortex and ventral striatum. Decreased binding in thalamus, dorso-lateral and medial prefrontal, medial temporal and cerebellar cortex and vermis were accounted for by the global changes.

The significantly decreased benzodiazepine receptor binding is consistent with the idea that PD is due to a deficiency in brain inhibition that leads to, or allows, paroxysmal elevations in anxiety during panic attacks. The peak decreases in benzodiazepine binding are in anatomical areas (e.g. orbito-frontal cortex and insula) thought to be involved in the experience of anxiety in man, and could represent a primary pathology.

There are three major types of mechanisms which could account for the widespread reduction in binding. These are not mutually exclusive and are summarized in Figure 5.4 and Table 5.2. First, there is an alteration of the subunit composition of the benzodiazepine–GABA$_A$ complex that could indicate an *a priori* differential expression of GABA$_A$–benzodiazepine receptors in PD patients (e.g. an increase in the expression of α_4 or α_6 subunits to which flumazenil does not bind with high affinity) or an environmentally induced modification in receptor configuration secondary to changes in receptor subunits[124] or endocytic loop phosphorylation.[125] Secondly, the presence of endogenous benzodiazepine ligands,[126] increased GABA concentration[127] or neurosteroid inverse agonists[128] can lead to reduced binding of flumazenil, and may mediate the corticosteroid-dependent reduced binding observed with stress in mice.[129–131] Finally, changes in afferent noradrenergic or serotonergic tone could also produce this effect by regulating GABAergic neurons or, directly, GABA$_A$ receptors.[132–135] Other explanations are possible but less plausible: a global decrease due to grey-matter atrophy is very unlikely, and MRI

Table 5.2 Possible mechanisms inducing global reduction in flumazenil binding in the brain[a]

Site	Mechanism	
GABA$_A$ receptor	Subunit composition	Genetically different (6)
		Environmentally induced changes (3)
		Increased GABA
		Increased endogenous BZ
		Increased neurosteroids
		Other
	Subunit function	Phosphorylation changes (5)
	Kinetics	Decreased apparent B_{max} (3)
		Increased endogenous agonist
Ascending monoaminergic projections	Decreased serotonergic tone (1, 2)	
	Decreased noradrenergic tone (1)	
Adrenal glands (4)	Increased neurosteroid precursors	
	Increased corticosteroids	

[a]The numbering in the table refers to sites of action as pictured in Figure 5.4.

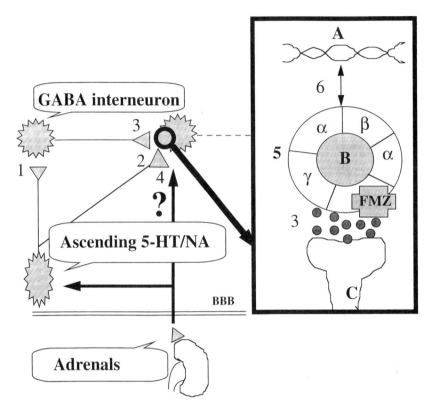

Figure 5.4 Schematic representation of possible mechanisms influencing benzodiazepine binding in the brains of patients with panic disorder. For further explanation see Table 5.2.

and [18]FDG-PET studies of PD have found only minimal changes, mostly in the temporal lobe.[105,112] Decreased binding due to occupancy by an anxiogenic endogenous inverse agonist is also unlikely to explain these findings, because the pure antagonist flumazenil would then be anxiolytic and not panicogenic, as previously demonstrated.[79]

The reduction in binding not only explains some of the known features of benzodiazepine receptor function in PD but also is congruent with animal data showing that chronic stress decreases benzodiazepine binding[129–131] and that animal strains that are more responsive to stress also have decreased benzodiazepine binding.[136] It is thus possible that this finding could be the result of experiencing repeated panic attacks or the consequence of one or more of the aetiological factors such as genetic predisposition or life events.

Response to challenge

Despite considerable evidence for lactate transport into the brain and the fact that the proposed mechanism of action was inconsistent with the known biochemistry of L-lactate, it had been argued that the effects of lactate infusion were mediated by changes in pCO_2. Dager et al,[137] using MR spectroscopy, have demonstrated that patients with PD who are lactate-sensitive have a greater and more prolonged elevation in cerebral lactate after the infusion of L-lactate.

Conclusions

A number of pharmacological abnormalities have been demonstrated in PD, although it is questionable whether any are absolutely specific to this disorder or whether they are more general manifestations of inappropriate chronic and/or severe anxiety. As pharmacological probes become more specific, it should be possible to dissect the psychopharmacology of PD with more clarity. We believe that alterations at benzodiazepine– $GABA_A$ receptors are going to be central to the understanding of the neurobiology of this disorder, but that useful information will also come from serotonergic and noradrenergic probes. However, the most significant future advances will come from the use of the various imaging techniques that are now becoming available to detect physiological and biochemical changes in the human brain in vivo, as demonstrated so far by preliminary results. As such, the time is now ripe to invest a great deal of methodological effort in order to develop paradigms that will allow us to make full use of these techniques in the future.

Acknowledgement

ALM is a Wellcome Training Fellow.

References

1. Nutt D, Lawson C, Panic attacks. A neurochemical overview of models and mechanisms. *Br J Psychiatry* 1992; **160**: 165–78.
2. Balon R, Pohl R, Yeragani VK et al, Follow up study of control subjects with lactate and isoproterenol induced panic attacks. *Am J Psychiatry* 1988; **145**: 238–41.
3. Jensen CF, Keller TW, Peskind ER et al, Behavioral and neuroendocrine responses to sodium lactate infusion in subjects with post-traumatic stress disorder. *Am J Psychiatry* 1997; **154**: 266–8.
4. Liebowitz MR, Fyer AJ, Gorman JM, et al. Specificity of lactate infusions in social phobia versus panic disorders. *Am J Psychiatry* 1985; **142**: 947–50.
5. Liebowitz MR, Coplan JD, Martinez J, Effects of intravenous diazepam pretreatment on lactate-induced panic. *Psychiatry Res* 1995; **58**: 127–38.
6. Pohl R, Balon R, Berchov R et al, Lactate induced anxiety after imipramine and diazepam treatment. *Anxiety* 1994; **1**: 54–63.
7. Coplan JD, Liebowitz MR, Gorman JM et al, Noradrenergic function in panic disorder. Effects of intravenous clonidine pretreatment on lactate induced panic. *Biol Psychiatry* 1992; **31**: 135–46.
8. Reschke AH, Mannuzza S, Chapman TF et al, Sodium lactate response and familial risk for panic disorder. *Am J Psychiatry* 1995; **152**: 277–9.

9. Coplan JD, Sharma T, Rosenblum LA et al, Effects of sodium lactate infusion on cisternal lactate and carbon dioxide levels in nonhuman primates. *Am J Psychiatry* 1992; **149**: 1369–73.

10. Dager SR, Rainey JM, Kenny MA et al, Central nervous system effects of lactate infusion in primates. *Biol Psychiatry* 1990; **27**: 193–204.

11. George DT, Lindquist T, Nutt DJ et al, Effect of chloride or glucose on the incidence of lactate-induced panic attacks. *Am J Psychiatry* 1995; **152**: 692–7.

12. Gorman JM, Battista D, Goetz RR et al, A comparison of sodium bicarbonate and sodium lactate infusion in the induction of panic attacks. *Arch Gen Psychiatry* 1989; **46**: 145–50.

13. Bissonette JM, Hohimer AR, Chao CR, Unidirectional transport of glucose and lactate into brain of foetal sheep and guinea pig. *Exp Physiol* 1991; **76**: 515–23.

14. La Manna JC, Harrington JF, Vendel LM et al, Regional blood brain lactate influx. *Brain Res* 1993; **614**: 164–70.

15. Lear JL, Kasliwal RK, Autoradiographic measurement of cerebral lactate transport rate constants in normal and activated conditions. *J Cereb Blood Flow Metab* 1991; **11**: 576–80.

16. Knudsen GM, Paulson OB, Hertz MM, Kinetic analysis of the human blood brain transport of lactate and its influence by hypercapnia. *J Cereb Blood Flow Metab* 1991; **11**: 581–6.

17. Fontaine S, Ontiveros A, Fontaine R, Elie R, Panic disorder: vascular evaluation with transcranial Doppler ultrasonography. *Can Assoc Radiol J* 1991; **42**: 412–16.

18. George DT, Nutt DJ, Walker WV et al, Lactate and hyperventilation substantially attenuate vagal tone in normal volunteers. A possible mechanism of panic provocation? *Arch Gen Psychiatry* 1989; **46**: 153–6.

19. Yeragani VK, Srinivasan K, Pohl R et al, Sodium lactate increases sympathovagal ratios in normal control subjects: spectral analysis of heart rate, blood pressure, and respiration. *Psychiatry Res* 1994; **54**: 97–114.

20. Yeragani VK, Srinivasan K, Balon R et al, Lactate sensitivity and cardiac cholinergic function in panic disorder. *Am J Psychiatry* 1994; **151**: 1226–8.

21. Wikander I, Roos T, Stakkestad A et al, Sodium lactate elicits a rapid increase in blood pressure in Wistar rats and spontaneously hypertensive rats. Effect of pretreatment with the antipanic drugs clomipramine and alprazolam. *Neuropsychopharmacology* 1995; **12**: 245–50.

22. Koenigsberg HW, Pollak CP, Fine J et al, Cardiac and respiratory activity in panic disorder: effects of sleep and sleep lactate infusions. *Am J Psychiatry* 1994; **151**: 1148–52.

23. Griez E, de Loof C, Pols H et al, Specific sensitivity of patients with panic attacks to carbon dioxide inhalation. *Psychiatry Res* 1990; **31**: 193–9.

24. Perna G, Bertani A, Arancio C et al, Laboratory response of patients with panic and obsessive compulsive disorders to 35% CO_2 challenges. *Am J Psychiatry* 1995; **152**: 85–9.

25. Harrington PJ, Schmidt NB, Telch MJ, Prospective evaluation of panic potentiation following 35% CO_2 challenge in nonclinical subjects. *Am J Psychiatry* 1996; **153**: 823–5.

26. Papp LA, Klein DF, Martinez J et al, Diagnostic and substance specificity of carbon dioxide induced panic. *Am J Psychiatry* 1993; **150**: 250–7.

27. Sanderson WC, Wetzler S, Asnis GM, Alprazolam blockade of CO_2 provoked panic in patients with panic disorder. *Am J Psychiatry* 1994; **151**: 1220–2.

28. Perna G, Brambilla F, Arancio C et al, Menstrual cycle related sensitivity to 35% CO_2 in panic patients. *Biol Psychiatry* 1995; **37**: 528–32.

29. Perna G, Cocchi S, Bertani A et al, Sensitivity to 35% CO_2 in healthy first degree relatives of patients with panic disorder. *Am J Psychiatry* 1995; **152**: 623–5.

30. Perna G, Bertani A, Caldirola D et al, Family history of panic disorder and hypersensitivity to CO_2 in patients with panic disorder. *Am J Psychiatry* 1996; **153**: 1060–4.

31. Haxhiu MA, Yung K, Erokwu B et al, CO_2 induced c fos expression in the CNS catecholaminergic neurons. *Respir Physiol* 1996; **105**: 35–45.

32. Elam M, Yao T, Thoren P et al, Hypercapnia and hypoxia: chemoreceptor mediated control of locus coeruleus neurons and splanchnic,

sympathic nerves. *Brain Res* 1981; **222:** 373–81.

33. Concas A, Sanna E, Cuccheddu T et al, Carbon dioxide inhalation, stress and anxiogenic drugs reduce the function of GABAA receptor complex in the rat brain. *Prog Neuropsychopharmacol Biol Psychiatry* 1993; **17:** 651–61.

34. Cuccheddu T, Floris S, Serra M et al, Proconflict effect of carbon dioxide inhalation in rats. *Life Sci* 1995; **56:** 321–4.

35. Pols H, Griez E, Verburg K et al, Yohimbine premedication and 35% CO_2 vulnerability in healthy volunteers. *Eur Arch Psychiatry Clin Neurosci* 1994; **244:** 81–5.

36. Gurguis GN, Uhde TW, Plasma 3-methoxy-4-hydroxyphenylethylene glycol (MHPG) and growth hormone responses to yohimbine in panic disorder patients and normal controls. *Neuropsychopharmacology* 1990; **13:** 65–73.

37. Charney DS, Heninger GR, Breier A, Noradrenergic function in panic anxiety. Effects of yohimbine in healthy subjects and patients with agoraphobia and panic disorder. *Arch Gen Psychiatry* 1984; **41:** 751–63.

38. Charney DS, Woods SW, Goodman WK et al, Neurobiological mechanisms of panic anxiety: biochemical and behavioral correlates of yohimbine induced panic attacks. *Am J Psychiatry* 1987; **144:** 1030–6.

39. Charney DS, Woods SW, Krystal JH et al, Noradrenergic neuronal dysregulation in panic disorder: the effects of intravenous yohimbine and clonidine in panic disorder patients. *Acta Psychiatr Scand* 1992; **86:** 273–82.

40. Goddard AW, Woods SW, Sholomskas DE et al, Effects of the serotonin reuptake inhibitor fluvoxamine on yohimbine induced anxiety in panic disorder. *Psychiatry Res* 1993; **48:** 119–33.

41. Charney DS, Heninger GR, Abnormal regulation of noradrenergic function in panic disorders. Effects of clonidine in healthy subjects and patients with agoraphobia and panic disorder. *Arch Gen Psychiatry* 1986; **43:** 1042–54.

42. Nutt DJ, Increased central alpha 2 adrenoceptor sensitivity in panic disorder. *Psychopharmacology* 1986; **90:** 268–9.

43. Nutt DJ, Altered central alpha 2 adrenoceptor

sensitivity in panic disorder. *Arch Gen Psychiatry* 1989; **46:** 165–9.

44. Schittecatte M, Ansseau M, Charles G et al, Growth hormone response to clonidine in male patients with panic disorder untreated by antidepressants. *Psychol med* 1992; **22:** 1059–62.

45. Abelson JL, Glitz D, Cameron OG et al, Endocrine, cardiovascular, and behavioral responses to clonidine in patients with panic disorder. *Biol Psychiatry* 1992; **32:** 18–25.

46. Tancer ME, Stein MB, Black B et al, Blunted growth hormone responses to growth hormone releasing factor and to clonidine in panic disorder. *Am J Psychiatry* 1993; **150:** 336–7.

47. Brambilla F, Perna G, Garberi A et al, Alpha 2 adrenergic receptor sensitivity in panic disorder: I. GH response to GHRH and clonidine stimulation in panic disorder. *Psychoneuroendocrinology* 1995; **20:** 1–9.

48. Tancer ME, Stein MB, Uhde TW, Growth hormone response to intravenous clonidine in social phobia: comparison to patients with panic disorder and healthy volunteers. *Biol Psychiatry* 1993; **34:** 591–5.

49. Coplan JD, Papp LA, Pine D et al, Clinical improvement with fluoxetine therapy and noradrenergic function in patients with panic disorder. *Arch Gen Psychiatry* 1997; **54:** 643–8.

50. Pohl R, Yeragani VK, Balon R et al, Isoproterenol induced panic attacks. *Biol Psychiatry* 1988; **24:** 891–902.

51. Nesse RM, Cameron OG, Curtis GC et al, Adrenergic function in patients with panic anxiety. *Arch Gen Psychiatry* 1984; **41:** 771–6.

52. Middleton HC, Ashby M, Robbins TW, Reduced plasma noradrenaline and abnormal heart rate variability in resting panic disorder patients. *Biol Psychiatry* 1994; **36:** 847–9.

53. Middleton HC, Ashby M, Clinical recovery from panic disorder is associated with evidence of changes in cardiovascular regulation. *Acta Psychiatr Scand* 1995; **91:** 108–13.

54. Mavissakalian MR, Perel JM, The relationship of plasma imipramine and N-desmethylimipramine to response in panic disorder. *Psychopharmacol Bull* 1996; **32:** 143–7.

55. Boyer W, Serotonin uptake inhibitors are

superior to imipramine and alprazolam in alleviating panic attacks: a meta analysis. *Int Clin Psychopharmacol* 1995; **10**: 45–9.

56. Graeff FG, Guimaraes FS, De Andrade TG et al, Role of 5HT in stress anxiety and depression. *Pharmacol Biochem Behav* 1996; **54**: 129–41.

57. Charney DS, Heninger GR, Serotonin function in panic disorders. The effect of intravenous tryptophan in healthy subjects and patients with panic disorder before and during alprazolam treatment. *Arch Gen Psychiatry* 1986; **43**: 1059–65.

58. Kahn RS, Westenberg HG, Verhoeven WM et al, Effect of a serotonin precursor and uptake inhibitor in anxiety disorders, a double blind comparison of 5-hydroxytryptophan, clomipramine and placebo. *Int Clin Psychopharmacol* 1987; **2**: 33–45.

59. Den Boer JA, Westenberg HG, Behavioral, neuroendocrine, and biochemical effects of 5-hydroxytryptophan administration in panic disorder. *Psychiatry Res* 1990; **31**: 267–78.

60. Westenberg HG, den Boer JA, Serotonin function in panic disorder: effect of 1,5-hydroxytryptophan in patients and controls. *Psychopharmacology* 1989; **98**: 283–5.

61. Goddard AW, Sholomskas DE, Walton KE et al, Effects of tryptophan depletion in panic disorder. *Biol Psychiatry* 1994; **36**: 775–7.

62. Targum SD, Marshall LE, Fenfluramine provocation of anxiety in patients with panic disorder. *Psychiatry Res* 1989; **28**: 295–306.

63. Germine M, Goddard AW, Sholomskas DE et al, Response to *meta*-chlorophenylpiperazine in panic disorder patients and healthy subjects: influence of reduction in intravenous dosage. *Psychiatry Res* 1994; **54**: 115–33.

64. Kahn RS, Wetzler S, Asnis GM et al, Effects of m chlorophenylpiperazine in normal subjects: a dose response study. *Psychopharmacology Berl* 1990; **100**: 339–44.

65. Kahn RS, Asnis GM, Wetzler S et al, Neuroendocrine evidence for serotonin receptor hypersensitivity in panic disorder. *Psychopharmacology* 1988; **96**: 360–4.

66. Kahn RS, Wetzler S, van Praag HM et al, Behavioral indications for serotonin receptor hypersensitivity in panic disorder. *Psychiatry Res* 1988; **25**: 101–4.

67. Lesch KP, Wiesmann M, Hoh A et al, 5 HT1A receptor effector system responsivity in panic disorder. *Psychopharmacology* 1992; **106**: 111–17.

68. Den Boer JA, Westenberg HG, Serotonin function in panic disorder: a double blind placebo controlled study with fluvoxamine and ritanserin. *Psychopharmacology* 1990; **102**: 85–94.

69. Guimaraes FS, Mbaya PS, Deakin JFW, Ritanserin facilitates anxiety in a simulated public speaking paradigm. *J Psychopharmacology* 1997; **11**: 225–31.

70. Hensman R, Guimaraes FS, Wang M et al, Effects of ritanserin on aversive classical conditioning in humans. *Psychopharmacology* 1991; **104**: 220–4.

71. Yoshioka M, Matsumoto M, Togashi H et al, Effect of conditioned fear stress on dopamine release in the rat prefrontal cortex. *Neurosci Lett* 1996; **209**: 201–3.

72. Coco ML, Kuhn CM, Ely TD et al, Selective activation of mesoamygdaloid dopamine neurons by conditioned stress: attenuation by diazepam. *Brain Res* 1992; **590**: 39–47.

73. Pitchot W, Ansseau M, Gonzalez Moreno A et al, Dopaminergic function in panic disorder: comparison with major and minor depression. *Biol Psychiatry* 1992; **32**: 1004–11.

74. Pitchot W, Hanserme M, Gonzalez-Moreno A et al, Growth hormone response to apomorphine in panic disorder: comparison with major depression and normal controls. *Eur Arch Psychiatr Clin Neurosci* 1995; **245**: 306–8.

75. Dorow R, Horowski R, Paschelke G et al, Severe anxiety induced by FG7142 a b carboline ligand for benzodiazepine receptors. *Lancet* 1983; **ii**: 98–9.

76. Petersen EN, Jensen LH, Proconflict effect of benzodiazepine receptor inverse agonists and other inhibitors of GABa function. *Eur J Pharmacol* 1984; **133**: 309–17.

77. Ninan PT, Insel TH, Cohen RM et al, Benzodiazepine receptor mediated experimental anxiety in primates. *Science* 1982; **218**: 1332–4.

78. Roy-Byrne PP, Cowley DS, Greenblatt DJ et al, Reduced benzodiazepine sensitivity in panic disorder. *Arch Gen Psychiatry* 1990; **47**: 259–72.

79. Nutt DJ, Glue P, Lawson C et al, Flumazenil

provocation of panic attacks. *Arch Gen Psychiatry* 1990; **47**: 917–25.

80. Woods SW, Charney DS, Delgado PL et al, The effect of long term imipramine treatment on carbon dioxide induced anxiety in panic disorder patients. *J Clin Psychiatry* 1990; **51**: 505–7.

81. Randall PK, Bremner JD, Krystal JH et al, Effects of the benzodiazepine antagonist flumazenil in PTSD. *Biol Psychiatry* 1995; **38**: 319–24.

82. Rodin EA, Calhoun HD, Metrazol tolerance in a 'normal' volunteer population. A ten year follow up report. *J Nerv Ment Dis* 1970; **150**: 438–43.

83. Hoehn-Saric R, Effects of THIP on chronic anxiety. *Psychopharmacology* 1983; **80**: 338–41.

84. File SE, Lister RG, Do the reductions in social interaction produced by picrotoxin and pentylenetetrazole indicate anxiogenic actions? *Neuropharmacology* 1984; **23**: 793–6.

85. Corbett R, Fielding S, Cornfeldt M et al, Amimetic agents display anxiolytic like effects in the social interaction and elevated plus maze procedures. *Psychopharmacology* 1991; **104**: 312–16.

86. Klein E, Zohar J, Geraci MF et al, Anxiogenic effects of m-CPP in patients with panic disorder: comparison to caffeine's anxiogenic effects. *Biol Psychiatry* 1991; **30**: 973–84.

87. DeMet E, Stein MK, Tran C et al, Caffeine taste test for panic disorder: adenosine receptor supersensitivity. *Psychiatry Res* 1989; **30**: 231–42.

88. Bradwejn J, Koszycki D, Annable L et al, A dose ranging study of the behavioral and cardiovascular effects of CCK tetrapeptide in panic disorder. *Biol Psychiatry* 1992; **32**: 903–12.

89. Bradwejn J, Koszycki D, Payeur R et al, Replication of action of cholecystokinin tetrapeptide in panic disorder: clinical and behavioral findings. *Am J Psychiatry* 1992; **149**: 962–4.

90. Bradwejn J, Koszycki D, Shriqui C, Enhanced sensitivity to cholecystokinin tetrapeptide in panic disorder. Clinical and behavioral findings. *Arch Gen Psychiatry* 1991; **48**: 603–10.

91. Bradwejn J, Koszycki D, Meterissian G,

Cholecystokinin tetrapeptide induces panic attacks in patients with panic disorder. *Can J Psychiatry* 1990; **35**: 83–5.

92. Abelson JL, Nesse RM, Vinik AI, Pentagastrin infusions in patients with panic disorder. II. Neuroendocrinology. *Biol Psychiatry* 1994; **36**: 84–96.

93. Abelson JL, Nesse RM, Pentagastrin infusions in patients with panic disorder. I. Symptoms and cardiovascular responses. *Biol Psychiatry* 1994; **36**: 73–83.

94. van Megen HJ, Westenberg HG, den Boer JA et al, Pentagastrin induced panic attacks: enhanced sensitivity in panic disorder patients. *Psychopharmacology Berl* 1994; **114**: 449–55.

95. Bradwejn J, Koszycki D, Couetoux du Tertre A et al, The panicogenic effects of cholecystokinin tetrapeptide are antagonized by L 365,260, a central cholecystokinin receptor antagonist, in patients with panic disorder. *Arch Gen Psychiatry* 1994; **51**: 486–93.

96. Bradwejn J, Koszycki D, Paradis M et al, Effect of CI 988 on cholecystokinin tetrapeptide induced panic symptoms in healthy volunteers. *Biol Psychiatry* 1995; **38**: 742–6.

97. Bradwejn J, Koszycki D, Couetoux de Tertre A et al, Effects of flumazenil on cholecystokinin tetrapeptide induced panic symptoms in healthy volunteers. *Psychopharmacology Berl* 1994; **114**: 257–61.

98. Rapoport MH, Risch SC, Gillin JC, The effects of physostigmine infusion on patients with panic disorder. *Biol Psychiatry* 1991; **29**: 658–64.

99. Liebowitz MR, Gorman JM, Fyer AJ et al, Effects of naloxone on patients with panic attacks. *Am J Psychiatry* 1984; **141**: 995–7.

100. Charney DS, Heninger GR, Alpha 2-adrenergic and opiate receptor blockade. Synergistic effects on anxiety in healthy subjects. *Arch Gen Psychiatry* 1986; **43**: 1037–41.

101. Roland PE, Friberg L, The effect of the GABA A agonist THIP on regional cortical blood flow in humans. A new test of hemispheric dominance. *J Cereb Blood Flow Metab* 1988; **8**: 314–23.

102. Peyron R, Cinotti L, Le Bars D et al, Effects of $GABA_A$ receptors activation on brain glucose metabolism in normal subjects and temporal lobe epilepsy (TLE) patients. A positron emission tomography (PET) study. Part II: The

focal hypometabolism is reactive to GABA_A agonist administration in TLE. *Epilepsy Res* 1994; **19**: 55–62.

103. Tagamets MA, Horwitz B, A computationally based account of GABA_A agonist in human brain imaging studies. *Neuroimage* 1997; **5**: S386.

104. Ontiveros A, Fontaine R, Breton G et al, Correlation of severity of panic disorder and neuroanatomical changes on magnetic resonance imaging. *J Neuropsychiatry Clin Neurosci* 1989; **1**: 404–8.

105. Fontaine R, Breton G, Dery R et al, Temporal lobe abnormalities in panic disorder: an MRI study. *Biol Psychiatry* 1990; **27**: 304–10.

106. Dantendorfer K, Prayer D, Amering M et al, Increased vulnerablility to panic disorder: panic disorder associated with brain abnormalities. *Behav Pharmacol* 1995; **6** (suppl 1): 142.

107. Reiman EM, Raichle ME, Butler FK et al, A focal brain abnormality in panic disorder, a severe form of anxiety. *Nature* 1984; **310**: 683–5.

108. Drevets WC, Videen TQ, MacLeod AK et al, PET images of blood flow changes during anxiety: correction. *Science* 1992; **256**: 1696.

109. Reiman EM, Raichle ME, Robins E et al, The application of positron emission tomography to the study of panic disorder. *Am J Psychiatry* 1986; **143**: 469–77.

110. Reiman EM, Raichle ME, Robins E et al, Neuroanatomical correlates of a lactate induced anxiety attack. *Arch Gen Psychiatry* 1989; **46**: 493–500.

111. Stewart RS, Devous MD Sr, Rush AJ et al, Cerebral blood flow changes during sodium lactate induced panic attacks. *Am J Psychiatry* 1988; **145**: 442–9.

112. Nordahl TE, Semple WE, Gross M et al, Cerebral glucose metabolic differences in patients with panic disorder. *Neuropsychopharmacology* 1990; **3**: 261–72.

113. De Cristofaro MT, Sessarego A, Pupi A et al, Brain perfusion abnormalities in drug-naive, lactate-sensitive panic patients: a SPECT study. *Biol Psychiatry* 1993; **33**: 505–12.

114. Malizia AL, Cunningham VJ, Bell CM et al, Decreased brain GABA_A-benzodiazepine Receptor Binding in Panic Disorder. *Arch Gen Psychiatry* 1998; (in press).

115. Woods SW, Koster K, Krystal JK et al, Yohimbine alters regional cerebral blood flow in panic disorder [letter]. *Lancet* 1988; **iii**: 678.

116. Rauch SL, Savage CR, Alpert NM et al, The functional neuroanatomy of anxiety: a study of three disorders using positron emission tomography and symptom provocation. *Biol Psychiatry* 1997; **42**: 446–52.

117. Malizia AL, Imaging in human anxiety and anxiety disorders. Abstracts of the Fifth Symposium of the International Society for Neuroimaging in Psychiatry. *Brain Res* 1998; (in press).

118. Middleton FA, Strick PL, Anatomical evidence for cerebellar and basal ganglia involvement in higher cognitive function. *Science* 1994; **266**: 458–61.

119. Schlegel S, Steinert H, Bockisch A et al, Decreased benzodiazepine receptor binding in panic disorder measured by iomazenil SPECT. A preliminary report. *Eur Arch Psychiatry Clin Neurosci* 1994; **244**: 49–51.

120. Kuikka JT, Pitkanen A, Lepola U et al, Abnormal regional benzodiazepine receptor uptake in the prefrontal cortex in patients with panic disorder. *Nucl Med Commun* 1995; **16**: 273–80.

121. Kaschka W, Feistel H, Ebert D, Reduced benzodiazepine receptor binding in panic disorders measured by iomazenil SPECT. *J Psychiatr Res* 1995; **29**: 427–3.

122. Onishi Y, Yonekura Y, Tanaka F, Delayed image of iodine-123 iomazenil as a relative map of benzodiazepine receptor binding: the optimal scan time. *Eur J Nucl Med* 1996; **23**: 1491–7.

123. Malizia AL, Cunningham VJ, Nutt DJ, Flumazenil delivery changes in panic disorder at rest. *Neuroimage* 1997; **5**(4, Part 2): S302.

124. Primus RJ, Gallager DW, GABAA receptor subunit mRNA levels are differentially influenced by chronic FG 7142 and diazepam exposure. *Eur J Pharmacol* 1992; **226**: 21–8.

125. Moss SJ, Smart TG, Blackstone CD et al, Functional modulation of GABA_A receptors by cAMP dependent protein phosphorylation. *Science* 1992; **257**: 661–5.

126. Kang I, Miller LG, Decreased GABA_A receptor subunit mRNA concentrations following chronic lorazepam administration. *Br J Pharmacol* 1991; **103**: 1285–7.

127. Maloteaux JM, Octave JN, Gossuin A et al, GABA induces down regulation of the benzodiazepine GABA receptor complex in the rat cultured neurons. *Eur J Pharmacol* 1987; **144:** 173–83.

128. Demirgoren S, Majewska MD, Spivak CE et al, Receptor binding and electrophysiological effects of dehydroepiandrosterone sulfate, an antagonist of the GABA$_A$ receptor. *Neuroscience* 1991; **45:** 127–35.

129. Weizman R, Weizman A, Kook KA et al, Repeated swim stress alters brain benzodiazepine receptors measured in vivo. *J Pharmacol Exp Ther* 1989; **249:** 701–7.

130. Weizman A, Weizman R, Kook KA et al, Adrenalectomy prevents the stress induced decrease in in vivo [³H]Ro15 1788 binding to GABA$_A$ benzodiazepine receptors in the mouse. *Brain Res* 1990; **519:** 347–50.

131. Inoue O, Akimoto Y, Hashimoto K et al, Alterations in biodistribution of [³H]Ro 15–1788 in mice by acute stress: possible changes in in vivo binding availability of brain benzodiazepine receptor. *Int J Nucl Med Biol* 1985; **12:** 369–74.

132. Doudet D, Hommer D, Higley JD et al, Cerebral glucose metabolism, CSF 5-HIAA levels, and aggressive behavior in rhesus monkeys. *Am J Psychiatry* 1995; **152:** 1782–7.

133. Huidobro Toro JP, Valenzuela CF, Harris RA, *Neuropharmacology* 1996; **35:** 1355–63.

134. Medina JH, Novas ML, Parallel changes in brain flunitrazepam binding and density of noradrenergic innervation. *Eur J Pharmacol* 1983; **88:** 377–82.

135. Doble A, Iversen LL, Bowery NG et al, 6-Hydroxydopamine decreases benzodiazepine but not GABA receptor binding in rat cerebellum. *Neurosci Lett* 1981; **27** 199–204.

136. Commissaris RL, Harrington GM, Altman HJ, Benzodiazepine anti conflict effects in Maudsley reactive (MR/Har) and non reactive (MNRA/Har) rats. *Psychopharmacology* 1990; **100:** 287–92.

137. Dager SR, Strauss WL, Marro KI et al, Proton magnetic resonance spectroscopy investigation of hyperventilation in subjects with panic disorder and comparison subjects. *Am J Psychiatry* 1995; **152:** 666–72.

6

The current status of respiration in panic disorder

Eric Griez and Kees Verburg

Introduction

This chapter discusses the role of respiration in the pathophysiology and etiology of panic disorder (PD). It will deal especially with recent findings on the comorbidity between PD and respiratory diseases, including findings on some lung-function parameters in PD. Next, recent laboratory research using panic provocation techniques and measurements of carbon dioxide (CO_2) sensitivity will be reviewed. Finally, some theoretical considerations will be made, with a particular emphasis on Klein's hypothesis of false suffocation alarms. Some suggestions will be given for future research.

Panic disorder and respiratory diseases

Difficulty with breathing during panic attacks (PA) is a common clinical observation. This observation has led to a long history of research into a possible relationship between a malfunctioning of the respiratory system and anxiety. This research most often took place within the theoretical framework of the so-called hyperventilation syndrome.[1] In this conceptual model 'bad breathing habits' caused bursts of hyperventilation and respiratory alkalosis, which elicited typical physical symptoms (such as dizziness, shaking and palpitations), causing fear and anxiety.[2] The hyperventilation literature is very large and will not be reviewed in detail here.

A large number of studies on the specific relationship between PD and the respiratory system have been published especially in the last 10–15 years. Most of these studies were either epidemiological or experimental.

A strong argument in favor of a relationship between PD and a malfunctioning of the respiratory system is the fact that patients with respiratory disorder often report panic-like experiences. Kinsman et al[3] showed that panic occurred frequently (42%) in a group of asthma patients. The increased incidence of PAs and PD in patients suffering with asthma compared with rates in the general population has been confirmed by other investigators.

Yellowlees et al[4] compared 13 patients who had suffered a near-miss death of asthma with 36 other asthma patients. They did not find a difference between those two groups. All asthma patients had a higher than expected level of psychiatric morbidity. Shavitt et al[5] found 14 patients with agoraphobia and 7 PD patients (respectively 13.1% and 6.1%) in 107 outpatients with asthma. In a study by Butz and Alexander[6] two-thirds of children with asthma reported 'panic' at the beginning of an asthma attack. The idea of a possible link between anxiety states and asthma attacks is supported by a single case study by Hibbert and Pilsbury.[7] Using transcutaneous pCO_2 monitoring, they showed that hyperventilation, accompanied by an anxious mood, preceded exacerbation of asthma.

Patients with chronic obstructive pulmonary disease (COPD) also show a high prevalence of anxiety disorders. Yellowlees et al[8] and Karajgi et al[9] both investigated 50 patients with chronic airflow obstruction. They found that respectively 24% and 8% of the patients suffered with PD. The difference between the two studies can be explained by the fact that the sample of Yellowlees and co-workers consisted of hospitalized patients, while the subjects of Karajgi and co-workers were outpatients. Pollack et al[10] examined 115 patients who were referred for pulmonary function testing. Forty-one percent of these patients reported PAs and 17% met screening criteria for PD. Patients with COPD had the highest rate of PD (six out of nine patients).

Van Peski-Oosterbaan et al[11] confirm that the relationship between PD and pulmonary disorders is not specific for asthma, but that the rate of PD is equal in all subjects referred for pulmonary function tests (9%). Despite very comparable results on the lung function tests, PD patients perceived higher levels of breathlessness. This confirms the results of Carr et al[12] and Porzelius et al[13] that, respectively in asthma and COPD, patients with a comorbid PD have more negative cognitions than patients without a comorbid PD, although their lung functions are equally impaired.

Apparently, the presence of a respiratory disease increases the risk of developing panic symptoms. This risk is not related to the objective severity of the respiratory pathology, although patients who develop panic do perceive their respiratory symptoms as being more severe.

In daily (psychiatric) clinical practice the relationship between PD and diseases of the respiratory system is not very obvious. Virtually none of the patients referred to anxiety clinics have impairment in their pulmonary functions. One study[14] suggests that there may be some subclinical anomalies in the lung functions of PD patients, but this is at odds with other studies.[15,16] One study[17] even demonstrated that the airways of PD patients, either with or without asthma, are chronically more dilated in both stressful and nonstressful conditions.

As acute respiratory diseases are rarely seen in anxiety clinics, our group investigated whether PD patients show an increased prevalence of respiratory pathology before they develop PD.[18] While point prevalence of respiratory disorders was equal to the controls, lifetime prevalence was significantly higher in PD patients. This finding has been replicated by others. Perna et al[19] found a lifetime prevalence of respiratory diseases of 29% in 102 PD patients, compared with 14% in a group of 101 patients with obsessive compulsive disorder (OCD). Spinhoven et al[20] found relatively low rates of 16% in 100 PD patients and 5% in a control group of 100 DSM IIIR 'V-code' patients. In this latter study, depressive patients had an intermediate score of 9%. However, lifetime comorbidity between depression and

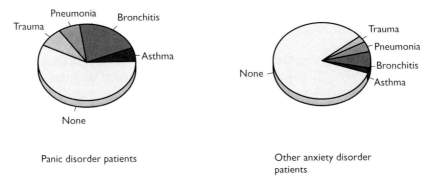

Figure 6.1   History of respiratory disorders. (From Verburg et al[21])

PD may have influenced the results. Our group did a second study in 82 PD patients and 68 other anxiety disorder patients.[21] We confirmed the results of our first study. The rates of respiratory disorders before the onset of the anxiety disorder were 42.7% and 16.2% respectively. This study also showed that PD patients most frequently report a childhood history of chronic bronchitis. PD patients with more severe respiratory symptoms during their PAs reported bronchitis significantly more often than PD patients with less severe respiratory-like panic symptoms (Figure 6.1). It is noteworthy that in all the above studies there appears to be a time gap between the respiratory disease and the onset of the PD.

All these studies confirm that respiratory diseases increase the risk of developing PD later in life (odds ratio = 3.9[21]). They suggest that in up to 40% of PD patients respiratory mechanisms could be a contributing factor.

Experimental panic and ventilatory control

The striking symptomatological resemblance between PD and the so-called hyperventilation syndrome led Gorman and co-workers[22] to investigate the effects of forced hyperventilation in subjects with PD. The authors hypothesized that hyperventilation may be a causal factor in the pathogenesis of PAs. A group of patients with a PD diagnosis voluntarily hyperventilated in an experimental laboratory environment. As a control condition for the resulting hypocapnic respiratory alkalosis, the authors administered a mixture with 5% CO_2, which was intended to cause hyperpnea but no hypocapnia. Surprisingly, not the hyperventilation but the control condition triggered PAs. Other studies soon followed, supporting the view that, in carefully controlled conditions, hyperventilation is devoid of any significant panicogenic properties. In our laboratory, panic patients who were hyperventilating for several minutes, lowering their baseline alveolar pCO_2 by more than 100%, failed to report any significant increase in subjective anxiety.[23] In another experiment, a group of PD patients were not affected by voluntary hyperventilation: in contrast, the same subjects report an instantaneous dramatic increase in anxiety when administered a single breath of 35% CO_2 mixture.[24] Recently, ambulant transcutaneous monitoring of pCO_2 clearly established that real-life PAs are not accompanied by any significant drop in pCO_2.[25]

After the finding by Gorman and co-workers,[22] it was repeatedly confirmed that subjects with PD, in contrast with healthy controls, develop a PA after about 10 minutes of breathing a mixture that is 5% hypercapnic. Despite large methodological differences across different studies, experiments from several laboratories have contributed to the evidence that subjects with PD are hypersensitive to breathing CO_2.[26] The specificity of CO_2 vulnerability has been thoroughly investigated in two different laboratories using the so-called 35% CO_2 challenge.[27,28] In this case, one single inhalation of a 35% CO_2/65% O_2 mixture is taken through a self-administration mask. The effect is immediate, and wanes in a matter of a minute. In healthy volunteers, a 35% CO_2 challenge has been shown to result in a brief respiratory stimulation with automatic symptoms similar to a PA.[29,30] In PD patients, however, the challenge induces a sharp rise in anxiety, which has been equated with a real-life PA.[27]

CO_2 susceptibility acted as a marker of PD amongst a mixed group with various anxiety disorders: although all patients had high ratings on anticipatory anxiety before CO_2, only those with a PD diagnosis reported a change in anxiety upon the challenge.[31] When administered to patients with OCD, CO_2 failed to affect their anxiety level, in contrast to PD subjects.[32,33] Patients with generalized anxiety disorder also responded with little increase in subjective anxiety, although the increase in autonomic panic symptoms was comparable to the response of PD patients.[34] We administered a 35% CO_2 challenge to 28 patients with a specific phobia, making a distinction between animal and situational phobics. This distinction is based on both clinical and epidemiological data, which suggest that situational phobias, such as claustrophobia, may belong to a panic spectrum of diseases.[33] The 35% CO_2 challenge

did not affect animal phobics. In keeping with the above spectrum idea, situational phobics as a group had a CO_2-induced reaction that tended to resemble that of PD subjects.[35] The case of social phobia is less clear. According to one study,[36] social phobics may be CO_2-sensitive. However, our group, applying conservative diagnostic criteria, was unable to replicate these findings.[37] In sum, it appears that, amongst DSM IV anxiety disorders, only patients suffering with panic-type anxiety are vulnerable to CO_2. An analysis of 135 of these patients using receiver operating characteristics showed that the 35% CO_2 challenge discriminates between PD and normals with an 86% probability to classify them correctly depending on the anxiety triggered by CO_2.[38] The high discriminatory power of the 35% CO_2 challenge was recently confirmed in a larger sample of normals and patients suffering with various types of anxiety disorders (Figure 6.2).[39]

Thus, in PD, there is a specific vulnerability to CO_2. This hypersensitivity can be clinically evaluated in a reliable way.[40] Also, there is an interaction between this CO_2 hypersensitivity and drugs that are specifically active against panic. PD patients lose their CO_2 susceptibility after a clinically successful treatment. This has been demonstrated after six weeks of clonazepam therapy,[41] as well as after six weeks of fluvoxamine.[42] Moreover, an attenuation of CO_2 vulnerability has been shown to occur as soon as one week into pharmacotherapy.[43–45] The latter early effect of antipanic drugs on the CO_2 challenge might be predictive of a favorable clinical response to the treatment.

Finally, CO_2 vulnerability may be a marker of a constitutional predisposition to develop panic. In a study by Perna and co-workers,[46] 23 first-degree relatives of patients with a PD underwent a 35% CO_2 challenge. Twenty-two of them had a PA reaction under CO_2, though they were free of clinical panic. In a study that is underway at

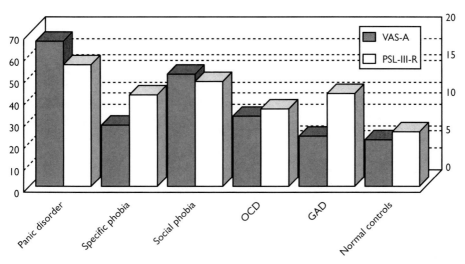

Figure 6.2 Vulnerability to 35% CO_2 panic provocation challenge in anxiety disorder patients, scores on the Visual Analogue Scale for Anxiety (VAS-A) and the Panic Sympton List (PSL-III-T). (From Verburg et al[39])

our laboratory, preliminary results confirm that first-degree relatives of PD patients present some degree of hypervulnerability to CO_2 inhalation. Also, CO_2 susceptibility showed a higher concordance ratio in a group of monozygotic twins compared with dizygotics.[47]

CO_2 vulnerability seems to be, at least in part, controlled by serotonergic pathways. In healthy subjects[48] as well as in panic patients,[49,50] CO_2 vulnerability appeared to increase after experimental tryptophan depletion.

With CO_2 being a crucial factor in ventilation control, the above data most likely point to the neuronal control of ventilation as a key to the pathophysiology of panic. There are more arguments linking respiratory regulation to experimental panic induction. It was already known that lactate infusion produces respiratory effects, inducing a paradoxical hyperventilation, while it causes a systemic alkalosis.[51] In fact it was the lactate-induced hyperventilation

that prompted Gorman and co-workers[22] to start studying the effects of respiration in experimental panic. Besides lactate and CO_2, no other panicogenic agent has been better studied, as far as specificity, reliability and sensitivity are concerned, than cholecystokinin tetrapeptide (CCK4). CCK4 has been shown to reliably induce experimental panic both in healthy controls and in PD subjects. PD patients, however, panic at much lower doses than normals[52] (see also Chapter 5). Patients with OCD have no hypersensitivity to CCK (J Bradwejn, personal communication). The symptomatology induced by both a 35% CO_2 challenge and a CCK4 injection has been found to be similar, yielding prominent respiratory symptoms.[52] Most interestingly, CCK4 injected into healthy volunteers produced a noticeable respiratory stimulation.[53] CCK receptors have been identified in the brain, and some of these receptors have been associated with respiratory control.[54]

In summary, a quite impressive bulk of facts from experimental panic induction supports a close link between respiratory control mechanisms and panic. These data rely mainly on CO_2 vulnerability in PD subjects, but also on lactate and CCK studies.

Central chemosensitivity for CO_2

Two lines of evidence link panic attacks to the brainstem.[55] The first is the nature of the somatic symptoms that occur during panic attacks: they all can be explained by a surge of impulses originating in the autonomic nervous system. The second line of evidence is the provocation of panic attacks in a laboratory situation by various pharmacological agents.

CO_2 primarily acts on the brainstem, specifically on the respiratory center, located in the reticular substance of the medulla oblongata and pons.[56] In panic provocation with CO_2, the influence of the peripheral chemosensitive areas is diminished by using mixtures with high concentrations of oxygen.

Logically, investigators looked closely at the central chemosensitivity in PD patients. Initially, panic due to inhalation of CO_2 was thought to be caused by a hypersensitive respiratory center in PD patients. The sensitivity of the respiratory center in the brainstem can be tested using the Read rebreathing method[57] which measures the increase in ventilation due to inhalation of increasing concentrations of CO_2. One study seemed to confirm the hypothesis of a hypersensitive respiratory center in PD patients. Those patients showed a greater increase in ventilation due to inhalation of increasing concentration of CO_2 than normal controls.[58] Most studies using Read's rebreathing technique, however, have been nega-

tive.[59-62] Pain and co-workers[60] did find a difference in respiratory patterns, PD patients having a higher frequency of breathing and a lower tidal volume. Papp et al[63] used a steady-state canopy method to assess the ventilatory response to CO_2. Their study was also negative, but they did find a difference between male panic disorder patients and controls. Woods et al[59] and Pols et al[64] showed that treatment of panic disorder – respectively with alprazolam and clomipramine – decreases the ventilatory response to CO_2.

In conclusion, although there are some indications that the brainstem respiratory center is involved in PD, most studies do not show a clear relationship between PD and an increased sensitivity of the respiratory center. This does not necessarily mean that this relationship does not exist, but merely that the rather crude methods used so far did not succeed in finding it. Berkenbosch et al[65] compared Read's rebreathing method with the steady-state method to assess the ventilatory CO_2 sensitivity. They found that the results from the two methods differed, and that the values obtained with Read's rebreathing method are 1.40–2.59 times higher than those obtained with the steady-state method. They assume that in Read's method the increase in ventilation is a direct function of the pCO_2 of the brain tissue. This would make this method very suitable for psychiatric purposes. The downside is that they attribute the differences between the two methods to changes in arterial blood flow. Considering (1) that arterial blood flow has a marked influence on the results of these experiments, and (2) that, compared with normal controls, PD patients show a different response in cerebral blood flow on changes in arterial pCO_2,[66] close monitoring of cerebral blood flow is a prerequisite for studies on the ventilatory response to CO_2 in PD patients. Possible adaptive changes in the peripheral respiratory system[17] should also be taken into account.

Apart from these physiological considerations, other factors have to be considered. First, subjects undergoing an assessment of their central chemosensitivity should preferably be non-anxious and have a regular breathing pattern. PD patients are, by definition, anxious – especially when exposed to CO_2 – and have irregular breathing patterns, even during sleep.[67] Secondly, results from panic provocation studies with 35% CO_2 suggest a large number of possible confounders, i.e. sex and phase of the menstrual cycle,[68] presence of a comorbid mood disorder,[69] history of respiratory disorders,[70] and, for the control groups, history of spontaneous panic attacks[71] and presence of specific phobia.[35] The fact that depression influences the ventilatory response to inhalation of CO_2 had already been shown by Shershow et al[72] and Damas-Mora et al.[73] Shershow et al[74] also linked low ventilatory responses to CO_2 to depressive and introverted personality traits.

However, using the above considerations, it should be possible to design a study that would provide a more definite answer on the issue of hypersensitivity to CO_2 in PD patients.

Respiration and panic: conjectures and perspectives

In brief, the facts linking panic to the respiratory system may be summarized as follows.

First, up to 40% of patients with PD have a childhood history of respiratory disease, in particular bronchitis and asthma. This high respiratory morbidity is specific, since there are no reports of increased childhood morbidity for other somatic disorders in PD patients. Conversely, there is a higher than expected prevalence of PD amongst patients with COPD

and asthma. However, this latter relationship may not be specific, since a higher than expected prevalence of PD has been reported in other populations with somatic pathology, for instance in patients with heart disease.[75,76]

Secondly, patients with PD are hypersensitive to CO_2 inhalation. In contrast to those with other types of anxiety disorders, only PD subjects report significant anxiety after a challenge with 35% CO_2. Some studies suggest that PD patients have hypersensitive CO_2 chemoreceptors, but results at present are inconclusive. However, most of the other substances known to induce experimental PA in patients with a PD have a clear-cut activity on the respiratory system. Lactate induces hyperventilation. CCK4 activates respiration in laboratory animals as well as in man. In sum, both clinical data and experimental studies provide good evidence that PAs may be linked to some physiological mechanisms of respiratory control.

Klein[77] proposes a theory that tries to integrate the different findings on panic disorder, respiration and responses to panic-provoking substances. He hypothesizes that panic attacks are a misplaced fear of suffocation, leading to hyperventilation, panic and an urge to flee. This fear of suffocation would be elicited by activation of a suffocation alarm system. Klein states that panic attacks result from false alarms from this hypothetical suffocation monitor. He gives the following arguments to support his theory.

Fear of, and during, suffocation occur in healthy individuals, and is extremely adverse. The existence of an inborn suffocation monitor is proved by the existence of the congenital central hypoventilation syndrome. In this rare disease a suffocation monitor is not present, and these children breathe while awake, but tend to stop breathing when they fall asleep. They can only survive with ventilatory support measures. A specific feature of panic attacks is the prominence of respiratory symptoms. Non-panic patients experience sweating and pounding heart as the most prominent symptoms in frightening situations. Panic attacks are also different from other forms of clinical and non-clinical anxiety in the sense that there is no activation of the hypothalamic–pituitary–adrenal (HPA) axis. Activation of the HPA axis does occur in emergency responses and on confrontation with (some) phobic stimuli. The False Suffocation Alarm theory also explains the panicogenic effects of lactate and CO_2 administration to PD patients. Lactate and carbon dioxide are metabolic end-products – a suffocation alarm would monitor the levels of these substances.

The False Suffocation Alarm theory evoked both support and criticism.

According to Klein, one of the strongest arguments in favor of the existence of a suffocation monitor is the fact that some people do not have one, i.e. children with the congenital central hypoventilation syndrome. Pine et al[78] assessed the presence of anxiety symptoms in 13 of these children, with the assumption that the absence of a suffocation monitor would decrease their vulnerability to anxiety symptoms or disorders. They were compared with a large community sample that included children with asthma and other chronic medical illnesses. The hypothesis was confirmed: children with the congenital central hypoventilation syndrome had the lowest rate of anxiety disorders, and, interestingly, children with asthma the highest.

Unfortunately, the above study is the only one we are aware of that constitutes a proper follow-up on the publication of this new theory. Namely, it tested new hypotheses that arise from this theory, using the new insights to design new research protocols. Other papers on the False Suffocation Alarm were merely replications of earlier studies, or were designed to prove the superiority of the author's own favorite theories. We shall mention the most interesting ones.

Asmundson and Stein[79] tested the False Suffocation Alarm theory by using a voluntary breath-holding procedure. PD patients had significantly lower durations of breath-holding than social phobia patients and normal controls. There were no differences in physiological responses between the three groups. They conclude that these results support the False Suffocation Alarm theory. Earlier, a similar study had been done by Zandbergen et al.[80] They did not find differences between PD patients and other anxiety disorder patients, but normal controls were able to hold their breath significantly longer. Van der Does[81] confirmed these results, but only after subjects took a maximal inhalation. After normal exhalation, no differences were found.

Schmidt et al[82] state that the above finding can be explained from the False Suffocation Alarm theory – but also from cognitive models of panic.[83] They designed a study to investigate whether markers of the hypothetical suffocation alarm – severity and frequency of dyspnea symptoms, respiration rate and pCO_2 levels – would predict the emotional response to challenges that affect the arterial pCO_2. They used a hyperventilation procedure and a 35% CO_2 test. Their conclusion is that none of the above markers predicted a difference in response to the two conditions.

Among some more questionable statements,[84] Ley raises one important issue: the matter of carbon monoxide poisoning, which is a form of suffocation where no anxiety occurs.[85] Klein[84] states that this is a matter for future research, but that the role of carbon monoxide as an inhibitory neurotransmitter within the carotid body is a possible explanation. Also, hypoxia does not provoke panic.

A key argument in questioning Klein's

hypothesis is that, to date, no suffocation detector has been identified within the central or peripheral nervous system. Yet, Klein's theory rests entirely on the existence of a suffocation detector. If a suffocation detector does exist, most probably it exists as a functional system linking some central (or peripheral) nervous system structures implicated in respiratory control to other neuronal structures responsible for anxiety. We posit that a suffocation detector does exist. We postulate that it consists of a functional circuit originating in the chemoreceptive areas, comprising as a key element the pontine locus ceruleus (LC) and projecting to the limbic system. The following analysis represents an attempt to substantiate our hypothesis.

The LC is the cornerstone of the above-postulated neuronal system. This small bilateral nucleus, located in the rostral pons, contains the highest density of noradrenergic cells in the CNS, accounting for more than half of all central noradrenergic neurons.[86] In the late 1970s Redmond and co-workers conducted a series of experiments in monkeys with implanted electrodes in the LC. They showed that electrical stimulation of the LC resulted in behaviors usually displayed in situations of impending aggression, or threatened attacks by humans. The same behaviors were elicited by administration of piperoxan, a drug that stimulates LC activity. Clonidine, which decreases LC activity, suppressed the above behaviors. These behaviors were interpreted as instances of fear, and LC stimulation was proposed as a model of anxiety.[87] However, a close examination of Redmond's experiments suggests that the animals' reactions may have been closer to behavioral activation and arousal than to anxiety. In fact, Redmond incorrectly proposed LC activation as a model of anxiety, but correctly stated that 'to call the LC an anxiety system ... is only partly correct, since anxiety requires

other areas (of the brain) and since anxiety is only a portion of this primitive neurophysiologically inhibitory system ... perhaps "alarm system" is a better name for the LC...'.[88]

Subsequent experimental evidence has clearly demonstrated that the LC is not involved in animal tests of anticipatory anxiety. Bilaterally LC lesioned rats had similar responses to controls in several models of anxiety.[89] Finally, LC stimulation in man is not necessarily associated with the experience of anxiety.[90]

Therefore it seems unlikely that LC activity by itself mediates anxiety. Yet, growing evidence supports the idea that the LC may be (part of) a biological alarm system. Within the CNS, the LC has a unique widespread efferent network, each individual LC neuron innervating large territories, amongst others in the limbic system and the cortex.[86,91] LC activation seems to increase the signal-to-noise ratio in the cells innervated by its network, namely in the cortex, hippocampus and cerebellum.[91] Accordingly, the LC has been attributed a general regulatory function, playing a role of facilitation in behavioral activation, vigilance and emotions.[86,92]

The LC is activated in the presence of external sensory stimuli that are associated with novelty and threat.[86] Elam and co-workers[93–97] have shown that LC activation also followed changes in internal state, such as hypercapnia, hypoxia, blood volume loss or dilatation of the digestive tract. Those changes representing a vital threat to the organism, i.e. hypercapnia, hypoxia and blood loss, induced the most dramatic LC activation.[97]

Further investigation has shown that, in sharp contrast to its widespread efferent network, the LC is under a limited afferent control. The vast majority of the impulses to the LC come from two nuclei in the rostral medulla – the nucleus prepositus hypoglossi and the nucleus paragigantocellularis, of which the latter is a crossroad for autonomic integration.[92] Also, electrical stimulation of the ventrolateral medulla causes increased firing in the LC.[91] It is worth noting that the central chemoreceptive area is situated in the ventral medulla. Thus current knowledge of the function of the LC, though based essentially on animal experimentation, is perfectly compatible with the notion that the LC represents an alarm system, monitoring stimuli from both the external and internal environments. This 'novelty detector'[94] is most sensitive to changes representing threats to the well-being of the organism. A suffocation detector as postulated in Klein's theory would fit perfectly as a functional part of the system. Gorman and co-workers[55] already postulated that panic may be due to hyperexcitable brainstem mechanisms, pointing to possible connections between structures in the medulla related to ventilatory control and the pontine LC. In their neuroanatomical model of PD, the above authors suggest a clear distinction between the locus of panic (the LC system) and the locus of (anticipatory) anxiety (the limbic system).

Probably, the difference is not that clear-cut. One must take into account the fact that the stimulation of the LC alarm system (and thus the suffocation monitor) does not appear to produce anxiety. Nor will a hypersensitive LC alarm system. Yet, LC stimulation produces activation in other brain structures that are innervated by its particular efferent system. Specifically, there is a rich efferent network from the LC to the limbic area, which has been demonstrated to be associated with the experience of anxiety.[98] Since the subjective experience of anxiety is an essential part of clinical panic, we propose that PAs consist of chemoreceptor-triggered, LC-driven, limbic activation. Possibly other triggers representing threats monitored by the LC system may act as prime movers as well, explaining the hetero-geneity of PD. We have mentioned that neurons innervated by LC efferents, when stimulated by noradrenaline, display a reduction of background activity, and more effective signal processing.[91] This phenomenon, at cortical as well as limbic level, may help explaining why PD patients display a remarkable capacity to discriminate interoceptive cues representing potential threats.[99]

Future research

Future research will confirm or refute the above hypotheses. If the LC system contains an anatomically and physiologically identifiable suffocation monitor, the next step will be to show why and how this system may become hypersensitive in PD subjects. The epidemiological findings described earlier in this chapter may provide some clues. It is striking that CO_2 vulnerability may be almost entirely accounted for by the high childhood prevalence of respiratory disorders in PD.[70] If confirmed, this finding may suggest that repeated exposure to hypercapnic and hypoxic episodes during infancy, as occur in asthma and bronchitis, may interact with the maturation of the LC system, causing it to become hyperexcitable. Others have speculated that immaturity of the LC system plays a role in some ventilation control disorders, such as the sudden infant death syndrome.[86] Sudden infant death, like the congenital hypoventilation syndrome, may represent an under-responsive suffocation alarm system.

Repeated evidence has been found showing that adult PD patients have, more often than others, suffered from respiratory disorders during childhood. One wonders whether PD subjects with a history of respiratory disorder present with symptomatological or biological differences compared with other PD patients.

Finally, according to the above findings of

Elam and colleagues, the LC system represents a biological alarm that monitors different types of internal vital parameters – not only CO_2. Klein already suggested that the suffocation system may monitor oxygen and lactate as well. One other stimulus to which the LC alarm is apparently very sensitive is acute loss of blood volume. Suffocation and metabolic disturbances, beside acute blood loss, obviously represent other types of fundamental vital threat. Is the LC system to be regarded as a more general inborn survival alarm? If so, may dysregulation of different parts of that system reflect different types of panic anxiety?

References

1. Lum LC, Hyperventilation: the tip and the iceberg. *J Psychosom Res* 1975; **19**: 375–83.
2. Magarian GJ, Hyperventilation syndromes: a frequently unrecognized common expression of anxiety and stress. *Medicine* 1982; **61**: 219–36.
3. Kinsman RA, Luparello T, O'Banion K, Spector S, Multidimensional analysis of the subjective symptomatology of asthma. *Psychosom Med* 1973; **35**: 250–67.
4. Yellowlees PM, Alpers JH, Bowden JJ et al, Psychiatric morbidity in patients with chronic airflow obstruction. *Med J Aust* 1987; **146**: 305–7.
5. Shavitt RG, Gentil V, Mandetta R, The association of panic/agoraphobia and asthma: contributing factors and clinical implications. *Gen Hosp Psychiatry* 1992; **14**: 420–3.
6. Butz AM, Alexander C, Anxiety in children with asthma. *J Asthma* 1993; **30**: 199–209.
7. Hibbert G, Pilsbury D, Demonstration and treatment of hyperventilation causing asthma. *Br J Psychiatry* 1988; **153**: 687–9.
8. Yellowlees PM, Haynes S, Potts N, Ruffin RE, Psychiatric morbidity in patients with life-threatening asthma: initial report of a controlled study. *Med J Aust* 1988; **149**: 246–9.
9. Karajgi B, Rifkin A, Doddi S, Kolli R, The prevalence of anxiety disorders in patients with chronic obstructive pulmonary disease. *Am J Psychiatry* 1990; **147**: 200–1.
10. Pollack MH, Kradin R, Otto MW et al, Prevalence of panic in patients referred for pulmonary function testing at a major medical center. *Am J Psychiatry* 1996; **153**: 110–13.
11. Van Peski-Oosterbaan AS, Spinhoven P, Van der Does AJW et al, Is there a specific relationship between asthma and panic disorder? *Behav Res Ther* 1996; **34**: 333–40.
12. Carr RE, Lehrer PM, Rausch L, Hochron SM, Anxiety sensitivity and panic attacks in an asthmatic population. *Behav Res Ther* 1994; **32**: 411–18.
13. Porzelius J, Vest M, Nochomovitz M, Respiratory function, cognitions, and panic in chronic obstructive pulmonary patients. *Behav Res Ther* 1992; **30**: 75–7.
14. Perna G, Marconi C, Battaglia M et al, Subclinical impairment of lung airways in patients with panic disorder. *Biol Psychiatry* 1994; **36**: 601–5.
15. Carr RE, Lehrer PM, Hochron SM, Panic symptoms in asthma and panic disorder: a preliminary test of the dyspnea–fear theory. *Behav Res Ther* 1992; **30**: 251–61.
16. Verburg K, De Leeuw M, Pols H, Griez E, No dynamic lungfunction abnormalities in panic disorder patients. *Biol Psychiatry* 1997; **41**: 834–6.
17. Carr RE, Lehrer PM, Hochron SM, Jackson A, Effect of psychological stress on airway impedance in individuals with asthma and panic disorder. *J Abnorm Psychology* 1996; **105**: 137–41.
18. Zandbergen J, Bright M, Pols H et al, Higher lifetime prevalence of respiratory diseases in panic disorder? *Am J Psychiatry* 1991; **148**: 1583–5.
19. Perna G, Bertani A, Diaferia G et al, Prevalence of respiratory diseases in patients with panic and obsessive compulsive disorders. *Anxiety* 1994; **1**: 100–1.
20. Spinhoven P, Ros M, Westgeest A, Van der Does AJM, The prevalence of respiratory disorders in panic disorder, major depressive disorder and V-code patients. *Behav Res Ther* 1994; **32**: 647–9.

21. Verburg K, Griez E, Meijer J, Pols H, Respiratory disorders as a possible predisposing factor in panic disorder. *J Affect Disord* 1995; **33**: 129–34.
22. Gorman JM, Askanazi J, Liebowtiz MR et al, Response to hyperventilation in a group of patients with panic disorder. *Am J Psychiatry* 1984; **141**: 857–61.
23. Griez E, Zandbergen J, Lousberg H, van den Hout MA, Effects of low pulmonary CO_2 on panic anxiety. *Compr Psychiatry* 1988; **29**: 490–7.
24. Zandbergen J, Lousberg H, Pols H et al, Hypercarbia versus hypocarbia in panic disorder. *J Affect Disord* 1990; **18**: 75–81.
25. Garssen B, Buikhuisen M, van Dyck R, Hyperventilation and panic attacks. *Am J Psychiatry* 1996; **153**: 513–18.
26. Sanderson WC, Wetzler S, Five percent carbon dioxide challenge: valid analogue and marker of panic disorder? *Biol Psychiatry* 1990; **27**: 689–701.
27. Griez E, Lousberg H, van den Hout MA, van der Molen GM, CO_2 vulnerability in panic disorder. *Psychiatry Res* 1987; **20**: 87–95.
28. Perna G, Battaglia M, Garberi A et al, 35% CO_2/65% O_2 inhalation test in panic patients. *Psychiatry Res* 1994; **52**: 159–71.
29. Griez E, van den Hout MA, Effects of carbon dioxide–oxygen inhalations on subjective anxiety and some neurovegetative parameters. *J Behav Ther Exp Ther* 1982; **13**: 27–32.
30. van den Hout MA, Griez E, Panic symptoms after inhalation of carbon dioxide. *Br J Psychiatry* 1984; **144**: 503–7.
31. Griez E, Zandbergen J, Pols H, de Loof C, Response to 35% carbon dioxide as a marker of panic in severe anxiety. *Am J Psychiatry* 1990; **147**: 796–7.
32. Griez E, de Loof C, Pols H et al, Specific sensitivity of patients with panic attacks to carbon dioxide inhalation. *Psychiatry Res* 1990; **31**: 193–9.
33. Perna G, Bertani A, Arancio C et al, Laboratory response of patients with panic and obsessive compulsive disorders to 35 CO_2 challenges. *Am J Psychiatry* 1995; **152**: 85–9.
34. Verburg K, Griez E, Meijer J, Pols H, Discrimination between panic disorder and generalized anxiety disorder by 35% carbon diox-

ide challenge. *Am J Psychiatry* 1995; **152**: 1081–3.
35. Verburg K, Griez E, Meijer J, A 35% carbon dioxide challenge in simple phobias. *Acta Psychiatr Scand* 1994; **90**: 420–3.
36. Caldirola D, Perna G, Arancio C et al, The 35% CO_2 challenge test in patients with social phobia. *Psychiatry Res* 1997; **71**: 41–8.
37. Verburg K, Pols H, Hauzer R et al, The 35% carbon dioxide challenge in social phobia. Submitted for publication.
38. Battaglia M, Perna G, The 35% CO_2 challenge in panic disorder: optimization by Receiver Operating Characteristic (ROC) analysis. *J Psychiat Res* 1995; **29**: 111–19.
39. Verburg K, Perna G, Bellodi L, Griez E, The 35% CO_2 panic provocation challenge as a diagnostic test for panic disorder. Submitted for publication.
40. Verburg K, Pols H, De Leeuw M, Griez E, Reliability of the 35% carbon dioxide panic provocation challenge. *Psychiatry Res* in press.
41. Pols H, Zandbergen J, De Loof C, Griez E, Attenuation of carbon dioxide-induced panic after clonazepam treatment. *Acta Psychiatr Scand* 1991; **84**: 585–6.
42. Pols H, Hauzer RC, Meijer JA et al, Fluvoxamine attenuates panic induced by 35% CO_2 challenge. *J Clin Psychiatry* 1996; **57**: 539–42.
43. Perna G, Cochi S, Bertani A et al, Pharmacological effect of toloxatone on reactivity to 35% CO_2 challenge: a single blind, random, placebo controlled study. *J Clin Psychopharmacol* 1994; **14**: 414–18.
44. Bertani A, Perna G, Arancio C et al, Pharmacological effect of imipramine, paroxetine and sertraline on 35% carbon dioxide hypersensitivity in panic patients: a double blind, random, placebo-controlled study. *J Clin Psychopharmacol* 1996; **17**: 97–101.
45. Perna G, Bertani A, Modification of 35% carbon dioxide hypersensitivity across one week of treatment with clomipramine and fluvoxamine: a double-blind, randomized, placebo-controlled study. *J Clin Psychopharmacol* 1997; **17**: 173–8.
46. Perna G, Cocchi S, Bertani A et al, 35% CO_2 challenge in healthy first degrees relatives of patients with panic disorder. *Am J Psychiatry* 1995; **152**: 623–5.

47. Arancio C, Perna G, Caldirola D et al, Carbon dioxide-induced panic in twins: preliminary results. *Eur Neuropsychopharmacol* 1995; **5**: 368.

48. Klaassen T, Klumperbeek J, Doutz N et al, Effects of tryptophan depletion on anxiety and on carbon dioxide provoked panic. *Psychiatry Res* in press.

49. Kent JM, Coplan JD, Martinez J et al, Ventilatory effects of tryptophan depletion in panic disorder: a preliminary report. *Psychiatry Res* 1996; **64**: 83–90.

50. Schruers K, Pols J, Klaassen T et al, Tryptophan depletion and 35% CO_2 challenge in panic patients: preliminary results. *Biol Psychiatry* 1997; **42**(Suppl): 1S–17S.

51. Liebowitz MR, Gorman J, Fyer M, Lactate provocation of panic attacks. *Arch Gen Psychiatry* 1984; **41**: 764–70.

52. Bradwejn J, Koszycki D, Shriqui C, Enhanced sensitivity to cholecystokinin tetrapeptide in panic disorder: clinical and behavioral findings. *Arch Gen Psychiatry* 1991; **48**: 603–10.

53. Bradwejn J, Legrand JM, Koszycki D et al, Effects of cholecystokinin-tetrapeptide on respiratory function in healthy volunteers. *Am J Psychiatry* 1998; **155**: 280–2.

54. Bourin M, Malinge M, Vasar E, Bradwejn J, Two faces of cholecystokinin: anxiety and schizophrenia. *Fundam Clin Pharmacol* 1996; **10**: 116–26.

55. Gorman JM, Liebowitz MR, Fyer AJ, Stein J, A neuroanatomical hypothesis for panic disorder. *Am J Psychiatry* 1989; **146**: 148–61.

56. Guyton AC, *Textbook of Medical Physiology.* Philadelphia: WB Saunders, 1981.

57. Read DJ, A clinical method for assessing the ventilatory response to carbon dioxide. *J Int Med Aust NZ* 1967; **16**: 20–32.

58. Lousberg H, Griez E, van den Hout MA, Carbon dioxide chemosensitivity in panic disorder. *Acta Psychiatr Scand* 1988; **77**: 214–18.

59. Woods SW, Charney DS, Loke J et al, Carbon dioxide sensitivity in panic disorder: ventilatory and anxiogenic responses to carbon dioxide in healthy subjects and patients with panic anxiety before and after alprazolam treatment. *Arch Gen Psychiatry* 1986; **43**: 900–9.

60. Pain MCF, Biddle N, Tiller JWG, Panic disorder, the ventilatory response to carbon dioxide and respiratory variables. *Psychosom Med* 1988; **50**: 541–8.

61. Zandbergen J, Pols H, De Loof C, Griez E, Ventilatory response to CO_2 in panic disorder. *Psychiatry Res* 1991; **39**: 13–19.

62. Papp LA, Martinez JM, Klein DF et al, Rebreathing tests in panic disorder. *Biol Psychiatry* 1995; **38**: 240–5.

63. Papp LA, Goetz R, Cole R et al, Hypersensitivity to carbon dioxide in panic disorder. *Am J Psychiatry* 1989; **146**: 779–81.

64. Pols H, Lousberg H, Zandbergen J, Griez E, Panic disorder patients show decrease in ventilatory response to CO_2 after clomipramine treatment. *Psychiatry Res* 1993; **47**: 295–6.

65. Berkenbosch A, Bovill JG, Dahan A et al, The ventilatory CO_2 sensitivities from Read's rebreathing method and the steady-state method are not equal in man. *J Physiol* 1989; **411**: 367–77.

66. Gibb DM, Hyperventilation-induced cerebral ischemia in panic disorder and effect of nimodipine. *Am J Psychiatry* 1992; **149**: 1589–91.

67. Stein MB, Millar TW, Larsen DK, Kryger MH, Irregular breathing during sleep in patients with panic disorder. *Am J Psychiatry* 1995; **152**: 1168–73.

68. Perna G, Brambilla F, Arancio C, Bellodi L, Menstrual cycle-related sensitivity in 35% CO_2 in panic patients. *Biol Psychiatry* 1995; **37**: 528–32.

69. Verburg K, Klaassen T, Pols H, Griez E, Comorbid depressive disorder increases vulnerability to the 35% carbon dioxide (CO_2) challenge in panic disorder patients. *J Affect Disord* in press.

70. Verburg K, Griez E, A history of respiratory disorders predicts the response to the 35% carbon dioxide panic provocation: a preliminary study. Submitted for publication.

71. Perna G, Gabariele A, Caldirola D, Bellodi L, Hypersensitivity to inhalation of carbon dioxide and panic attacks. *Psychiatry Res* 1996; **57**: 267–73.

72. Shershow JC, Kanarek DJ, Kazemi H, Ventilatory response to carbon dioxide inhalation in depression. *Psychosom Med* 1976; **38**: 282–7.

73. Damas-Mora J, Jenner FA, Sneddon J, Addis WD, Ventilatory response to carbon dioxide in syndromes of depression. *J Psychosom Res* 1978; **22**: 473–6.

74. Shershow JC, King A, Robinson S, Carbon dioxide sensitivity and personality. *Psychosom Med* 1973; **35**: 155–60.

75. Chignon JM, Lépine JP, Adès J, Panic disorder in cardiac out-patients. *Am J Psychiatry* 1993; **150**: 780–5.

76. Griez E, Mammar N, Bouhour J, Panic disorder in cardiac plant candidates. Submitted for publication.

77. Klein DF, False suffocation alarms, spontaneous panics, and related conditions. *Arch Gen Psychiatry* 1993; **50**: 306–17.

78. Pine DS, Weese-Mayer DE, Silvestri JM et al, Anxiety and congenital central hypoventilation syndrome. *Am J Psychiatry* 1994; **151**: 864–70.

79. Asmundson GJG, Stein MB, Triggering the false suffocation alarm in panic disorder by using a voluntary breath holding procedure. *Am J Psychiatry* 1994; **151**: 264–6.

80. Zandbergen J, Strahm M, Pols H, Griez EJL, Breath-holding in panic disorder. *Compr Psychiatry* 1992; **33**: 47–51.

81. Van der Does AJW, Voluntary breath holding: not a suitable probe of the suffocation alarm in panic disorder. *Behav Res Ther* 1997; **35**: 779–84.

82. Schmidt NB, Telch MJ, LaNae Jaimez T, Biological challenge manipulation of PCO_2 levels: a test of Klein's suffocation alarm theory of panic. *J Abnorm Psychol* 1996; **105**: 446–54.

83. Clark DM, A cognitive approach to panic. *Behav Res Ther* 1986; **24**: 441–70.

84. Klein DF, In reply to Ley. *Arch Gen Psychiatry* 1996; **53**: 83–5.

85. Ley R, The 'suffocation alarm' theory of panic attacks: a critical commentary. *J Behav Ther Exp Psychiatry* 1994; **24**: 269–73.

86. Svensson TH, Brain norepinephrine neurons in the locus coeruleus and the control of arousal and respiration: implications for sudden infant death syndrome. In: *Neurobiology of the Control of Breathing* (van Euler C, Lagercrantz H, eds). New York: Raven Press, 1987: 297–301.

87. Redmond DE Jr, Huang YH, Snyder DR et al, Hyperphagia and hyperdipsia after locus coeruleus lesions in the stumptailed monkey. *Life Sci* 1977; **20**: 1619.

88. Redmond DE Jr, Alternations in the function of the nucleus locus couruleus: a possible model for studies of anxiety. In: *Animal Models in Psychiatry and Neurology* (Hanin I, Usdin E, eds). New York: Pergamon Press, 1977, 293–305.

89. File SE, Vellucci SV, Studies on the role of stress hormones and of 5-HT in anxiety using an animal model. *J Pharm Pharmacol* 1978; **30**: 105–110.

90. Kaitin KI, Bliwise DL, Gleason C et al, Sleep disturbance produced by electrical stimulation of the locus coeruleus in a human subject. *Biol Psychiatry* 1986; **21**: 710–16.

91. Saper CB, Function of the locus coeruleus. *TINS* 1987; **10**: 343–4.

92. Aston Jones G, Ennis M, Pieribone VA et al, The brain nucleus locus coeruleus: restricted afferent control of a broad efferent network. *Science* 1986; **234**: 734–7.

93. Elam M, Yao T, Thorén P, Svensson TH, Hypercapnia and hypoxia: chemoreceptor-mediated control of locus coeruleus neurons and splanchnic sympathetic nerves. *Brain Res* 1981; **222**: 373–81.

94. Elam M, Yao T, Svensson TH, Thorén P, Regulation of locus coeruleus neurons and splanchnic, sympathetic nerves by cardiovascular afferents. *Brain Res* 1984; **290**: 281–7.

95. Elam M, Svensson TH, Thorén P, Differential cardiovascular afferent regulation of locus coeruleus neurons and sympathetic nerves. *Brain Res* 1985; **358**: 77–84.

96. Elam M, Thorén P, Svensson TH, Locus coeruleus neurons and sympathetic nerves: activation by visceral afferents. *Brain Res* 1986; **375**: 117–25.

97. Elam M, Yao T, Svensson TH, Thorén P, Locus coeruleus neurons and sympathetic nerves: activation by cutaneous sensory afferents. *Brain Res* 1986; **366**: 254–61.

98. Kuhar MJ, Neuroanatomical substrates of anxiety: a brief survey. *TINS* 1986; **9**: 307–11.

99. Ehlers A, Morgaf J, Roth WT et al, Anxiety induction by false heart rate feed back in patients with panic disorder. *Behav Res Ther* 1988; **26**: 2–11.

7

Psychological theories of panic disorder

George R Thorn, Anne Chosak, Sandra L Baker and David H Barlow

CONTENTS • Introduction • Psychoanalytic theory • Psychodynamic theory • Behavioral theories • Cognitive theories • Discussion and conclusions

Introduction

In recent years, the psychological literature has seen a proliferation of research on panic and anxiety, making these disorders among the most extensively investigated emotional disorders.[1] In the context of these research findings, much debate has focused on the etiology of panic and anxiety. Although models have been suggested from a variety of theoretical perspectives, no one theory has yet succeeded in providing an empirically based model of panic disorder that is widely accepted, although data are beginning to accumulate on the validity of parts of some theories.

In this chapter, we provide a brief review and critique of major psychoanalytic/dynamic, behavioral and cognitive theories of panic. We then examine the overlapping features of the theories and provide directions for future research in this area.

Psychoanalytic theory

Although central to psychoanalytic theory, very little empirical research has been conducted from this perspective on the nature of anxiety. Thus, classic psychoanalytic notions of anxiety and panic have changed very little over the decades, but will be briefly presented here as a backdrop for more recent psychological theories. Freud,[2] in his early psychoanalytic theory of anxiety, viewed anxiety as both a cause and result of unconscious underlying defense mechanisms. As Josephs[3] has noted, Freud's toxic theory of anxiety includes a metapsychological theory and clinical theory. In his metapsychological theory, Freud viewed anxiety as resulting from pent-up and repressed libido. Unexpressed sexual wishes confined by defense mechanisms led to a frustrated libido, which in turn led to the biochemical building up and imbalance of toxic material, which subsequently brought on anxiety. However, Freud's metapsychological theory has been viewed as weak because of its inability to universally explain all manifestations of anxiety (i.e. those with and without sexual frustration experienced anxiety), as well as the lack of empirical support for the biochemical correlates of the libido.

Freud's[2] clinical theory viewed anxiety as a fear of the expression of repressed emotions associated with traumatic experiences. In Freud's view, primary defenses were triggered to prevent the revelation of an unconscious wish and minimize intrapsychic conflict within the individual. Failure of defense mechanisms created the possibility of the expression of trauma-related emotions and triggered an alternative emotional response of anxiety. In order to preclude the distressing emotions from entering into conscious awareness, secondary and tertiary defense mechanisms were implemented to re-repress the disturbing emotions. Failure in these superimposed defense mechanisms then led to additional anxiety, ultimately culminating in an anxiety attack. Freud substantiated his clinical theory through his personal observations that anxiety was alleviated following abreaction of the traumatic experience. However, he subsequently revised his theory because this method provided only temporary symptom relief.

Freud's[4] signal theory of anxiety viewed anxiety as a cause and trigger of defense mechanisms, in contrast to his previous theory, which only viewed anxiety as a result of failure in defense mechanisms. In this later elaboration, anxiety served as a signal for danger, which in turn prompted the activation of defense mechanisms. Failure in defense mechanisms to repress traumatic emotions resulted in an anxiety attack. Perceived danger was not necessarily the consequence of a truly dangerous environment, but arose from unconscious intrapsychic conflict between desires or wishes and their opposing forces. Defense mechanisms were triggered to prevent the relevation of the wish or to avoid entering a situation whereby

the wish might be fulfilled. Thus anxiety was not only related to an affective fear of the repressed emotions, but also to a cognitive fear of experiencing the traumatic situation again, along with the distressing emotions with which it was associated. Freud's model was then able to account for the reason why abreaction alone was insufficient for complete alleviation of symptoms; previous conceptualizations did not incorporate the cognitive component of fearing repetition of the event. However, Freud's theory was still limited in that it de-emphasized the role of environmental context in triggering anxiety in certain situations, assuming that unconscious intrapsychic conflicts signaled danger, as opposed to perceptions of danger in the environment.

Psychodynamic theory

According to Nemiah,[5] psychodynamic theory generally holds that anxiety is experienced by the ego in response to either an external threat of danger or an internal instinctual drive. In addition, anxiety not only is a reaction to underlying psychological conflict, but also prompts specific defenses that influence the expression of the psychological disorder. Panic occurs when an individual reacts with feelings of helplessness in response to a traumatic situation, which may be caused by the threat of an environmental stressor, the expression of an innate drive, or some combination.

Shear et al[6] proposed a psychodynamic model of panic disorder (Figure 7.1) based on overlapping themes from interviews with nine patients. Their model is based on an intrinsic neurophysiological irritability that predisposes the individual to be fearful early on. This biological vulnerability is influenced by the commonly reported critical, controlling and fear-provoking behaviors of their parents.

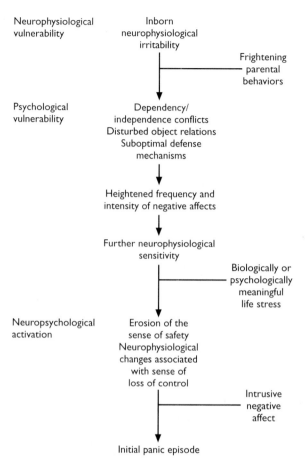

Neurophysiological vulnerability — Inborn neurophysiological irritability

Frightening parental behaviors

Psychological vulnerability — Dependency/ independence conflicts
Disturbed object relations
Suboptimal defense mechanisms

Heightened frequency and intensity of negative affects

Further neurophysiological sensitivity

Biologically or psychologically meaningful life stress

Neuropsychological activation — Erosion of the sense of safety
Neurophysiological changes associated with sense of loss of control

Intrusive negative affect

Initial panic episode

Figure 7.1 Psychodynamic model of panic disorder. (From Shear et al[6])

Conflicts between dependence and independence are consequently fostered in the patient, in which concerns of separation from the parents or of maintaining a sense of independence are prominent. These concerns ultimately culminate in a weak sense of self versus others anda disruption in the development of object relations. Unconscious or conscious fantasies of abandonment or of being trapped are readily activated, leading to increased negative affect,

threat and additional increases in anxiety. Neurophysiological sensitivity in the brain is further magnified by the inherent neurophysiological predisposition along with increased exposure to negative affect. This process is additionally exacerbated by stressful life events, which lead to an increased sense of uncontrollability and a diminished sense of security. A vicious cycle between fear and increased physiological symptomatology begins, ultimately resulting in an episode of panic. Finally, as a consequence of the avoidance associated with panic disorder, the patient never fully develops mature coping and defense mechanisms.

In a later study, Busch et al[7] investigated the nature of defense mechanisms specific to panic disorder versus dysthymia, speculating that individuals with panic disorder would use particular defenses to ward off negative affect. They found that individuals with panic disorder used defense mechanisms such as reaction formation (substituting opposing feelings, impulses and behaviors to those initially stated) and undoing (stating specific emotions and then retracting or contradicting original statements) significantly more than individuals with dysthymia. Busch and colleagues asserted that their findings were supportive of their 1993 model of panic disorder, which posited that individuals with panic disorder used defense mechanisms to evade feelings of negative affect perceived as threatening.

Shear and colleagues[6] articulated the similarities and differences between their psychodynamic theory of panic disorder and other competing theories. First, they do not support the neurobiological view of panic attacks as being spontaneous and not involving psychological content, but view panic attacks as always triggered by thoughts, images or sensations. However, their theory also differs from the cognitive–behavioral views in that they posit the role of fearful fantasies (unconscious or conscious) based on feelings of being trapped or isolated from powerful others as triggering panic.

Additional research is needed to further explore the psychodynamic model of panic disorder due to Shear et al.[6] In particular, a larger sample coupled with a control group is necessary to tease out whether the overlapping themes they found are specific to panic disorder or whether they also may be common in other psychological disorders, for example other anxiety or mood disorders. Further, Busch and colleagues noted that their 1995 study could not determine the causal direction of whether the defense mechanisms preceded or developed as a consequence of panic disorder. Further research is therefore required to identify factors that may predispose individuals to develop panic disorders, as well as variables that may be targeted for treatment and relapse prevention strategies.

Behavioral theories

Classical conditioning theory

Early behavioral explanations of panic focused on the role of classical or Pavlovian conditioning[8] in the etiology of the disorder. Although conditioning theories explaining the etiology of panic have been described differently in the literature,[9–12] generally these models involve the pairing of physiological sensations (conditioned stimulus, CS) such as heart palpitations with hyperventilation or lactation (unconditioned stimulus, UCS), which triggers panic/anxiety (unconditioned response/conditioned response, UCR/CR).

Evidence supporting conditioning theory has been drawn largely from research on the induction of fear in laboratory animals. The study of classical fear conditioning in humans gained its

popularity with the seminal work of Watson and Rayner,[13] who demonstrated the conditioning of fear in a young child. Classical fear conditioning in humans has received some support from earlier research by Rachman and Teasdale[14] and the more recent work of Ohman[15] and Baker et al.[16] During an investigation of Seligman's[17] preparedness theory, Ohman[15] found that it is possible to produce conditioned fear in humans in the laboratory, although the responses were of small magnitude and were extinguished after only a few trials.

More clear evidence of conditioned fear responses has been shown in oncology patients undergoing chemotherapy,[18,19] and in earlier studies on respiratory paralysis.[20,21] Patients undergoing chemotherapy were found to develop moderate to severe nausea reactions to neutral stimuli associated with the administration of chemotherapy, such as sights, sounds and strong smells. The studies on respiratory paralysis showed that conditioning reactions can occur very rapidly in humans when injected with succinylcholine, a drug that produces respiratory paralysis in a matter of seconds. The likely cause of such dramatic conditioning reactions as those reported above was the powerfulness of the UCSs – succinylcholine and chemotherapy (Barlow[1]).

Several criticisms have been levied against conditioning theories of panic. For example, Wolpe and Rowan[12] criticized the theory for assuming that all panic attacks are due to classical conditioning. They distinguish between the first panic attack, which, according to them, may be either biologically or psychologically based, and recurrent attacks that comprise panic disorder, which are due to conditioning. They propose that drugs such as amphetamines, cocaine and lysergic acid diethylamide (LSD), toxins, medical conditions such as hyperthyroidism and hypoglycemia, or severe stress precipitate the first panic attack, while recurrent attacks are likely due to conditioning.

Interoceptive conditioning theory

According to Wolpe and Rowan[12] and van den Hout,[22] panic disorder most likely reflects interoceptive conditioning (see Figure 7.2). In this model, anxiety becomes associated with physiological symptoms caused by low-intensity hyperventilation. After repeated pairings, the physiological symptoms that are caused by

hyperventilation begin to evoke panic as a conditioned response. Wolpe and Rowan also hold that panic can develop as a conditioned response to external stimuli, such as airplanes, public transportation, or other places and situations where a quick escape is difficult. This model treats the catastrophic misinterpretations of the feared physical sensations emphasized by Clark[23-25] as cognitions that arise after the panic attack in an attempt to rationalize or explain the experience.

The interoceptive conditioning theory of panic[12,22] is consistent with Goldstein and Chambless'[11] earlier interoceptive conditioning model explaining the etiology of agoraphobia. Goldstein and Chambless[6] cited studies by Razran[26] to describe how interoceptive conditioning involves the pairing of low levels of anxiety or arousal (CS) with higher levels of anxiety or arousal (UCS). According to this model, after an initial panic attack that involves intense arousal and anxiety, the individual becomes hypervigilant to physiological sensations. They then interpret even mild feelings of anxiety or arousal as predicting the onset of a panic attack. This sequence increases their level of anxiety, triggering the feared panic attack. The interoceptive conditioning theory has been criticized, however, as circular and conceptually confusing because anxiety serves as the CS, the UCS, the CR and the UCR.[27,28] Reiss stated that anxiety has too many roles in the interoceptive conditioning process. This, in Reiss' view, would mean that anxiety becomes conditioned to itself, which is conceptually confusing.

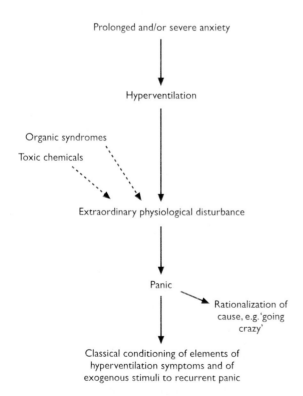

Figure 7.2 Flowchart of development of panic disorder. (From Wolpe and Rowan[12])

Modified conditioning theories

Various components have been added to conditioning theory to address criticisms of the model. For example, the classical conditioning theory of panic has been criticized for not providing an adequate explanation of why panic is not extinguished after numerous extinction trials where arousal is not followed by panic.[29] The theory has also been criticized because it does not explain why some fears are more easily conditioned than others. For example, earlier studies by English[30] and Bregman[31] showed that fear was more easily conditioned to animals and furry objects than to wooden objects, shapes and clothes. Seligman's[17] theory of evolutionary preparedness helps to explain this phenomenon. According to the preparedness principle, certain types of situations or objects (i.e. situations or objects with significant potential for danger, such as heights, animals or heart palpitations) are highly prepared for learning because this learning facilitates the survival of the species. Seligman[29] went on to state that when a biologically related CS and UCS co-occur, such as heart palpitations and panic, a blind association occurs that is learned in one trial and it is difficult to extinguish. Furthermore, it does not track the contingencies of the world, it is not conscious, and it is carried out in lower brain areas. The preparedness theory was partially supported in studies by Ohman[15] and Mineka,[32] but this modification to classical conditioning theory continues to be insufficient in its explanation of panic disorder. Specifically, the theory does not explain how the biologically related CSs and UCSs, such as heart palpitations and panic, co-occur to facilitate conditioning, nor why panic and learning occurs in some persons who experience heart palpitations and not in others.

Neo-conditioning or information processing theories

According to Rachman,[33] weaknesses in conditioning theory's explanations of panic and fear acquisition caused some researchers to abandon the model in favor of more cognitive explanations and further modification of conditioning theory models. Perhaps the most substantial revisions or modifications to the classical conditioning theory of panic disorder involve the consideration of cognition and information processing. Dickinson stated: 'even the simplest forms of conditioning ... involve cognitive processes, that learning can occur without reinforcement ... strict contiguity between the responses or stimulus and the reinforcer is neither necessary nor sufficient for conditioning' (Dickinson,[34] pp 57–8). The information processing theory holds that conditioning involves learning about the relationship between events, and not just the simple temporal contiguity of pairs of stimuli.[35] According to this theory, conditioning can occur even when the stimuli are not paired in time.

Experiments on learned taste aversion, where there is strong aversion for foods eaten as much as several hours earlier,[36,37] provide some evidence supporting noncontiguous conditioning. Furthermore, studies have reported that many people cannot recall a traumatic event to account for the development of their fear or phobia.[38,39] This is particularly true in persons with panic disorder.[1] Although these findings have been used to criticize traditional conditioning theories, Rachman[33] views them as examples supporting neo-conditioning, where noncontiguous conditioning may have taken place.

Barlow[1] provided another hypothesis to account for the conditioning of fear in persons with panic and other phobic disorders who have not experienced a traumatic event. He described a system of alarms that occurs in all human beings (this theory will be explained in more detail below). Although Barlow's alarm theory is not entirely based on a behavioral model, some discussion is warranted here. According to Barlow, panic attacks are false alarms that occur in the absence of real threat or danger. These alarms are marked by feelings of apprehension and impending doom. In persons with panic disorder, repeated occurrence of false alarms can become associated with internal or external cues and cause learned alarms. In Barlow's words, 'the occurrence of a false alarm may be one of the missing links in a traumatic conditioning etiology of some phobias' (Barlow,[1] p 228).

The neo-conditioning theory still does not completely account for the etiology of panic disorder. For example, the theory does not adequately explain why some individuals develop panic disorder subsequent to a panic attack, and others do not. Cognitive theories of panic disorder have produced interesting research that addresses criticisms of the behavioral theories of panic and adds to our understanding of the disorder. Interested readers are referred to Rachman[33] and Rescorla[35] for more in-depth reviews of conditioning and neo-conditioning theories.

Cognitive theories

Clark's cognitive theory

Clark's[23–25] model emphasizes the importance of catastrophic misinterpretations of feared physical sensations in the cycle of panic (see also Chapter 8). Individuals with panic disorder have a tendency to catastrophically misinterpret a range of somatic sensations. These somatic sensations may be anxiety-related (palpitations) or natural fluctuations in bodily processes (fullness after eating). The attack is triggered by an initial stimulus, which may be external (e.g. a feared situation or activity) or internal (cognitions or somatic sensations).

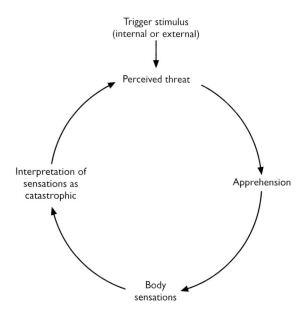

Figure 7.3 A cognitive approach to panic. (From Clark[23])

This initial stimulus provokes a perception of an immediate threat or impending danger (Figure 7.3). Rapid heartbeats, for example, may be misinterpreted as signs of an imminent heart attack.

Apprehension as a result of catastrophic misinterpretation causes an increase in arousal and further sensations, which are again interpreted as dangerous and imminently threatening. The misinterpretation of symptoms as indicating impending danger increases the perception of threat, and the cycle continues, causing a panic attack.

Panic attacks versus panic disorder
Experiencing a panic attack without necessarily developing the disorder is possible within this model. An individual with a relatively benign

cognitive style might not attend to an isolated panic attack at all once it has passed. An individual with a tendency to interpret autonomic events in a catastrophic manner would, however, be likely to develop panic disorder once he or she has experienced a panic attack. Such a cognitive style may have been learned or modeled, for example by a parent frequently calling attention to physical symptoms in an anxious way. A catastrophic cognitive style could also develop or be magnified by reinforcing events subsequent to a first panic attack, such as attention from family members, significant others, medical staff, etc.

Maintenance of panic disorder

From Clark's perspective, misinterpreting somatic sensations leads to additional tendencies that can maintain panic disorder. Because the individual fears particular sensations, he or she may become vigilant and focus attention internally to detect sensations. This internal focus promotes an over-sensitivity and over-awareness of normal bodily sensations. Chronic vigilance and attentiveness to physical sensations make it more likely that the cycle of panic may be triggered by an internal event or sensation, which leads to apprehension, further physical sensations of arousal, misinterpretation of those sensations, and subsequent panic.

In addition, avoidance tendencies may further contribute to the maintenance of panic disorder. Individuals with panic may begin to avoid activities like exercise or physical labor because those activities may lead to feared sensations. The avoidance of these activities is believed to help prevent the feared consequences of the sensations, but the individual is in fact prevented from learning that the exercise and associated physical symptoms are benign. Instead, avoidance and subsequent relief reinforce the notion that some catastrophe has been averted.

Empirical evidence supporting Clark's cognitive model comes from tests of predictions generated by the model, and, indirectly, from studies of cognitive treatment for panic disorder. In his papers on the cognitive model of panic, Clark[23-25] described four predictions following from his model that are currently supported with empirical data. First, individuals with panic disorder are more likely than nonpanickers to catastrophically misinterpret physical sensations.[40,41] Second, activating catastrophic interpretations of somatic sensations leads to increased anxiety and panic in individuals with panic disorder.[24,42] Third, biologically induced panic attacks can be averted if catastrophic misinterpretations are reduced or prevented.[40,43-45] Fourth, to maintain gains from treatment (including medication), cognitive change must take place during treatment.[46] Finally, the success of cognitive treatments of panic disorder[46-48] is consistent with a cognitive model of panic disorder.

There have been a number of critiques of Clark's cognitive model. One major challenge is the occurrence of noncognitive and nocturnal panic attacks. Clark[25] has suggested, however, that noncognitive attacks may be attacks in which the crucial misinterpretations are so quick and automatic as to be almost undetectable. Nocturnal attacks may occur because individuals with panic disorder continue to be vigilant for internal sensations even during sleep. Little empirical evidence is available to evaluate these issues.

Seligman[29] has commented that the cognitive theory of panic is not parsimonious, does not generate differential predictions from other theories, and is not anchored in the language of basic science. Furthermore, Ballenger[49] has questioned whether cognitive theories adequately account for the first attack or for the development of full-blown panic disorder. Barlow[50] similarly has commented that univariate models may not be able to account fully for the phenomenology of panic disorder. These concerns are criticism of cognitive theories of panic in general rather than of Clark's model per se; however, it may be that Clark's model does not sufficiently account for all aspects of the phenomenology of panic. It should be emphasized that Clark's model has had considerable heuristic value for research and practice and is the most influential primarily cognitive theory of panic in use today.

Anxiety sensitivity theory

Anxiety sensitivity is characterized by a belief that, beyond any immediate physical discomfort, anxiety and its associated symptoms may cause deleterious physical, psychological or social consequences.[51–53] Thus an individual who has high anxiety sensitivity would, for example, believe that palpitations were an impending sign of a heart attack, that feelings of derealization were an indication of insanity, or that dizziness was a sign of fainting and subsequent embarrassment. In contrast, an individual low on anxiety sensitivity would interpret these as unpleasant yet inconsequential bodily sensations.

McNally[54] clearly differentiates anxiety sensitivity from other theoretical explanations of panic disorder. First, anxiety sensitivity differs from interoceptive conditioning in that the former does not refer to a conditioned response pattern to physical sensations, but to the individual's belief that the anxiety symptoms are harmful. In addition, one does not need to personally experience panic to have beliefs that physical sensations are dangerous, despite the fact that panic may intensify anxiety sensitivity; thus conditioning is not necessary for anxiety sensitivity. Second, anxiety sensitivity is distinguished from catastrophic misinterpretations of anxiety. Although individuals with panic disor-

der may be inclined to make such misinterpretations, they may be fully aware of the causes of their sensations, and still hold an inherent belief that the sensations alone are dangerous.

One of the most common measures of anxiety sensitivity is the Anxiety Sensitivity Index (ASI),[52] a 16-item self-report measure of fear of the physical sensations of anxiety, which has undergone behavioral validation.[55] Although the ASI asks about a fear of and beliefs about the harmfulness of physical sensations, it has been shown to be factorially independent of actual panic symptomatology.[56] In general, anxiety sensitivity has been found to be normally distributed in the population, suggesting that it is a dimensional construct[52,57] in which the greater the anxiety sensitivity, the more strongly the individual believes in the harmful consequences.[28] Individuals with panic disorder and agoraphobia have been found to score higher on measures of anxiety sensitivity than individuals with other anxiety disorders, who in turn score higher than normal controls.[52] Individuals without such disorders who experience unexpected bodily sensations generally do not respond with anxiety or uneasiness.[58] More recently, Taylor, Koch and McNally[59] compared anxiety sensitivity in DSM-III-R diagnoses of panic disorder, post-traumatic stress disorder (PTSD), social phobia, generalized anxiety disorder (GAD), obsessive–compulsive disorder (OCD) and specific phobia. Individuals with anxiety disorders, other than specific phobia, scored higher on anxiety sensitivity than normal controls. Further, individuals with panic disorder scored higher than those with other anxiety disorders, although not significantly higher than individuals with PTSD.

Anxiety sensitivity is thought to put an individual at increased risk for developing anxiety disorders in general, and in particular panic disorder and agoraphobia.[51,60] Increased levels of anxiety sensitivity lead to greater overall anxiety levels due to increased worry over the anxiety itself, which additionally may lead to decreased tolerance for stress.[28] However, in the development of panic disorder and/or agoraphobia, although an individual may experience increased anxiety as a result of a panic attack, a panic attack alone may not be sufficient to induce panic disorder or agoraphobia. Here, the individual may need to have originally high anxiety sensitivity to develop the disorder. In fact, anxiety sensitivity does not necessarily develop through personal experience with panic, but may precede the first panic attack.[61] However, specificity may be limited in identifying individuals with an anxiety disorder based on high anxiety sensitivity alone; although one may sensitively rule out the likelihood of an anxiety disorder based on low anxiety sensitivity, not all individuals with high anxiety sensitivity develop an anxiety disorder.[51]

Several criticisms have been levied against the anxiety sensitivity theory. McNally and Lorenz[51] maintain that trait anxiety and anxiety sensitivity are theoretically dissimilar, in that, although individuals with panic disorder may have a general tendency to respond anxiously to situational stressors, they may also have an added fear of the sensations themselves. To support their theory, they argue that anxiety sensitivity has predictive validity over and above measures of general trait anxiety,[51,52] and that individuals with high anxiety sensitivity tend to respond more to a biological hyperventilation challenge.[62] However, debate has surrounded the question whether anxiety sensitivity is conceptually distinct from trait anxiety.[63–66] Most recently, Taylor[66] concluded that anxiety sensitivity appeared to be distinct from trait anxiety, possibly in accordance with a hierarchical model proposed by Lilienfeld et

al[64] in which anxiety sensitivity was viewed as a dimension of trait anxiety, which in turn was thought to be a component of a larger overall negative emotionality factor.

In addition, controversy has surrounded the factor structure of the ASI, with some investigators arguing that it is unidimensional[52,59,67] and others arguing that it is multidimensional.[68–70] Based on current findings, Taylor[66] concluded that anxiety sensitivity appears to be unidimensional, yet may consist of lower-order factors such as somatic, psychological or social harm.

Future research is needed to determine the causal direction of anxiety sensitivity and panic disorder, as well as to further explore its relationship to other anxiety disorders. In addition, confirmatory factor analyses need to be conducted to provide support for the hierarchical model proposed by Lilienfeld et al[64] and to explore other potential models of anxiety sensitivity. Developmental aspects of anxiety sensitivity should also be explored, which may contribute to our understanding of anxiety sensitivity as a dimensional construct. Finally, it has been shown that anxiety sensitivity changes across behavioral treatment;[51] the influence of pharmacological treatment on anxiety sensitivity also deserves investigation. The reader is referred to Lilienfeld et al[64] and Taylor[66] for detailed reviews of methodological and theoretical issues surrounding anxiety sensitivity.

Barlow's false alarm theory

Barlow's[1,50] model incorporates concepts and empirical support from a number of independent areas, including the biological, emotional, learning, and cognitive realms of basic science. He describes panic as the basic emotion of fear, which is an acute reaction to perceived imminent danger, with one crucial difference: no danger is present. In contrast, anxiety describes an apprehensive state oriented toward the possibility of a future threat. Barlow identifies three types of alarms: true alarms (immediate danger present), false alarms (panic attacks) and learned alarms (conditioned panic attacks). In panic, there are physiological, cognitive and behavioral components mobilizing the individual to act immediately – either to fight or to escape. Once again, when there is no objectively apparent source of danger, the reaction is a false alarm; this is the same as a panic attack.

Panic attack versus panic disorder

Many individuals experience a panic attack or false alarm. Panic attacks may be cued or uncued, although uncued attacks may be in reaction to specific internal or external triggers that are simply not noticed. Cued panic attacks are relatively common in the general population, but 'uncued' attacks are less common.[71] The mere occurrence of an initial false alarm

when under life stress is not sufficient to cause the development of panic disorder. Barlow hypothesizes that biology and stress, moderated by factors such as cognitive coping strategies and social support, may be necessary contributors to the development of panic disorder.

Development and maintenance of panic disorder

Barlow's[1] model of panic disorder (Figure 7.4) includes a biological diathesis, or propensity to experience arousal under stress. Another contributing factor is psychological vulnerability, influenced by factors such as early life events and parenting style.[72] Psychologically vulnerable individuals fail to develop a sense of competence with respect to the world and themselves, and typically experience poor predictability and control over life events such as

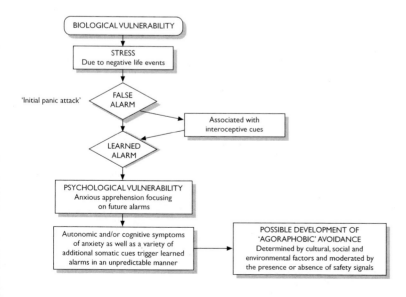

Figure 7.4 A model of the etiology of panic disorder. (From Barlow[1])

intense emotional states. For biologically and psychologically vulnerable individuals, an initial false alarm may be followed by arousal and self-focused attention (anxious apprehension) centering on the possibility of experiencing further panic attacks and the belief that the attacks are dangerous.

In addition, internal somatic or cognitive cues and sensations can become associated with the experience of false alarms (interoceptive conditioning), such that the experience of somatic symptoms reliably triggers a panic attack. Such interoceptively cued attacks are learned alarms. Interoceptive sensitivity and anxious apprehension may contribute to avoidance of activities and situations associated with somatic sensations and cues. The avoidance then becomes negatively reinforced, since the individual believes that an attack has been averted owing to escape or avoidance.

As Barlow's[1,50] model draws from research in areas such as basic emotion theory, biology and learning, a comprehensive discussion of empirical literature bearing on his model is outside the scope of this chapter. Generally, family and twin studies support the possibility of a biological and heritable vulnerability toward anxious apprehension.[71] From learning theory come the conceptualizations of learned alarms and interoceptive sensitivity. Another significant component of the model is the role of cognitions in the maintenance of panic, which is supported by the types of studies discussed in the earlier section on Clark's cognitive model. Barlow's[1,50] distinction between anxiety and panic is supported by emotion theory literature concerning the specificity and organization of panic as compared with that of anxiety.[73] The interested reader is referred to Barlow[1] and Barlow et al[72] for a more thorough examination of the empirical literature relevant to this model of panic.

Criticisms of Barlow's model have concerned his distinction between panic and anxiety, conflicting models (e.g. Klein's biological model[74]), and Barlow's extension of his theories to the emotional disorders. With respect to panic versus anxiety, it has been suggested that they are similar in terms of symptoms experienced and that they differ only in severity.[23] Conflicting models, such as more biologically oriented theories, attempt to account for the phenomena of panic more parsimoniously (see Chapter 3). For the issue of expansion of Barlow's theories to the emotional disorders, the interested reader is again referred to Barlow.[1,50]

Discussion and conclusions

Psychological theories of panic and anxiety are in the early developmental stage. Much the same can be said for biological theories. This is due to the explosion of data in the last decade, which has irrevocably changed our views of the nature and etiology of panic and anxiety. Classical psychoanalytic theories, relatively unchanged for nearly 100 years, seem dated at this point in time, as is evident from the discussion at the beginning of this chapter. More modern psychodynamic theories, some of them incorporating important elements from early psychoanalytic theory, may have more relevance, particularly as articulated by Shear et al.[6] In fact, data are beginning to accumulate on the importance of the contribution of parenting styles and early experiences to psychological vulnerabilities for anxiety and, perhaps, panic, consistent with some notions from attachment theory.[72,75] But theories in the end are no more nor less than useful tools that serve as organizing principles for emerging data. Thus these theories can and should change and evolve as new data appear, and this is just what is happening as we learn more about the nature of anxiety and panic.

As theories develop in any area of inquiry, one sees a progression from one-dimensional linear model to more satisfactory multidetermined causal sequences organized in a systemic fashion. Thus this may be among the last chapters devoted exclusively to psychological theories of panic and panic disorder. Ultimately, any satisfactory theory will have to incorporate biological vulnerabilities and sensitivities interacting in an integral way with psychological factors. This development will not be fully realized until both psychological and biological investigators become more intimately familiar with evolving data in each other's area, which is one of the goals of this volume.

Returning to exclusively psychological theories for a moment, little attention has been paid to a sharp analysis of important similarities and differences among these models. But only this kind of analysis, complete with hypothesis-generating exercises, will uncover what is truly unique to some of these notions versus what is basically the same hypothesis restated with slightly different terminology. For example, beyond the superficial differences noted in contrasting models of anxiety sensitivity and other cognitive theories, there is much that is very similar. Both models propose a fundamental cognitive vulnerability predating the development of the panic disorder that affects the processing of information emanating from objective physiological or environmental events. A fruitful exercise would be to determine if differential predictions could be made from these closely related models that could ultimately be tested. Admirably, David M Clark has attempted differential predictions in the context of his own model – but only in the service of providing a gross contrast with more fundamental and linear biological models. Others have not even progressed this far. This type of exercise is best accomplished in a collaborative fashion, and proponents of varying psychological models may well benefit from collaborating on a set of sharp predictions. Surely this would advance the field.

Another clear trend is found in the beginnings of attempts to move away from predictions that focus on current state in those presenting with panic disorder, either before or after treatment, to predictions concerned with more distal vulnerabilities for developing disorder, and the development of these vulnerabilities. For example, investigators are beginning to focus on discovering the nature of psychological vulnerabilities that predate the development of disorder. This is a difficult question to address, ultimately requiring prospective studies. But such studies are beginning to appear in the area of depression,[76] and it is very likely that similar efforts will uncover the origins of psychological vulnerabilities in the closely related states of anxiety and panic. As noted above, both behavioral and psychodynamic investigators are re-examining attachment theory, early parenting styles and the occurrence of stressful events early in childhood as possible precursors to anxiety and related disorders. Presumably these vulnerabilities would have to line up correctly with biological vulnerabilities to provide a substantial diathesis, but this too needs evaluation. To take one (rather radical) possible outcome of this trend, perhaps the variety of cognitive and emotional phenomena associated with the presentation of panic disorder are simply trivial epiphenomena of the disorder itself (e.g. catastrophic misinterpretations, anxiety sensitivity, interoceptive conditioning) and that crucial factors contributing to psychological theories of panic disorder may be found elsewhere. (One example might be fundamental constructions of controllability over negative life events emerging from early experience.) Only prospective studies will ultimately make these determinations.

In conclusion, it can be said with some certainty that theoretical models of panic, from both biological, psychological and, ultimately, an integrative perspective, will be far more complex than the present focused linear models currently undergoing evaluation. It seems likely that both biological and psychological vulnerabilities may be nonspecific, and that the development of specific panic and anxiety disorders may involve a variety of experiences at different developmental stages to activate these nonspecific diatheses. Future theory building should emphasize an integrationist approach that takes development into consideration.

References

1. Barlow DH, *Anxiety and its Disorders: The Nature and Treatment of Anxiety and Panic.* New York: The Guilford Press, 1988.
2. Freud S. The neuropsychoses of defense. In: *The Standard Edition of the Complete Psychological Works of Sigmund Freud*, Vol 3 (Strachey J, ed. and trans.). London: Hogarth Press, 1962: 43–61. (Original work published in 1894.)
3. Josephs L, Psychoanalytic and related Interpretations. In: *Anxiety and Related Disorders: A Handbook* (Wolman BB, Stricker G, eds). New York: Wiley, 1994: 11–29.
4. Freud S, Inhibitions, symptoms and anxiety. In: *The Standard Edition of the Complete Psychological Works of Sigmund Freud*, Vol 20 (Strachey J, ed. and trans.). London: Hogarth Press, 1959: 77–174. (Original work published in 1926.)
5. Nemiah JC, The psychodynamic view of anxiety: an historical approach. In: *Handbook of Anxiety*, Vol 1: *Biological, Clinical and Cultural Perspectives* (Roth M, Noyes R Jr, Burrows GD, eds). New York: Elsevier, 1988: 277–303.
6. Shear MK, Cooper AM, Klerman GL et al, A psychodynamic model of panic disorder. *Am J Psychiatry* 1993; **150**: 859–66.
7. Busch FN, Shear MK, Cooper AM et al, An empirical study of defense mechanisms in panic disorder. *J Nerv Ment Dis* 1995; **183**: 299–303.
8. Pavlov IP, *Conditioned Reflexes.* London: Oxford University Press, 1927.
9. Eysenck HJ, A theory of the incubation of anxiety/fear response. *Behav Res Ther* 1968; **6**: 319–21.
10. Eysenck HJ, Incubation theory of fear/anxiety. In: *Theoretical Issues in Behavior Therapy* (Reiss S, Bootzin RR, eds). New York: Academic Press, 1985: 83–102.
11. Goldstein AJ, Chambless DL, A reanalysis of agoraphobia. *Behav Ther* 1978; **9**: 47–59.
12. Wolpe J, Rowan VC, Panic disorder: a product of classical conditioning. *Behav Res Ther* 1988; **26**: 441–50.
13. Watson JB, Rayner P, Conditioned emotional reactions. *J Exp Psychol* 1920; **3**: 1–14.
14. Rachman S, Teasdale J, *Aversion Therapy and the Behavior Disorders.* London: Routledge & Kegan Paul, 1969.
15. Ohman A, Evolution, learning and phobias. In: *Psychopathology* (Magnusson D, Ohman A, eds). New York: Academic Press, 1987: 5–28.
16. Baker TB, Cannon DS, Tiffany ST, Gino A. Cardiac response as an index of the effect of aversion therapy. *Behav Res Ther* 1984; **22**: 403–11.
17. Seligman MEP, Phobias and preparedness. *Behav Ther* 1971; **2**: 307–20.
18. Cella DF, Pratt A, Holland JC, Persistent anticipatory nausea, vomiting and anxiety in cured Hodgkin's disease patients after completion of chemotherapy. *Am J Psychiatry* 1986; **143**: 641–3.
19. Redd WH, Andrykowski MA, Behavioral interventions in cancer treatment: controlling aversion reactions to chemotherapy. *J Consult Clin Psychol* 1982; **50**: 1018–29.
20. Campbell D, Sanderson R, Laverty SG, Characteristics of a conditioned response in

human subjects during extinction trials following a single traumatic conditioning trial. *J Abnorm Soc Psychol* 1964; **66**: 627–39.

21. Sanderson R, Laverty S, Campbell D, Traumatically conditioned responses acquired during respiratory paralysis. *Nature* 1963; **196**: 1235–6.

22. van den Hout MA, The explanation of experimental panic. In: *Panic: Psychological Perspectives* (Rachman S, Maser JD, eds). Hillsdale, NJ: Erlbaum, 1988: 237–57.

23. Clark DM, A cognitive approach to panic. *Behav Res Ther* 1986; **24**: 461–70.

24. Clark DM, A cognitive model of panic. In: *Panic: Psychological Perspectives* (Rachman S, Maser JD, eds). Hillsdale, NJ: Erlbaum, 1988: 71–89.

25. Clark DM, Panic disorder: from theory to therapy. In: *Frontiers of Cognitive Therapy* (Salkovskis P, ed.). New York: The Guilford Press, 1996: 318–44.

26. Razran G, The observable unconscious and the inferable conscious in current Soviet psychophysiology: interoceptive conditioning, semantic conditioning, and orienting reflex. *Psychol Rev* 1961; **68**: 81–147.

27. McNally RJ, Psychological approaches to panic disorder: a review. *Psychol Bull* 1990; **108**: 403–19.

28. Reiss S, Theoretical perspectives on the fear of anxiety. *Clin Psychol Rev* 1987; **7**: 585–96.

29. Seligman MEP, Competing theories of panic. In: *Panic: Psychological Perspectives* (Rachman S, Maser JD, eds). Hillsdale, NJ: Erlbaum, 1988: 321–9.

30. English HB, Three cases of the 'conditioned fear response'. *J Abnorm Soc Psychol* 1929; **34**: 221–5.

31. Bregman E, An attempt to modify the emotional attitudes of infants by the conditioned response technique. *J Genet Psychol* 1934; **45**: 169–96.

32. Mineka S, The Role of fear in the theories of avoidance learning, flooding and extinction. *Psychol Bull* 1979; **86**: 985–1010.

33. Rachman S, Neo-conditioning and the classical theory of fear acquisition. *Clin Psychol Rev* 1991; **11**: 155–73.

34. Dickinson A, Animal conditioning and learning theory. In: *Theoretical Foundations of Behaviour Therapy* (Eysenck HJ, Marin I, eds). New York: Plenum Press, 1987: 45–61.

35. Rescorla RA, Pavlovian conditioning: It's not what you think it is. *Am Psychol* 1988; **43**: 151–60.

36. Garcia J, Ervin F, Koelling R, Learning with prolonged delay of reinforcement. *Psychonomic Sci* 1966; **5**: 121–2.

37. Garcia J, Koelling D, Relation of cue to consequence in avoidance. *Psychonomic Sci* 1966; **4**: 123–4.

38. Murray EJ, Foote F, The origins of fear and snakes. *Behav Res Ther* 1979; **17**: 489–93.

39. Rimm DC, Janda LH, Lancaster DW et al, An exploratory investigation of the origin and maintenance of phobias. *Behav Res Ther* 1977; **15**: 231–38.

40. Harvey JM, Richards JC, Dziadosz T, Swindell A, Misinterpretations of ambiguous stimuli in panic disorder. *Cognitive Ther Res* 1993; **17**: 235–48.

41. McNally RJ, Foa EB, Cognition and agoraphobia: bias in the interpretation of threat. *Cognitive Ther Res* 1987; **11**: 567–81.

42. Ehlers A, Margraf J, Roth WT et al, Anxiety produced by false heart rate feedback in patients with panic disorder. *Behav Res Ther* 1988; **26**: 1–11.

43. Clark DM, Cognitive mediation of panic attacks induced by biological challenge tests. *Adv Behav Res Ther* 1993; **15**: 75–84.

44. Rapee R, Mattick R, Murrell E, Cognitive mediation in the affective component of spontaneous panic attacks. *J Behav Ther Exp Psychiatry* 1986; **17**: 245–53.

45. Sanderson WC, Rapee RM, Barlow DH, The influence of an illusion of control on panic attacks induced via inhalation of 5.5% carbon dioxide enriched air. *Arch Gen Psychiatry* 1989; **46**: 157–62.

46. Clark DM, Salkovskis PM, Hackmann A et al, A comparison of cognitive therapy, applied relaxation, and imipramine in the treatment of panic disorder. *Br J Psychiatry* 1994; **164**: 759–69.

47. Margraf J, Schneider S, Outcome and active ingredients of cognitive–behavioral treatments for panic disorder. Paper presented at the Annual Conference of the Association for Advancement of Behavior Therapy, New York, 1991.

48. Ost L-G, Westling B, Applied relaxation vs. cognitive therapy in the treatment of panic disorder. *Behav Res Ther* 1995; **33**: 145–58.

49. Ballenger JC, Toward an integrated model of panic disorder. *Am J Orthopsychiatry* 1989; **59**: 284–93.

50. Barlow DH, Disorders of emotion. *Psychol Inquiry* 1991; **2**: 58–71.

51. McNally RJ, Lorenz M, Anxiety sensitivity in agoraphobics. *J Behav Ther Exp Psychiatry* 1987; **18**: 3–11.

52. Reiss S, Peterson RA, Gursky DM, McNally RJ, Anxiety sensitivity, anxiety frequency and the prediction of fearfuln ess. *Behav Res Ther* 1986; **24**: 1–8.

53. Taylor S, Koch WJ, McNally RJ, Crockett DJ, Conceptualizations of anxiety sensitivity. *Psychol Assess* 1992; **4**: 245–50.

54. McNally RJ, *Panic Disorder: A Critical Analysis*. New York: The Guilford Press, 1994.

55. Maller RG, Reiss S, A behavioral validation of the Anxiety Sensitivity Index. *J Anxiety Disord* 1987; **1**: 265–72.

56. Cox BJ, Endler NS, Swinson RP, Anxiety sensitivity and panic attack symptomatology. *Behav Res Ther* 1995; **33**: 833–6.

57. Rapee RM, Psychological factors in panic disorder. *Adv Behav Res Ther* 1993; **15**: 85–102.

58. Rapee RM, Ancis JR, Barlow DH, Emotional reactions to physiological sensations: panic disorder patients and non-clinical Ss. *Behav Res Ther* 1988; **26**: 265–9.

59. Taylor S, Koch WJ, McNally RJ, How does anxiety sensitivity vary across the anxiety disorders? *J Anxiety Disord* 1992; **6**: 249–59.

60. Reiss S, Expectancy model of fear, anxiety, and panic. *Clin Psychol Rev* 1991; **11**: 141–53.

61. Donnell CD, McNally RJ, Anxiety sensitivity and panic attacks in a nonclinical population. *Behav Res Ther* 1990; **28**: 83–5.

62. Holloway W, McNally RJ, Effects of anxiety sensitivity on the response to hyperventilation. *J Abnor Psychol* 1987; **96**: 330–4.

63. Lilienfeld SO, Jacob RG, Turner SM, Comment on Holloway and McNally's (1987) effects of anxiety sensitivity on the response to hyperventilation. *J Abnor Psychol* 1989; **98**: 100–2.

64. Lilienfeld SO, Turner SM, Jacob RG, Anxiety sensitivity: an examination of theoretical and methodological issues. *Adv Behav Res Ther* 1993; **15**: 147–83.

65. McNally RJ, Is anxiety sensitivity distinguishable from trait anxiety? Reply to Lilienfeld, Jacob, and Turner (1989). *J Abnorm Psychol* 1989; **98**: 193–4.

66. Taylor S, Anxiety sensitivity: theoretical perspectives and recent findings. *Behav Res Ther* 1995; **33**: 243–58.

67. Taylor S, Koch WJ, Crockett DJ, Anxiety sensitivity, trait anxiety, and the anxiety disorders. *J Anxiety Disord* 1991; **5**: 293–311.

68. Peterson RA, Heilbronner RL, The Anxiety Sensitivity Index: construct validity and factor analytic structure. *J Anxiety Disord* 1987; **1**: 117–21.

69. Telch MJ, Shermis MD, Lucas JA, Anxiety sensitivity: unitary personality trait or domain-specific appraisals? *J Anxiety Disord* 1989; **3**: 25–32.

70. Wardle J, Ahmad T, Hayward P, Anxiety sensitivity in agoraphobia. *J Anxiety Disord* 1990; **4**: 325–33.

71. Carter M, Barlow DH, Learned alarms: the origins of panic. In: *Theories of Behavior Therapy: Exploring Behavior Change* (O'Donahue W, Krasner L, eds). Washington, DC: American Psychological Association, 1995: 209–28.

72. Barlow DH, Chorpita B, Turovsky J, Fear, panic, anxiety, and disorders of emotion. In: *Nebraska Symposium on Motivation* (Hope D, ed.). Lincoln, NE: University of Nebraska–Lincoln Press, 1996: 251–328.

73. Gray JA, Fear, panic, and anxiety: What's in a name? *Psychol Inquiry* 1991; **2**: 77–8.

74. Klein DF, Gorman JM, A model of panic and agoraphobia development. *Acta Psychiatr Scand* 1987; **76**: 87–95.

75. Bowlby J, *Attachment and Loss*, Vol 1: *Attachment*. New York: Basic, 1969.

76. Nolen-Hoeksema S, Girgus JS, Seligman MEP, Learned helplessness in children: a longitudinal study of depression, achievement, and attributional style. *J Pers Soc Psychol* 1986; **51**: 435–42.

8

Medical aspects of panic disorder and its relationship to other medical conditions

David France Jakubec and C Barr Taylor

CONTENTS • **Introduction** • **Recognizing panic disorder in the medical setting** • **Cardiovascular system** • **Endocrine disorders** • **Neurologic disorders** • **Pulmonary diseases** • **Gastrointestinal disorders** • **Medication** • **Conclusions**

Introduction

The relationship of panic disorder (PD) to medical conditions is complex and at times puzzling. PD presents with symptoms that mimic many other medical problems, and medical problems interact with PD to make its symptoms worse. In this chapter we review studies that have examined the medical aspects of PD. Along the way, we present recommendations for evaluating the medical status of PD patients.

Recognizing panic disorder in the medical setting

The separation of PD from physical disease is difficult because many of the symptoms of PD mimic those of other medical disorders (Table 8.1).[1] Patients experiencing panic attacks for the first time are frightened and bewildered by their symptoms, and will often go to an emergency room or see their physician. Because of the somatic nature of this illness, these patients

are often seen for long periods of time in medical practices other than psychiatry, resulting in improper diagnosis and incorrect or inadequate treatment.

It has been estimated that 6–10% of patients seen by primary care or family practice physicians and 10–14% seen by cardiologists actually suffer from PD.[2] Fleet et al[3] found that only 2% of emergency room patients with panic disorder were given the correct diagnosis.

Determining the true prevalence of panic disorder in medical settings and with medical problems is complicated by the fact that some patients have panic attacks with atypical features or presentation. Most notably, Beitman and colleagues[4] found that a large number of patients with chest pain and 'normal coronary arteries' have a constellation of symptoms very characteristic of panic attacks but without 'fear'. Such patients do not present significant differences compared with patients with PD.[5] The diagnosis of such events will be discussed in the cardiovascular section below.

Patients with PD are high consumers of medical services[6] and may have more medical

Table 8.1 Differential diagnosis: symptoms of anxiety and of medical disorders[a]

Acute anxiety symptom	Possible medical condition	Characteristic of medical symptom
Shortness of breath, smothering sensation	Congestive heart failure	Rapid, shallow breathing, worse on lying down
	Pneumonia, pleuritis	Fever, cough
	Asthma	Wheezing on expiration, cough
	Chronic obstructive pulmonary disease	Chronic cough, history of smoking, yellow sputum
Dizziness, unsteady feelings, or faintness	Orthostatic hypotension, anemia	Worse upon standing up
	Benign positional, vertigo	Triggered by rotation of head, jogging, stopping
Palpitations or accelerated heart rate	Paroxysmal atrial or supraventricular tachycardia	Sudden onset of rapid heart rate; rate > 120 bpm
	Mitral-valve prolapse	Systolic click or late systolic murmur
	Ventricular ectopic beats	Feeling of the heart flopping or turning over
	Tumors of the adrenal medulla	Episodes of hypertension with tachycardia developing rapidly
	Thyrotoxicosis, hyperthyroidism	Fine tremor, excessive sweating, heat intolerance
	Hypoglycemia	Symptoms 2–4 hours after a meal
Sweating, flushes, or chills	Menopause	Female sex, appropriate age
Nausea or abdominal distress	Innumerable	
Depersonalization or derealization	Temporal lobe epilepsy	Perceptual distortions, hallucinations
Numbness or tingling	Hyperventilation	Rapid, shallow breathing
Chest pain or discomfort	Angina pectoris	Precipitated by physical exercise, emotions, sex, or heavy meals
	Myocardial infarction	Severe pressing, constricting chest pain and pain radiating into left arm
	Costal chondritis	Tender spots in costochondral junctions
	Pleuritis, pneumonia	Fever, cough

[a]Reprinted with permission from Taylor and Arnow.[1]

problems than the public at large. For instance, Rogers et al,[7] comparing the medical history of 527 PD patients with a control population from the Rand Health Insurance Experiment, found significantly higher rates of ulcer disease and angina in males with PD and higher rates of ulcer and thyroid disease in females with PD.

Much as primary care physicians may overlook the diagnosis of panic attacks, psychiatrists often fail to recognize physical illness.[8] Anxiety may occur as a manifestation of a primary psychiatric disorder or secondarily to either a medical illness or the medications prescribed for treatment. Many medical illnesses, such as anemia, angina, asthma and endocrine disorders, present with anxiety.[9] Thus we recommend that both new patients and current patients who develop new panic-like symptoms have a medical examination.

While, in almost all cases, the diagnosis becomes apparent with careful history and continued observation, many physicians are not afforded this luxury and appropriately rely on tests. On the other hand, the index of suspicion should always remain high when patients present with symptoms characteristic of PD.

Cardiovascular system

The most common PD symptoms are cardiologic. In one sample of patients, 87% reported palpitations, 75% reported shortness of breath and 61% reported chest pain.[1] In cardiac clinics, as many as 50% of patients referred by general practitioners with signs of palpitation or chest pain may not receive a cardiac or other major physical diagnosis.[10] Up to 23% of such patients have a current PD.[11]

Mitral valve prolapse

Mitral valve prolapse (MVP) is a disorder in which a proportion of the mitral valve bellows into the left atrium of the heart when blood is being ejected. It is a common condition, occurring in approximately 4–6% of the population, but has been described in as many as 17%.[12] Psychological symptoms have long been associated with the physical findings of MVP. Da Costa[13] described the syndrome of 'irritable heart' in American Civil War soldiers, and reported hearing occasional clicks and apical murmurs. In 1941, Wood[14] noted that Da Costa's syndrome was most common in young women, and described symptoms of palpitations, dyspnea, chest pain, fatigue and anxiety. In known MVP patients, palpitations occur in 50% and chest pain in 30–50% of patients.

In recent times, Gorman et al[15] were among the first to report an association between MVP and PD (10 of 20 PD patients had MVP). Since then, researchers have found a high rate of PD (8–20%) in patients with MVP; conversely, 7–34% of patients with PD have MVP.[16] These studies are strongly affected by selection bias. Patients with PD are sensitive to symptoms and are likely to seek an evaluation when unusual symptoms occur. Studies that attempted to control for this bias examined both MVP and PD in families, or MVP compared with a cardiac control group, and have not found any significant difference in the prevalence of PD between MVP and cardiac controls.[17] Taken together, these studies do not suggest that MVP and PD are comorbid conditions, although they may share common features, in particular autonomic dysfunction,[18] connective tissue abnormalities (joint hypermobility syndrome),[19] palpitations,[11] chest pain,[20] and presyncope or syncope. It is of note that the DSM-IV indicates that a diagnosis of MVP does not preclude a diagnosis of PD.

Patients with syncope and other symptoms of MVP or PD require special attention. Sudden death may occur as an extremely rare complication of MVP, especially among women. Such patients have been found to have Q-T prolongation and/or ST-T abnormalities, premature beats or nonsustained ventricular tachycardia,[21] and may have a family history of sudden death.[12] We recommend that each patient who presents with signs of presyncope or syncope should be carefully examined and at least have an ECG.

Tachycardia

Patients with panic can sometimes have higher than normal resting heart rates, although usually less than 90 bpm. PD patients may have significantly elevated heart rates on tricyclic antidepressants (TCAs), even exceeding 100 bpm.[22] Medical causes, such as hyperthyroidism, should be excluded in PD patients with an elevated resting heart rate.

Arrhythmias

A variety of arrhythmias have been reported to occur with PD. Arrhythmias are abnormalities of the rate and the rhythm of the pulse. Several studies have shown that many panic attacks occur at heart rates disproportionate to physical activity; maximum heart rates ranged between 115 and 150 bpm. Although a variety of pathological conditions can produce such high rates, in panic patients, nonexertional heart rates in these ranges have usually been found to be sinus tachycardia. However, most physicians who have seen many PD patients have encountered a rare patient or two who presents with classic panic symptoms but turns out to have severe arrhythmias.

Despite many studies, it is not clear if patients with PD have a greater interoceptive acuity for pericardiac sensations.[23] After reviewing recent studies, Ehlers and Breuer[24] conclude that the majority of studies have found that PD patients show a better heartbeat perception than controls. Discrepant results are probably related to different instructions and differences in sample characteristics, such as the inclusion of patients on medication affecting the cardiovascular system. More accurate heartbeat perception may, however, be restricted to those patients who show agoraphobic avoidance behavior.

- *Recommendation* Patients with frequent panic episodes associated with nonexertional heart rates of over 125 bpm should be considered for evaluation by a cardiologist.

Cardiovascular disease

Many studies suggest that patients with PD have increased cardiovascular morbidity and mortality. Most impressively, Weissman and colleagues[25] found that the risk of stroke in persons with lifetime diagnoses of PD was over twice that in persons with other or no psychiatric disorders. In a recent prospective study of males, risk of sudden cardiac death was significantly related to anxiety: a multivariate odds ratio of 2.96 (95% CI: 1.02–8.55) for men who scored 1 on the Anxiety Symptom Scale compared with men who scored 0, and 4.46 (95% CI: 0.92–21.6) for men who scored 2 or higher.[26] However, variations in methodology and inconsistency of results across studies limit clear conclusions (Table 8.2).[38] For instance, the association between mortality and PD may be more related to depression than to panic, which has been clearly associated with increased morbidity and mortality and is highly comorbid with panic.

Table 8.2 Studies reporting cardiovascular mortality or morbidity in patients with anxiety disorders[a]

Author	Sample size and sex	Sample type[b]	Design[c]	Control for known cardiovascular disease risk factors	Estimated relative risk[d]
Panic disorder only					
Coryell et al[27]	42 F, 71 M	Instit	Retro	No	2 F; 2 M*
Weissman et al[25]	60 M and F	Comm	Cross	No	OR = 4,5*
Anxiety disorders					
Sims and Prior[28]	1982 M and F	Instit	Retro	No	1.7*
Martin et al[29]	60 M and F	Instit	Retro	No	–
Coryell et al[30]	155 M and F	Instit	Retro	No	–, + M only
Allgulander and Lavori[31]	685 F, 255 M	Instit	Retro	No	1.0 F; 1.2 M
Anxiety scales					
Paffenbarger et al[32]	41 266 M	Comm	Pros	No	1.6*
Thorne et al[33]	7685 M	Comm	Pros	No	–
Medalie et al[34]	10 059 M	Comm	Pros	No	2*
Thiel et al[35]	50 M	Instit	Retro	No	–,* +
Wardwell and Banson[36]	114 M	Instit	Retro	No	–
Haines et al[37]	1457 M	Comm	Pros	Yes	3.77*
Kawachi et al[26]	33 999 M	Comm	Pros	Yes	2.5*

[a] Adapted with permission from Hayward.[38]
[b] Comm = community; Instit = institution.
[c] Pros = prospective; Cross = cross-sectional; Retro = retrospective.
[d] * = significant at $p < 0.05$; – = negative finding with relative risk not determinable; + = positive finding with relative risk not determinable.

Cardiovascular risk factors

A number of authors have attempted to determine how PD might be related to increasing cardiovascular disease (CVD) morbidity and mortality. Atherosclerosis, the main cause of CVD, is strongly affected by a number of factors, including smoking, hypertension, high low density lipoprotein (LDL) cholesterol and low levels of physical activity. Psychosocial and psychological factors are also important.

Hypertension

The few studies of hypertension and anxiety disorders report a positive association.

Furthermore, PD patients may have an increased risk of antidepressant-induced hypertension.[39] Todd and colleagues[40] demonstrated that hyperventilation significantly increases blood pressure of healthy subjects.

Alcoholism

Excessive alcohol use is a risk factor for CHD. Panic patients also have high rates of alcohol abuse.[41,42] It is of note that alcohol intake is positively related to systolic and diastolic blood pressure in men.[43]

Smoking

Smoking rates have generally been found to be higher in anxiety patients compared with controls.[38,44] In one study,[45] smoking prevalence for female patients with PD was found to be significantly higher than that of control subjects (40% versus 25%).

High cholesterol

A few studies suggest that high cholesterol levels could be associated with PD patients but not with patients with major depression.[46] Recently, Shiori and colleagues[47] found that total cholesterol was significantly reduced in 45 PD patients treated with pharmacotherapy compared with age-matched controls in a controlled trial. However, Taylor et al[48] observed no change in total, LDL or high density lipoprotein (HDL) levels in patients treated with alprazolam, imipramine or placebo.

Exercise

Low levels of exercise are associated with increased CVD risk. Many PD subjects are exercise-avoidant. In fact, it was Pitts' and McClure's[49] speculation that the panic attacks reported by patients during exercise were related to high levels of lactate acid that led to the use of lactate infusion to induce panic attacks. Some studies have found higher resting heart rates in PD patients compared with controls, which might be accounted for by poor physical conditioning. However, no study has systematically examined physical activity patterns in PD patients compared with controls.

Psychosocial risk factors

Psychosocial factors have also been implicated as risk factors for heart disease in both men and women.[50] In particular, depression and social isolation have consistently been found to increase morbidity and mortality in post-myocardial-infarction patients.[51]

Patients with PD frequently demonstrate social isolation. Noyes et al,[52] investigating social functioning both in patients with PD and in normal controls, found that PD patients were rated as having more social maladjustment than normal controls in the areas both of work and of social and marital adjustment. Phobic avoidance often leads to social isolation. However, it is unknown whether this type of social isolation is similar to that reported in the epidemiologic studies that have related it to increased CVD mortality.

The well-known comorbidity between depression and PD is high: up to 60% of PD patients may suffer from depression.[2] It is possible that this comorbidity, or depression itself, may account for the increased risk.

Chest pain

About 60% of panic patients complain of chest pain associated with the panic attacks. Chest pain may be a sign of serious heart disease. Angina pectoris, one type of chest pain, occurs when the need for oxygen exceeds the supply, usually because the coronary artery vessels are constricted.

Margraf et al[53] had patients with panic attacks but no apparent heart disease and patients with documented myocardial infarctions (MIs) but no PD draw the pattern of their chest pain on body silhouettes. Cardiologists examining the figures were more likely to classify the panic attacks as MIs than vice versa. The pattern of angina is usually similar from one episode to the next, whereas the symptoms change from one episode to the next in patients with panic attacks. We examined ambulatory ECG in 10 patients who reported panic attacks accompanied by chest pain. In this largely young, female and therefore at low risk of heart disease population, we did not find any episodes of ischemia occurring with panic attacks accompanied by chest pain.[54]

Patients can have both panic attacks and angina, as illustrated by the following case.

- Mark was a 42-year-old male who presented for treatment of a reoccurrence of his panic attacks, which had first begun at around age 18. He reported that he lived with his panic and avoidance during his early 20s; then the symptoms just went away. About six months before presentation, he began to have 2–3 panic attacks a week, usually accompanied by palpitations and shortness of breath. His attacks were occasionally accompanied by chest pain. He had a history of hypertension treated with antidiuretics for the previous five years, he was overweight and had a high cholesterol level. With psychotherapy and antidepressant medication, his panic attacks resolved within six months, and medication was discontinued. He returned to therapy two years later following being laid off from his work. The frequency and presentation of his panic attacks were indistinguishable from before, although he was complaining of more chest pain. He also had episodes of exertional chest pain, which were followed by panic-like feelings.

He was encouraged to consult a cardiologist, who recommended an exercise treadmill. The exercise treadmill revealed ischemia at relatively low work-loads, and Mark was scheduled for coronary angiography. At angiography, he was found to have several blocked coronary arteries, and an angioplasty was performed. Post procedure, his exertional chest pain disappeared and he had fewer panic attacks, but they did not disappear entirely.

This patient clearly had angina and panic attacks, and the two were not easy to distinguish. Given his high cardiovascular risk profile (history of hypertension, being overweight) and the chest pain, a cardiologic consultation was obviously warranted. The diagnosis of angina can often be made on the basis of clinical signs and symptoms, ECG changes characteristic of ischemia, and rapid relief by taking sublingual nitroglycerin. However, the clinician treating a patient with panic disorder, particularly one with cardiovascular risk factors, needs to be constantly aware of such medical problems.

To complicate the picture, anxiety affects the self-report of angina. In a long-term follow-up study,[55] patients with nonspecific chest pain and psychiatric illness are more likely to complain of chest pain and to continue to seek treatment on a regular basis. In an emergency room, up to 25% of patients complaining of chest pain met criteria for PD.[3] Furthermore, many patients with chest pain but normal coronary arteries met criteria for current PD[56] or have atypical panic attacks.[7] The long-term course of patients with these problems is not known, although at least one treatment study has found that patients remain symptomatic.[57]

- *Recommendation* Patients with symptoms of angina deserve close observation and further work-up if the diagnosis is not clear.

Endocrine disorders

The links between endocrine disorders (ED) and PD have received relatively little investigation, but some tantalizing links have been noted. We omit discussion of PD and endocrine disorders, such as phenochromocytomas and hypoparathyroidism, because only a few cases have been described.

Thyroid disease

Excessive levels of thryoid hormones can produce severe anxiety symptoms. The excessive levels can occur because of various diseases or result from overtreatment of hypothyroidism. Lindemann et al[58] found that about 11% of patients with panic attacks reported a history of thyroid disease, compared with less than 1% of the general population. Using a structured interview, Kathol et al[59] found that 23 of 29 consecutively evaluated hyperthyroid patients had symptoms of significant anxiety. Also, 21 of the 23 patients with anxiety displayed complete resolution of these symptoms with antithyroid therapy.

The diagnosis of hyperthyroidism is usually straightforward and depends on a careful clinical history. Combined serum T4 and T3 assays are a highly accurate combination of initial tests for assessing thryoid status.

A survey of medical problems in a large cohort of panic patients being followed longitudinally found an increased rate of thyroid disease.[5] A recent case report indicates that PD may not only be a consequence of Graves' disease but may precede its onset and potentially predispose to its development.[60]

- *Recommendation* Serum T3, T4 and TSH should be routinely obtained on anxious patients who have any signs or symptoms of thryoid disease on history or clinical examination.

Hypoglycemia

Hypoglycemia occurs when there is an abnormally low blood glucose level. The condition falls into two categories: reactive hypoglycemia, which occurs in response to a meal, specific nutrients or drugs, and spontaneous hypoglycemia. In reactive hypoglycemia, most of the symptoms develop 2–4 hours after eating. Spontaneous hypoglycemia is rare, and results either from excessive glucose utilization or deficient glucose production.

The diagnosis is made by a documented low plasma glucose (<50 mg/dl), specifically associated with objective signs or subjective symptoms that are relieved by the ingestion of sugar or other food. Once the diagnosis is suspected, a series of subsequent tests can be performed to pinpoint the diagnosis. However, hypoglycemia is a rare condition, and probably overdiagnosed.[61,62] Recently, Gold and colleagues[63] described an increase in tension and profound changes in mood during acute hypoglycemia. There is, however, little evidence that hypoglycemia occurs at a higher rate in panic patients than with other patient groups.

- *Recommendation* Only when panic attacks are associated with hunger should hypoglycemia be considered. The best time to obtain diagnostic laboratory tests with spontaneous hypoglycemia is at presentation. The goal is to assess plasma insulin level and counterregulatory hormone response while the plasma glucose is low (a glucose tolerance test is no longer used).[64,65]

Sex hormones

Some female PD patients report increased premenstrual rates of PD. Building on such observations, Fachinetti and colleagues[66] found that premenstrual syndrome (PMS) patients have an increased rate of lactate-infusion-induced panic attacks. Fava and his team[67] found that patients with confirmed late luteal phase dysphoric disorder (LLPDD) are more likely to suffer from concurrent anxiety or mood disorders: 8 of 32 LLPDD patients had a current PD diagnosis. Perna et al[68] found, on the basis of a sample of 10 women with PD, that patients had stronger reactivity to 35% CO_2 during the early follicular than during the midluteal phases compared with controls who did not present such a phenomenon. Furthermore, some case reports describe PD resulting from oral contraceptives.[69] Such findings suggest that fluctuations of hormones in the menstrual cycle may play a role in the modulation of PD.

Growth hormone

Despite the characteristic spectrum of behavioral and cognitive disabilities resulting from a growth hormone deficiency during childhood (such children are described as being immature, dependent, shy, withdrawn and socially isolated),[70] very little is known about links between growth hormone and anxiety or panic disorder. A recent study found that the hypothalamic–GH–somatomedin axis was normal in PD.[71]

Neurologic disorders

Vestibular abnormalities

Vestibular abnormalities can produce symptoms that are identical to panic attacks. The most common symptoms are dizziness and vertigo, and these two symptoms usually dominate the clinical picture. The symptom of dizziness can be categorized into[72]

(1) rotational sensation;
(2) loss of balance without head sensations (e.g. being pulled to the left);

(3) feelings like fainting or losing consciousness;
(4) ill-defined 'light-headedness'.

The first two symptoms more strongly implicate neurological or vestibular pathology, whereas the fainting variety usually signifies a vagal or cardiovascular origin.[73] The most common vestibular abnormality is benign paroxysmal positional vertigo triggered by head rotation or sometimes linear acceleration. Driving and even jogging can precipitate this problem.

It remains controversial whether or not vestibular abnormalities are common among PD patients.[74] A recent study suggests that subclinical vestibular dysfunction may contribute to the phenomenology of PD patients, especially with agoraphobia.[75] Complaints of dizziness have been associated more with symptoms of phobic avoidance than have complaints of hearing loss.[76]

• *Recommendation* Patients with a clinical history consistent with vestibular abnormalities should be worked up for the problem. Simple, in-office tests of autonomic dysfunction, such as the patient's heart rate and blood pressure response to standing, should be considered in patients with dizziness, postural instability and normal otological function.

Seizures

Psychiatric disorders are frequent (65%) among patients with seizures.[77] Patients with PD seem to have higher prevalences of EEG abnormalities than depressed patients.[78]

Edlund and colleagues[79] found that panic attack patients with abnormal EEGs differed from the usual panic attack patients in several ways. First, the panic attacks were usually associated with severe derealization and sometimes unusually severe autonomic symptoms, such as tachycardia with a heart rate of over 125 bpm. Second, immediately before, during or after panic attacks, the patients became either highly irritable or overtly aggressive. In no case was the panic associated with avoidance or loss of consciousness. The EEG abnormalities involved the temporal lobes.

- Mr B, 21 years old, reported panic attacks 'as long ago as I can remember'. By his early teens, he was experiencing circumscribed episodes of palpitations, sweating, increased respiration, feelings of impending doom, and marked depersonalization and derealization. He found that these attacks were made worse by marijuana and improved by alcohol. After some attacks he would 'blow up' and smash things. Results of a neurological examination were normal; an EEG showed brief runs of left temporal sharp slowing.[79]

There may be a common neurophysiological substrate linking temporal lobe epilepsy and PD. A recent study[80] comparing psychosensorial phenomena in panic and epileptic disorders, using instruments specially constructed for evaluating psychosensorial phenomena, found that PD patients and complex partial epilepsy (CPE) patients record no significant differences of frequency for experiences of depersonalization–derealization (63% versus 48%). Furthermore, one-third of PD patients without depersonalization–derealization reported phenomena considered temporal lobe features such as déjà vu, déjà vécu, hypersensitivity to sounds, hypersensitivity to light and panoramic memory. Toni and colleagues[80] hypothesized that an increased excitability or kindling of limbic structures could be a pathophysiological mechanism in PD.

Partial seizures have also been associated with panic attacks. Partial seizures begin with specific motor, sensory or psychomotor focal phenomena. Partial seizures leading to focal symptoms without involving motor movement are rare, but have been reported.

In the absence of any of these features, the diagnosis of temporal lobe epilepsy is unlikely, and routine EEG studies are not warranted. The diagnosis of partial seizures requires an EEG.

Nighttime panic attacks can occur with hypogenic paroxysmal dystonia, a rare condition thought to be the result of abnormal epileptiform discharges in deep, mesial regions of the brain. These attacks usually occur during non-REM sleep, and are characterized by the sudden onset of twisting, dystonic movements of the limbs that may last from 15 to 45 seconds.

- A 22-year-old single woman presented for evaluation of 'anxiety attacks'. Her first attack was spontaneous and occurred during the day, but six months after the first attack, the attacks became exclusively nocturnal. Each attack lasted 30–60 seconds, and she was having 3–4 attacks a night. There was no loss of consciousness nor any nightmares. A daytime EEG with nasopharyngeal leads was normal. However, the patient was started on carbamazepine, 400 mg at night, and the attacks were promptly relieved. It is of interest that a trial of imipramine also relieved her panic attacks after two weeks of treatment. A videotape obtained during one of her episodes when she was off all medication showed 'tonic extension of the left arm and hand, flexion of the right arm, and flexion of the right wrist in a "drawn" position', suggesting the diagnosis of hypogenic paroxysmal dystonia.[81]

A recent case report describes the same features.[82]

Enoch et al[83] found that a heritable EEG trait, the low-voltage alpha (LV), is significantly associated with PD or generalized anxiety disorder (GAD) (only 7/19 subjects with PD or GAD were normal alpha compared to 64/70 subjects without an anxiety disorder). They hypothesized that LV may be an EEG phenotype underlying a vulnerability factor for anxiety disorders.

These studies suggest that the clinician should remain open to unusual seizure problems that might appear very similar to panic.

- *Recommendation* Patients with a history of altered consciousness, automatism, head injury, other seizures, characteristics of temporal lobe epilepsy, and neurological deficits on examination should be evaluated with a sleep-deprived EEG and other neurological tests.[84]

Migraine

PD has been associated with migraine in several studies. Breslau and Davis,[85] in a prospective study of a random sample of 1007 adults, found that subjects with a history of migraine at baseline had significantly increased rates of first-incidence major depression and PD. Marazetti et al[86] found that 42% of 17 patients with migraine without aura and 32% of 55 patients with migraine with aura had PD. PD rates were higher than for any other psychiatric condition.

Pulmonary diseases

Some theorists argue that the respiratory system plays a key role in panic attacks. Recently, Ley[87] suggested that the classic panic attack is characterized by uncontrollable dyspnea in conjunction with the fear of suffocation (hyper-ventilation theory). Klein[88] hypothesized that a physiologic misinterpretation by a suffocation monitor misfires an evolved suffocation alarm system (suffocation false alarm theory). It remains unclear, however, whether asthmatic and chronic obstructive pulmonary disease patients are associated with PD. A few studies indicate that pulmonary patients have high rates of PD.[89] Also, Smoller et al[90] found higher rates of panic attacks in COPD patients. Carr et al[91] found that 23% of 93 asthmatics had had panic attacks. However, in an elegant, carefully controlled study, van Peski-Oosterbaan et al[92] found no evidence for higher prevalence of PD and asthma, once selection bias had been accounted for.

One study found abnormal dynamic pulmonary function (e.g. abnormal peak expiratory flow rate) in panic patients,[93] but another did not.[94]

Gastrointestinal disorders

Despite a very old relationship between gastrointestinal (GI) and affective disorders, which is reflected in the etymology and the history of hypochondriasis (from the Greek *hupokhondria*, a region of the abdomen felt to be the site of melancholia), recent studies about this topic are rare. According to the Epidemiologic Catchment Area Study,[95] subjects who report gastrointestinal symptoms are more likely to have experienced lifetime episodes of major depression (2.5 times) or PD (3.5 times). Based on 13 537 subjects surveyed at four sites of the National Institute of Mental Health Epidemiological Catchment Area Project, Lydiard et al[96] found a 4.6 times greater risk for persons with PD to report nausea without vomiting than for persons without PD. There was also a 4.6 times greater risk for persons with PD to have irritable bowel syndrome-like composite symptoms (i.e. abdominal pain, diarrhea or constipation, and abdominal bloating) than persons without PD. It is of note that some authors have found high comorbidity between panic and eating disorders, suggesting a common diathesis for such disorders both in adolescents[97,98] and in adults.[99,100]

An intriguing new development is the recent discovery that a GI hormone receptor, the cholecystokinin B (CCK-B) receptor antagonist, possesses panic-inducing properties. A CCK-B receptor antagonist (L-365,260) is able to block CCK-induced panic attacks and reduce apprehension and anxiety. Nevertheless, Kramer and colleagues[101] did not find any significant differences between groups in a placebo-controlled trial of a CCK-B receptor antagonist. On the basis of a sample of 24 subjects, van Megen and colleagues[102] found that sodium-lactate-induced panic attacks were not blocked by a CCK-B receptor antagonist.

Medication

Intoxication or withdrawal syndromes may be associated with PD: for example, alcohol, amphetamines, benzodiazepines, caffeine and cocaine.[9]

From a psychiatric point of view, it can be useful to remember that treatments may induce panic. Not only can neuroleptics produce akathisia, which is easily mistaken for primary anxiety,[103] but they may also worsen a panic disorder[104,105] or even induce a panic attack.[106] Antidepressants are well known to sometimes precipitate panic attacks, especially when full doses are used early in treatment. For this reason, most people initiate a slow dose-rising regime.[107]

Conclusions

A variety of medical problems co-occur with PD. It is not clear, but appears unlikely, that these medical problems are inherently related to PD, and they may also worsen its symptoms and course. More likely, panic patients are sensitive to symptoms of a variety of diseases, and are more likely to seek treatment for them, particularly if they are depressed. The high rate of occurrence and, more generally, the high prevalence of medically unexplained symptoms in outpatient clinics and the underdiagnosis of medical and psychiatric problems in patients underscore the need to approach patients from both medical and psychiatric standpoints.

References

1. Taylor CB, Arnow B, *The Nature and Treatment of Anxiety Disorders*. New York: The Free Press, 1988.
2. Ballenger JC, Overview of panic disorder. *Trans Am Clin Climatol Assoc* 1993; **105**: 36–53.
3. Fleet RP, Dupuis G, Marchand A et al, Panic disorder in emergency department chest pain patients: prevalence, comorbidity, suicidal ideation, and physician recognition. *Am J Med* 1996; **101**: 371–80.
4. Beitman BD, Basha I, Flaker G et al, Non-fearful panic disorder: panic attack without fear. *Behav Res Ther* 1987; **25**: 487–92.
5. Beitman BD, Mukerji V, Russell JL, Grafing M, Panic disorder in cardiology patients: a review of the Missouri Panic/Cardiology Project. *J Psychiatr Res* 1993; **27**(Suppl 1): 35–46.
6. Katon WJ, Von Korff M, Lin E, Panic disorder: relationship to high medical utilization. *Am J Med* 1992; **92**: S7–11.

7. Rogers MP, White K, Warshaw MG et al, Prevalence of medical illness in patients with anxiety disorders. *Int J Psychiatry Med* 1994; **24:** 83–96.

8. Koran LM, Sox HC Jr, Marton KI et al, Medical evaluation of psychiatric patients. *Arch Gen Psychiatry* 1989; **46:** 733–40.

9. Reus VI, Anxiety disorders. In: *Harrison's Principles of Internal Medicine*, 14th edn (Fauci AS, Braunwald E, Isselbacher KJ et al, eds). New York: McGraw-Hill, 1998: 2486–90.

10. Mayou R, Bryant B, Forfar C, Clark D, Non-cardiac chest pain and benign palpitations in the cardiac clinic. *Br Heart J* 1994; **72:** 548–53.

11. Barsky AJ, Delamater BA, Clancy SA et al, Somatized psychiatric disorder presenting as palpitations. *Arch Intern Med* 1996; **156:** 1102–8.

12. Sternbach G, Varon J, Barlow J, Mitral valve prolapse. *J Emerg Med* 1993; **11:** 475–8.

13. Da Costa JM, On irritable heart: a clinical study of a form of functional cardiac disorder and its consequences. *Am J Med Sci* 1871; **61:** 17–52.

14. Wood PW, Da Costa's Syndrome (or Effort Syndrome). *Br Med J* 1941; *i:* 845–51.

15. Gorman JM, Fyer AF, Gliklich J et al, Effect of sodium lactate on patients with panic disorder and mitral valve prolapse. *Am J Psychiatry* 1981; **138:** 247–9.

16. Alpert MA, Sabeti M, Kushner MG et al, Frequency of isolated panic attacks and panic disorder in patients with the mitral valve prolapse syndrome. *Am J Cardiol* 1992; **69:** 1489–90.

17. Sivaramakrishnan K, Alexander PJ, Saharsarnamam N, Prevalence of panic disorder in mitral valve prolapse: a comparative study with a cardiac control group. *Acta Psychiatr Scand* 1994; **89:** 59–61.

18. Oki T, Fukuda N, Kawano T et al, Histopathologic studies of innervation of normal and prolapsed human mitral valves. *J Heart Valve Dis* 1995; **4:** 496–502.

19. Bulbena A, Duro JC, Porta M et al, Anxiety disorders in the joint hypermobility syndrome. *Psychiatry Res* 1993; **46:** 59–68.

20. Yingling KW, Wulsin LR, Arnold LM, Rouan GW, Estimated prevalence of panic disorder and depression among consecutive patients seen in an emergency department with acute chest pain. *J Gen Intern Med* 1993; **8:** 231–5.

21. Schaal SF, Ventricular arrhythmias in patients with mitral valve prolapse. *Cardiovasc Clin* 1992; **22:** 307.

22. Cameron OG, Smith CB, Nesse RM et al, Platelet alpha 2-adrenoreceptors, catecholamines, hemodynamic variables, and anxiety in panic patients and their asymptotic relatives. *Psychosom Med* 1996; **58:** 289–301.

23. Barsky AJ, Cleary PD, Sarnie MK, Ruskin JN, Panic disorder, palpitations, and the awareness of cardiac activity. *J Nerv Ment Dis* 1994; **182:** 63–71.

24. Ehlers A, Breuer P, How good are patients with panic disorder at perceiving their heart beats? *Biol Psychol* 1996; **42:** 165–82.

25. Weissman MM, Markowitz JS, Ouellette R et al, Panic disorder and cardiovascular/cerebrovascular problems: results from a community survey. *Am J Psychiatry* 1990; **147:** 1504–8.

26. Kawachi I, Sparrow D, Vokonas PS, Weiss ST, Symptoms of anxiety and risk of coronary heart disease: the Normative Aging Study. *Circulation* 1994; **90:** 2225–9.

27. Coryell W, Noyes R, Clancy J, Excess mortality in panic disorder: a comparison with unipolar depression. *Arch Gen Psychiatry* 1982; **39:** 701–3.

28. Sims A, Prior P, Arteriosclerosis-related deaths in severe neurosis. *Compr Psychiatry* 1982; **23:** 181–5.

29. Martin RL, Cloninger CR, Guze SB et al, Mortality in a follow-up of 500 psychiatric outpatients. II. Cause-specific mortality. *Arch Gen Psychiatry* 1985; **42:** 58–66.

30. Coryell W, Noyes R Jr, House JD, Mortality among outpatients with anxiety disorders. *Am J Psychiatry* 1986; **143:** 508–10.

31. Allgulander C, Lavori PW, Excess mortality among 3302 patients with 'pure' anxiety neurosis. *Arch Gen Psychiatry* 1991; **48:** 599–602.

32. Paffenbarger RS, Wolf PA, Notkin J et al, Chronic disease in former college students. I. Early precursors of fatal coronary heart disease. *Am J Epidemiol* 1996; **83:** 314–28.

33. Thorne MC, Wing AL, Paffenbarger RS Jr, Chronic disease in former college students. VII. Early precursors of nonfatal coronary heart disease. *Am J Epidemiol* 1968; **87:** 520–9.

34. Medalie JH, Snyder M, Groen JJ et al, Angina pectoris among 10,000 men: 5-year incidence and univariate analysis. *Am J Med* 1973; **55:** 583–94.

35. Thiel HG, Parker D, Bruce TA, Stress factors and the risk of myocardial infarction. *J Psychosom Res* 1973; **17:** 43–57.

36. Wardwell WI, Bahnson CB, Behavioral variables and myocardial infarction in the Southeastern Connecticut Heart Study. *J Chronic Dis* 1973; **26:** 447–61.

37. Haines AP, Imeson JD, Meade TW, Phobic anxiety and ischaemic heart disease. *Br Med J, Clin Res Ed* 1987; **295:** 297–9.

38. Hayward C, Psychiatric illness and cardiovascular disease risk. *Epidemiol Rev* 1995; **17:** 129–38.

39. Louie AK, Louie EK, Lannon RA, Systemic hypertension associated with tricyclic antidepressant treatment in patients with panic disorder. *Am J Cardiol* 1992; **70:** 1306–9.

40. Todd GPA, Chadwick IG, Yeo WW et al, Pressor effect of hyperventilation in healthy subjects. *J Hum Hypertens* 1995; **9:** 119–22.

41. Kushner MG, Mackenzie TB, Fiszdon J et al, The effects of alcohol consumption on laboratory-induced panic and state anxiety. *Arch Gen Psychiatry* 1996; **53:** 264–70.

42. Lepola U, Koponen H, Leinonen E, A naturalistic 6-year follow-up study of patients with panic disorder. *Acta Psychiatr Scand* 1996; **93:** 181–3.

43. Jones-Webb R, Jacobs DR Jr, Flack JM, Liu K, Relationships between depressive symptoms, anxiety, alcohol consumption, and blood pressure: results from the CARDIA Study (Coronary Artery Risk Development in Young Adults Study). *Alcohol Clin Exp Res* 1996; **20:** 420–7.

44. Patton GC, Hibbert M, Rosier MJ et al, Is smoking associated with depression and anxiety in teenagers? *Am J Public Health* 1996; **86:** 225–30.

45. Pohl R, Yeragani VK, Balon R et al, Smoking in patients with panic disorder. *Psychiatry Res* 1992; **43:** 253–62.

46. Bajwa WK, Asnis GM, Sanderson WC et al, High cholesterol levels in patients with panic disorder. *Am J Psychiatry* 1992; **149:** 376–8.

47. Shiori T, Fujii K, Someya T, Takahashi S, Effect of pharmacotherapy on serum cholesterol levels in patients with panic disorder. *Acta Psychiatr Scand* 1996; **93:** 164–7.

48. Taylor CB, Hayward C, King R et al, Cardiovascular and symptomatic reduction effects of alprazolam and imipramine in patients with panic disorder: results of a double-blind, placebo-controlled trial. *J Clin Psychopharmacol* 1990; **10:** 112–18.

49. Pitts FM, McLure JN, Lactate metabolism in anxiety neurosis. *N Engl J Med* 1967; **277:** 1329–36.

50. Brezinka V, Kittel F, Psychosocial factors of coronary heart disease in women: a review. *Soc Sci Med* 1996; **42:** 1351–65.

51. Taylor CB, Miller NH, Smith PM, DeBusk RF, The effect of a home-based case management multifactorial risk reduction program on reducing psychological distress in patients with cardiovascular disease. *J Cardiopulm Rehab* 1997; **17:** 157–62.

52. Noyes R Jr, Reich J, Christiansen J et al, Outcome of panic disorder: relationship to diagnostic subtypes and comorbidity. *Arch Gen Psychiatry* 1990; **47:** 809–18.

53. Margraf J, De Vries-Wehrhahn E, Sonnentag S, Myokardinfarkt, funktionelle Herzbeschwerden und Paniksyndrom. *Psychother Psychosom Med Psychol* 1991; **41:** 31–4.

54. Lint DW, Taylor CB, Fried-Behar L, Kenardy J, Does ischemia occur with panic attacks? *Am J Psychiatry* 1995; **152:** 1678–80.

55. Tew R, Guthrie EA, Creed FH et al, A long-term follow-up study of patients with ischaemic heart disease versus patients with nonspecific chest pain. *J Psychosom Res* 1995; **39:** 977–85.

56. Maddock RJ, Carter CS, Tavano-Hall L, Amsterdam EA, Hypocapnia associated with cardiac stress scintigraphy in chest pain patients with panic disorder. *Psychosom Med* 1998; **60:** 52–5.

57. Potts SG, Bass CM, Psychological morbidity in patients with chest pain and normal or near-normal coronary arteries: a long-term follow-up study. *Psychol Med* 1995; **25:** 339–47.

58. Lindemann CG, Zitrin CM, Klein DF, Thyroid dysfunction in phobic patients. *Psychosomatics* 1984; **25**: 603–6.

59. Kathol RG, Turner R, Delahunt J, Depression and anxiety associated with hyperthyroidism: response to antithyroid therapy. *Psychosomatics* 1986; **7**: 501–5.

60. Matsubayashi S, Tamai H, Matsumoto Y et al, Graves' disease after the onset of panic disorder. *Psychother Psychosom* 1996; **65**: 277–80.

61. Permutt MA, Is it really hypoglycemia? If so, what should you do. *Medical Times* 1980; **108**: 35–43.

62. Ford CV, Bray GA, Swerdloff RS, A psychiatric study of patients referred with a diagnosis of hypoglycemia. *Am J Psychiatry* 1976; **133**: 290–4.

63. Gold AE, MacLeod KM, Frier BM, Deary IJ, Changes in mood during acute hypoglycemia in healthy participants. *J Pers Soc Psychol* 1995; **68**: 498–504.

64. Stein MB, Panic disorder and medical illness. *Psychosomatics* 1986; **27**: 833–8.

65. Foster DW, Rubenstein AH, Hypoglycemia. In: *Harrison's Principles of Internal Medicine*, 14th edn (Fauci AS, Braunwald E, Isselbacher KJ et al, eds). New York: McGraw-Hill, 1998: 2081–7.

66. Facchinetti F, Romano G, Fava M, Genazzani AR, Lactate infusion induces panic attacks in patients with premenstrual syndrome. *Psychosom Med* 1992; **54**: 288–96.

67. Fava M, Pedrazzi F, Guaraldi GP et al, Comorbid anxiety and depression among patients with late luteal phase dysphoric disorder. *J Anx Disord* 1992; **6**: 325–35.

68. Perna G, Brambilla F, Arancio C, Bellodi L, Menstrual cycle-related sensitivity to 35% CO_2 in panic patients. *Biol Psychiatry* 1995; **37**: 528–32.

69. Wagner KD, Berenson AB, Norplant-associated major depression and panic disorder. *J Clin Psychiatry* 1994; **55**: 478–80.

70. Stabler B, Clopper RR, Siegel P et al, Links between growth hormone deficiency: adaptation and social phobia. *Horm Res* 1996; **45**: 30–3.

71. Pitchot W, Hansenne M, Moreno AG, Ansseau M, Growth hormone response to apomorphine in panic disorder: comparison with major depression and normal controls. *Eur Arch Psychiatry Clin Neurosci* 1995; **245**: 306–8.

72. Drachman DA, Hart CW, An approach to the dizzy patient. *Neurology* 1972; **22**: 323–4.

73. Jacob RG, Rapport MD, Panic disorder: medical and psychological parameters. In: *Behavioral Theories and Treatment of Anxiety* (Turner SM, ed.). New York: Plenum Press, 1984, 187–237.

74. Stein MB, Asmundson GJ, Ireland D, Walker JR, Panic disorder in patients attending a clinic for vestibular disorders. *Am J Psychiatry* 1994; **151**: 1697–700.

75. Jacob RG, Furman JM, Durrant JD, Turner SM, Panic, agoraphobia, and vestibular dysfunction. *Am J Psychiatry* 1996; **153**: 503–12.

76. Clark DB, Hirsch BE, Smith MG et al, Panic in otolaryngology patients presenting with dizziness or hearing loss. *Am J Psychiatry* 1994; **151**: 1223–5.

77. Blumer D, Montouris G, Hermann B, Psychiatric morbidity in seizure patients on a neurodiagnostic monitoring unit. *J Neuropsychiatry Clin Neurosci* 1995; **7**: 445–6.

78. Jabourian AP, Erlich M, Desvignes C, Panic attacks and 24-hour ambulatory EEG monitoring. *Annales Medico-Psychologiques* 1992; **150**: 240–4.

79. Edlund JE, Swan AC, Clothier J, Patients with panic attacks and abnormal EEG results. *Am J Psychiatry* 1987; **144**: 508–9.

80. Toni C, Cassano GB, Perugi G, Psychosensorial and related phenomena in panic disorder and in temporal lobe epilepsy. *Compr Psychiatry* 1996; **37**: 125–33.

81. Stoudemire A, Ninan PT, Wooten V, Hypogenic paroxysmal dystonia with panic attacks responsive to drug therapy. *Psychosomatics* 1987; **28**: 280–1.

82. Young GB, Chandarana PC, Blume WT et al, Mesial temporal lobe seizures presenting as anxiety disorders. *J Neuropsychiatry Clin Neurosci* 1995; **7**: 352–7.

83. Enoch MA, Rohrbaugh JW, Davis EZ et al, Relationship of genetically transmitted alpha EEG traits to anxiety disorders and alcoholism. *Am J Med Genet* 1995; **60**: 400–8.

84. Raj A, Sheehan DV, Medical evaluation of panic attacks. *J Clin Psychiatry* 1987; **48**: 309–13.

85. Breslau N, Davis GC, Migraine, physical health and psychiatric disorder: a prospective epidemiologic study in young adults. *J Psychiatr Res* 1993; **27**: 211–21.

86. Marazzeti D, Toni C, Pedri S et al, Headache, panic disorder and depression: comorbidity or a spectrum? *Neuropsychobiology* 1995; **31**: 125–9.

87. Ley R, The many faces of Pan: psychological and physiological differences among three types of panic attacks. *Behav Res Ther* 1992; **30**: 347–57.

88. Klein DF, False suffocation alarms, spontaneous panics, and related conditions: an integrative hypothesis. *Arch Gen Psychiatry* 1993; **50**: 306–17.

89. Pollack MH, Kradin R, Otto MW et al, Prevalence of panic in patients referred for pulmonary function testing at a major medical center. *Am J Psychiatry* 1996; **153**: 110–13.

90. Smoller JW, Pollack MH, Otto MW et al, Panic, anxiety, dyspnea, and respiratory disease. Theoretical and clinical considerations. *Am J Respir Crit Care Med* 1996; **154**: 6–17.

91. Carr RE, Lehrer PM, Rausch LL, Hochron SM, Anxiety sensitivity and panic attacks in an asthmatic population. *Behav Res Ther* 1994; **32**: 411–18.

92. van Peski-Oosterbaan AS, Spinhoven P, van der Does AJW et al, Is there a specific relationship between asthma and panic disorder? *Behav Res Ther* 1996; **34**: 333–40.

93. Perna G, Marconi C, Battaglia M et al, Subclinical impairment of lung airways in patients with panic disorder. *Biol Psychiatry* 1994; **36**: 601–5.

94. Spinhoven P, Onstein EJ, Sterk PJ, Pulmonary function in panic disorder: evidence against the dyspnea-fear theory. *Behav Res Ther* 1995; **33**: 457–60.

95. Walker EA, Katon WJ, Jemelka RP, Roy-Byrne PP, Comorbidity of gastrointestinal complaints, depression, and anxiety in the Epidemiologic Catchment Area Study. *Am J Med* 1992; **92**: S26–30.

96. Lydiard RB, Greenwald S, Weissman MM et al, Panic disorder and gastrointestinal symptoms: findings from the NIMH Epidemiologic Catchment Area Project. *Am J Psychiatry* 1994; **151**: 64–70.

97. Bradley SJ, Hood J, Psychiatrically referred adolescents with panic attacks: presenting symptoms, stressors, and comorbidity. *J Am Acad Child Adolesc Psychiatry* 1993; **32**: 826–9.

98. Valdisseri S, Kihlstrom JF, Abnormal eating and dissociation experiences: a further study of college women. *Int J Eat Disord* 1995; **18**: 145–50.

99. Yanovski SZ, Nelson JE, Dubbert BK, Spitzer RL, Association of binge eating disorder and psychiatric comorbidity in obese subjects. *Am J Psychiatry* 1993; **150**: 1472–9.

100. Brewerton TD, Lydiard RB, Herzog DB et al, Comorbidity of Axis I psychiatric disorders in bulimia nervosa. *J Clin Psychiatry* 1995; **56**: 77–80.

101. Kramer MS, Cutler NR, Banllenger JC et al, A placebo-controlled trial of L-365,260, a CCK_B antagonist, in panic disorder. *Biol Psychiatry* 1995; **37**: 462–6.

102. van Megen HJGM, Westenberg, HGM, den Boer JA, Effect of the cholecystokinin-B receptor antagonist L-365,260 on lactate-induced panic attacks in panic disorder patients. *Biol Psychiatry* 1996; **40**: 804–6.

103. Hughes DH, Medical causes of anxiety: a guide to recognition. In: *Integrative Treatment of Anxiety Disorders* (Ellison JM, ed.). Washington, DC: American Psychiatric Press, 1996, 249–74.

104. Argyle N, Panic attacks in chronic schizophrenia. *Br J Psychiatry* 1990; **157**: 430–3.

105. Hogarty GE, McEvoy JP, Ulrich RF et al, Pharmacotherapy of impaired affect in recovering schizophrenic patients. *Arch Gen Psychiatry* 1995; **52**: 29–41.

106. Bachmann KM, Modestin J, Neuroleptic-induced panic attacks in a patient with delusional depression. *J Nerv Ment Dis* 1987; **175**: 373–5.

107. Altshuler LL, Fluoxetine-associated panic attacks. *J Clin Psychopharmacol* 1994; **14**: 433–4.

9

Treatment of panic disorder with tricyclics and MAOIs

Raben Rosenberg

CONTENTS • Introduction • Tricyclic antidepressants (TCAs) • Monoamine oxidase inhibitors (MAOIs) • Conclusions

Introduction

Classical antidepressants such as the tricyclics (TCAs) and the irreversible monoamine oxidase inhibitors (MAOIs) have had an important position in the psychopharmacological treatment of panic disorder and for the pathophysiological conception of the disorder.

The benefit of imipramine treatment of panic attacks was demonstrated by Klein[1] in 1964 and the effect of MAOIs on anxiety symptoms in a series of studies from 1959 to 1981 (reviewed in references 2–4). In 1980 Sheehan et al[5] reported that patients with 'endogenous anxiety' (i.e. agoraphobia with panic attacks) improved markedly on treatment with phenelzine, a classical MAOI. Results from a series of controlled studies and a growing knowledge of the biology of panic disorder[6,7] have further substantiated the importance of antidepressants in the treatment of panic disorder.

According to the influential theory of Klein,[8] the core symptom of panic disorder is recurrent panic attacks, some of which are spontaneous while others are precipitated by phobic stimuli. Anticipatory anxiety and agoraphobia are suggested sequelae to recurrent panic attacks, which are eventually followed by depression as a demoralization phenomenon.[9] Accordingly, the most important target of antidepressants is the amelioration of panic attacks.[1,3,10] Improvement of other anxiety symptoms may eventually require additional psychotherapy according to cognitive–behavioral principles.[11,12]

The heuristic validity of panic disorder has been generally accepted. However, important issues with respect to the validity of the putative nosological entity still need clarification, including the efficacy of drug action on individual components of the clinical features in panic disorder.

Will the appearance of the selective serotonin reuptake inhibitors (SSRIs) and the reversible monoamine oxidase inhibitors type A (RIMAs) mean an end to the use of the TCAs and the irreversible MAOIs, or will there still be a place for these classical compounds in the treatment of panic disorder? A review of the large literature on TCA treatment of panic disorder and the more limited literature on the MAOIs may clarify this problem.

Tricyclic antidepressants (TCAs)

Previous reviews

Since the initial discovery of the antipanic activity of imipramine, several controlled studies of the efficacy of TCAs have been performed, and the literature has often been reviewed (see e.g. references 3 and 13–18). Most reviewers agree upon the efficacy of the TCAs on various clinical components of panic disorder. This same opinion is expressed in a 1993 report from a World Psychiatric Association task force on the treatment of panic anxiety.[19] However, not all agree. Thus to McNally imipramine seems to benefit panic disorder patients with agoraphobia only when combined with behavioral therapy (exposure).[20]

Quality issues

When selecting studies for review, some methodological aspects need to be considered. Most studies have, for evident experimental reasons, focused on short-term efficacy of the drugs, i.e. within 6–12 weeks, although the long-term efficacy of drug treatment may be more clinically relevant considering that panic disorder often takes a chronic course.[21,22] Several studies have allowed some kind of concomitant psychotherapy, and many influential studies have integrated psychotherapeutic methods in the experimental design (see e.g. references 23–26). This may be reasonable from a clinical point of view, but is a restraint on the interpretation of the experimental data

when evaluating drug efficacy, especially since cognitive–behavioral techniques have increasingly demonstrated their value in the treatment of panic disorder.[27]

Treatment studies vary considerably in other important experimental aspects, which makes it difficult to compare studies. Although randomized controlled designs are often applied, the number of subjects included in the studies are often fairly small, i.e. with less than 25 in each treatment cell. This may introduce type II errors, and does not allow for subgrouping of subjects according to clinical phenomenology, i.e. degree of avoidance behavior and depression.

Older studies do not all fulfill the modern requirement of standardized assessment of diagnoses (i.e. the DSM system[28] or ICD10[29]) of the rich clinical phenomenology of panic disorder. Only a few relevant outcome measures have been reported. Mixed groups of patients are sometimes studied.

A major issue of controversy is the definition of treatment outcome measures. Considering the importance of panic attacks in the conception of panic disorder, the number and severity of panic attacks are claimed as a primary outcome measure,[30] but panic attacks may show large intra- and interindividual variability. Thus van Vliet et al[4] have argued that other outcome measures are more important. However, most authors today agree that major outcome variables should include

- panic attacks,
- anticipatory anxiety,
- phobic avoidance and
- global improvement.

Studies also vary according to the rigor of the statistical analysis. As differences in attrition rates across treatment cells often appear in placebo-controlled studies, both intent-to-treat and completer analyses should be presented.

Considerable placebo responses have been reported in several recent studies.[31,32] These may be due to the rigorous assessments during the trial, which act as a kind of cognitive–behavior therapy, or the inclusion of patients who experience only a short-lived exacerbation of their chronic disease.[10] As not all groups observe a marked placebo response,[4] patients enrolled in controlled studies may be fairly heterogeneous, although fulfilling the diagnostic criteria for panic disorder.

Rigorous research methodologies have been applied in some recent multicenter studies (see below), including very large groups of patients. However, multicenter studies require extensive quality assurance with respect to interrater reliability and to minimization of selection biases.

In summary, a necessary requirement for considering a study for review will be the inclusion of a placebo control group. Furthermore, studies applying a modern clinical research methodology, large groups of patients and controlling for concomitant psychotherapy should be given more attention.

Placebo-controlled studies

Table 9.1 presents major short-term placebo-controlled studies of TCA treatment of panic disorder from 1980 to 1997. Studies including specific psychotherapeutic methods in the experimental design (see e.g. references 23–26) or special designs[33,34] are not reviewed.

Among TCAs, imipramine and clomipramine dominate the scene. The studies by Andersch et al,[35] CNCPS[31] and Lecrubier et al[32] are multicenter studies, the last two of which will be reviewed separately (see below).

In five out of seven studies, imipramine was superior to placebo, but surprisingly not consistently so when panic attacks are considered. Fairly high drop-out rates were observed in several studies in both the imipramine and

placebo groups. Two studies with clomipramine also suggested that this TCA is efficacious. Interestingly, the study of Modigh et al[36] suggested that clomipramine was superior to imipramine and better tolerated.

However, it should be noticed that some kind of psychotherapy or even concomitant drug therapy was allowed in some studies and that experimental groups were often fairly small.

Meta-analyses

The literature has recently also been reviewed applying meta-analytic techniques. Meta-analyses are statistical methods giving a systematic and quantitative approach to assessment. They have been increasingly used in psychiatry to summarize results from several treatment studies.

The quantitative approach may allow for much more detailed analysis of the influence of several experimental parameters that may be difficult to control when designing the studies. Thus Clum et al[37] have reported how calculated effect sizes depend on the percentage of agoraphobic patients in the studies, the duration of panic disorder, the type of assessment and the treatment modalities. They may also help to differentiate efficacies of individual treatment components in studies integrating different treatment modalities, e.g. drugs and psychotherapy.

Typically normalized effect sizes are calculated for the major outcome measure from the distribution of scores in treatment and control groups. Such effect sizes may be clinically more meaningful than p-values, which just test the null hypothesis, i.e. whether a significant difference exists between a drug and placebo. This matter is especially relevant when considering multicenter studies with many patients, since statistically significant findings may be

Table 9.1 Panic disorder: some placebo-controlled studies of TCAs

Study	Diagnosis[a]	TCA,[b] no. of drop-outs	Placebo, no. of drop-outs	Dose[b]	Duration (weeks)	Other therapy	Efficacy[b]	Comments[b]
Sheehan et al (1980)[5]	(PD ± AG)	IMI, 17[c] PHE, 18	22	IMI 150 mg PHE 45 mg	12	Supportive psychotherapy	IMI = PHE > P	Panic attacks not analyzed
Evans et al (1986)[26]	AG + PA	IMI, 19 (26%) ZIM, 16 (19%)	9 (22%)	IMI 150 mg ? ZIM 150 mg ?	6	Not given	ZIM > IMI = P	Small groups
Pohl et al (1989)[72]	PD ± AG	IMI, 14 (29%) BUS, 16 (31%)	14 (21%)	IMI 140 mg BUS	8	No psychotherapy	IMI = BUS = P	Small groups, high drop-out rates
Robinson et al (1989)[73]	PD	IMI, 28 (14%) BUS, 34 (24%)	29 (14%)	IMI 221 mg BUS 43 mg	8	Not given	IMI = BUS > P	Part of multicenter study; preliminary analysis; drugs not efficacious on panic attacks
Uhlenhuth et al (1989)[74]	PD ± AG	IMI, 20 (50%) ALZ 2 mg, 20 (35%) ALZ 6 mg, 21 (14%)	20 (60%)	IMI 225 mg ALZ 2 and 6 mg	8	Not given	ALZ 6 mg > ALZ 2 mg > IMI > P	Fixed doses; high dropout rates for IMI
Taylor et al (1990)[75]	PD	IMI, 26 ALP, 27	26	IMI 147 mg ALZ 3.7 mg	8	Not given	I = ALZ > P	Drugs not efficacious on panic attacks, ALZ > IMI at some measures
Andersch et al (1991)[35]	PD ± AG	IMI, 41 (27%) ALP, 41 (5%)	41 (54%)	IMI 170 mg ALZ 4.6 mg	8	No psychotherapy allowed	IMI = ALZ > P	Scandinavian sample of the CNCPS[d]
Fahy et al (1992)[49]	PD ± AG	CLO, 27 (33%) LOF, 26 (8%)	26 (8%)	CLO 100 mg LOF 140 mg	6 (+ follow-up protokol)	Behavioural counseling 1 h every 1–2 weeks	CLO = LOF > P	Short period: concomitant psychotherapy

Table 9.1 Continued

Study	Diagnosis[a]	TCA,[b] no. of drop-outs	Placebo, no. of drop-outs	Dose[b]	Duration (weeks)	Other therapy	Efficacy[b]	Comments[a]
Modigh et al (1992)[36]	PD ± AG	CLO, 29 (0%) IMI, 22 (18%)	17 (41%)	CLO 100 mg IMI 124 mg	12	Diazepam max. 15 mg/day	CLO > IM = P	IMI not better than placebc; reduction of diazepam for CLO
CNCPS[d] (1992)[31]	PD ± AG	IMI, 391 (30%) ALZ, 386 (17%)	391 (44%)	IMI 155 mg ALP 5.7 mg	8	No psychotherapy allowed	IMI = ALZ > P	High proportion of placebo responders
Gentil et al (1993)[60]	PD ± AG	CLO, 20 (12%) IMI, 20 (10%)	PLA, 20 (3.3%)	CLO 50 mg IMI 114 mg	8		CLO > IMI > PLA	Active placebo (propanteline) High proportion of placebo responders panic attacks not directly assessed
Lecrubier et al (1997)[32]	PD ± AG	CLO, 121 (36%) (PAR 27%)	123 (36%)	CLO (range 10–150 mg) (PAR range 10–60 mg)	12	Chloral hydrate p.n.	CLO = PAR > P	High proportion of placebo responders

[a] PD = panic disorder; PA = panic attacks; AG = agoraphobia.

[b] IMI = imipramine; CLO = clomipramine; ALP = alprazolam; BUS = buspirone; PAR = paroxetine; ZIM = zimeldine, P = placebo.

[c] Sheehan et al:[5] 'endogenous anxiety' = panic disorder; 21 out of 87 (24%) dropped out, no difference across groups; 9 patients had only specific phobia (analyzed separately).

[d] CNCPS = Cross-National Collaborative Panic Study.

Table 9.2 Panic disorder: meta-analysis of short-term TCA treatment trials

Study	N	Years	Double-blind placebo control only	Outcome: TCA > Placebo/ control	Comments
Mattick et al (1990)[40]	4	1980–1985	No	Yes	Few drug studies included; focus on psychotherapy
Wilkinson et al (1991)[38]	13	1964–1986	Yes	Yes	Comprehensive study; effect sizes calculated for major outcome measure
Cox et al (1992)[41]	5–7	1980–1989	No	No	Few drug studies included; included studies not stated
Clum et al (1993)[37]	3–5	1980–1988	No	Yes (phobias)	Few drug studies included; focus on psychotherapy
Boyer (1995)[39]	15	1980–1992	Yes	Yes	Panic-free was main outcome measure (four studies other anxiety measure); only completer analysis; clomipramine and SSRI combined
Gould et al (1995)[27]	43 (9)[a]	1980–1994	No	Yes	Comprehensive analyses of efficacy of drugs and psychotherapy; special analyses on antidepressants versus placebo; statistical testing of effect sizes

[a]Antidepressants vs placebo.

Table 9.3 Panic disorder: meta-analysis of treatment outcome of 19 placebo-controlled trials according to Wilkinson et al[38]

Variable	Antidepressants (effect size)	Benzodiazepines (effect size)
Panic attacks	0.27	0.45
Anxiety symptoms	0.62	0.57
Phobic symptoms	0.46	0.66
Social functioning	0.34	0.20
Global clinical improvement	0.73	0.53
Treatment medians	0.55	0.43

obtained for differences that are not clinically meaningful.

Table 9.2 presents the results from some meta-analyses of short-term treatment trials. Wilkinson et al[38] and Boyer[39] analyzed only placebo-controlled studies, while the other authors included a broader spectrum of studies – typically those including some kind of control groups (either another drug or a psychotherapeutic technique).[27,37,40,41] Hence, the number of papers included in the meta-analyses varied greatly across studies. The interpretations of meta-analyses are of course dependent on the quality of the studies included and on the number of patients in individual studies. Such important aspects are not addressed in the papers on meta-analyses of outcome for panic disorder. Nor are the markedly different sample sizes in the individual studies taken into consideration.

Wilkinson et al[38] calculated effect sizes for several important clinical parameters based on 13 studies on antidepressants (12 with imipramine) and 6 on benzodiazepines. The treatment median effect size for TCAs was 0.55, indicating moderate improvement (Table 9.3). The effect size for panic attacks was fairly low, but it should be mentioned that panic attacks were not systematically registered in all studies and that the effect sizes varied widely (i.e. from 0.002 to 0.76) on panic attacks in individual studies.

Similar effect sizes were obtained for benzodiazepines. In the psychotherapeutic outcome literature, higher overall effect sizes are generally reported.[27,40] However, such numerical differences must be interpreted with caution owing to methodological differences between studies.

Boyer[39] has calculated an improvement ratio, defined as the improvement on the active drug divided by that on placebo. For imipramine, the mean improvement ratio for 12 studies was 1.90 (range 1.00–2.97) and for clomipramine (3 studies) 2.43 (range 1.66–5.41). However, Boyer evaluated only efficacy for completers in the trials, and only considered one major outcome (i.e. panic attacks).

Boyer also analyzed results from trials with SSRIs. As clomipramine has a higher affinity for the serotonin reuptake inhibitor than imipramine, Boyer subsumed clomipramine under the concept of serotonin reuptake inhibitors. The meta-analysis demonstrated that serotonin reuptake inhibitors were significantly superior to both imipramine and alprazolam, another claimed reference drug for panic disorder.

Surprisingly, Cox et al[41] concluded that imipramine was not significantly effective for either panic or avoidance behavior, and was only marginally effective for depressed mood and global severity. However, this conclusion was based on only a few studies.

In their comprehensive meta-analysis Gould et al[27] provided statistical testing of calculated effect sizes. Based on nine studies with placebo control, an effect size of 0.55 was obtained for antidepressants, which is significantly different from zero ($p < 0.001$), but not different for the effect size calculated for benzodiazepines (0.40, 13 trials). Furthermore, effect sizes were calculated for both endpoint and completer analyses (4 studies), indicating that completer analyses may suppress the estimate for drug versus placebo-effect size. The effect size for cognitive–behavioral treatments yielded the highest effect size (0.68).

In summary, meta-analyses of placebo-controlled double-blind studies of TCAs (i.e. imipramine and clomipramine) support the view that imipramine and clomipramine are efficacious in the treatment of panic disorder. Patients improve on a variety of outcome measures. As evaluated by the statistical measure effect size, the magnitude of the clinical efficacy is moderate with respect to overall outcome. Clomipramine is suggested as being more efficacious than imipramine.

Multicenter studies

Two major multicenter studies have focused on the efficacy of TCAs in the treatment of panic disorder. They have been planned to fulfill many of the experimental aspects that are today considered important when studying a clinically complex disorder such as panic disorder. Inclusion of a large population of patients allows for analysis of important subgroups, i.e. patients with agoraphobia and affective symptoms.

Cross-National Collaborative Panic Study

Among the experimental advantages of the phase II of the Cross-National Collaborative Panic Study (CNCPS)[31] are the following:

- a randomized placebo-controlled double-blind design;
- 1112 patients were randomized to three treatment cells in an eight-week trial: imipramine, alprazolam and placebo;
- standardized diagnostic criteria (DSM-III) for inclusion and exclusion;
- a flexible dose regime up to 250 mg imipramine and 10 mg alprazolam;
- several standardized outcome measures (panic attacks, phobias, anticipatory anxiety, depression, social functioning and overall improvement, and others);
- assessment of adverse effects;
- explicit limitation of concomitant psychotherapy;
- statistical analysis of completer and endpoint data;
- quality assurance and supervision of project.

No previous studies in the literature on TCA efficacy in panic disorder have fulfilled similar strict criteria (see Table 9.1). The inclusion of quality assurance with respect to diagnostic and assessment procedures is an important aspect guarding against bias due to participation of many different raters. Centers from 15 countries participated in the trial. The rationale of the study is further described by Klerman.[42]

Affective symptoms are frequent in panic

Analysis	Group	Panic-free	Panic attacks[a]	Phobia[a]	Anticipatory anxiety[a]	Hamilton Depression Scale[a]	Global improvement[a]
Endpoint	Imipramine	70%	I = A > P	I = A > P	I = A > P	I = A > P	I = A > P
	Alprazolam	70%					
	Placebo	50%					
Completer	Imipramine	78%	I = A = P	I = A > P	I = A = P	I = A > P	I = A > P
	Alprazolam	74%					
	Placebo	68%					

Table 9.4 Cross-National Collaborative Panic Study (CNCPS)[31] Phase II: main results

[a] I = imipramine; A = alprazolam; P = placebo.

patients, but patients with current major depressive episode were excluded unless the depression was judged secondary to the anxiety disorder.

The major results of the CNCPS are shown in Table 9.4.

Efficacy of imipramine

The drop-out rates differed significantly across treatment cells. Thus 30% of imipramine, 17% of alprazolam and 44% of placebo-treated patients withdrew.

The mean dose of imipramine was 155 mg/24 h and for alprazolam 5.7 mg/24 h.

Table 9.4 demonstrates that imipramine was efficacious on a wide range of panic phenomenology, including panic attacks, anticipatory anxiety and phobic avoidance behavior. However, for completers of the trial, no differences were seen on the primary outcome measure, panic attack. Thus a striking finding was the high proportion of responders in the placebo group. As withdrawal in placebo often represents a lack of therapeutic gain, endpoint analyses are more relevant for evaluation of drug efficacy than completer analyses.

An important finding was that the efficacy of imipramine was not restricted to the amelioration of panic attacks, but comprised a spectrum of clinically relevant symptoms, including phobic avoidance behavior, even in the absence of concomitant psychotherapy. Further, as in the treatment of depression with TCAs, that improvement was gradual over weeks, while the benzodiazepine alprazolam had a faster mode of action.

Panic disorder subtypes and comorbidity

As a major proportion of panic disorder patients may have complicating affective symptoms, it has been questioned whether the efficacy of imipramine may be due to effects on affective symptoms (e.g. major depression or dysthymia).[43]

Affective symptoms

Among panic patients, 16% fulfilled criteria for current major depressive episodes, 16% for past major depressive episodes and 12% for dysthymia. Thus a substantial proportion of the patients had affective symptoms.

Deltito et al[44] analyzed a subgroup of patients (N = 312) from the CNCPS, applying strict criteria to rule out affective symptoms, i.e. current or previous affective episodes as well as dysphoria. They found that the clinical response to imipramine or alprazolam was independent of the presence of current or past affective symptoms. Analyses of the importance of current major depressive episodes relying on general linear models are in accordance with this conclusion.[45] Detailed analysis of panic patients with dysthymia did not suggest this syndrome to be of major clinical relevance for the outcome of drug treatment of panic disorder.[46]

Although patients with affective symptoms did improve significantly, patients with current major depressive episodes improved less, probably because of the higher scores at baseline on most anxiety and affective scales.[46] No significant differences were observed between imipramine and alprazolam considering subgroups defined by affective symptoms.

In summary, improvement of panic disorder by imipramine is not secondary to amelioration of coexisting affective symptoms. However, panic patients with current major depressive episodes tend to improve less.

Avoidance behavior

Twenty-two percent of the patients had uncomplicated panic disorder, 40% limited phobic avoidance and 36% had agoraphobia.

The role of avoidance behavior has been further analyzed, applying analysis of variance within the framework of a linear model to test the efficacy of active drugs in different subgroups of patients.[45,47] Patients with extensive avoidance behavior (agoraphobia) profited the most from treatment with active drugs, but, surprisingly, specific drug effects were most pronounced in avoidance behavior. Panic disorder uncomplicated by avoidance behavior responded nearly equally well to alprazolam, imipramine and placebo, while phobic avoidance was significantly improved by both drugs. A beneficial effect of imipramine could only be found if a certain degree of avoidance behavior was present, and it could be demonstrated in the absence of depression.

The results of these studies are compatible with the view proposed by the ICD-10 classification that agoraphobia with panic attacks is distinct from panic disorder. They are also in line with the meta-analysis of Wilkinson et al,[38] who found only a moderate efficacy of imipramine on panic attacks. They bring into question the oft-cited statement that panic attacks are the major target for antipanic drugs, and the abolishment of panic attacks is a prerequisite for improvements in avoidance behavior.[48] Furthermore, they may be of relevance in explaining the high degree of placebo response in some studies.

In summary, panic disorder patients improve on a spectrum of symptoms on short-term imipramine treatment, independently of comorbid affective or phobic symptoms. The improvement is gradual over several weeks. However, patients with agoraphobia may have a better response to drugs than patients with uncomplicated panic disorder.

Clomipramine multicenter study

Lecrubier et al[32] have recently published the results from a large multicenter study including 467 patients with panic disorder. The majority of patients had agoraphobia (about 80%). Clomipramine was compared with the specific serotonin reuptake inhibitor paroxetine in a double-blind placebo-controlled study. Thirty-nine centers from 13 countries participated. Panic attacks were the primary efficacy variable, but several other outcome measures were applied. Clomipramine doses ranged from 10 to 150 mg (with 47% <100 mg).

Twenty-seven percent in the clomipramine groups withdrew prematurely from the study, compared with 29% in the paroxetine and 36% in the placebo groups. As in the CNCPS, a significant percentage of placebo-treated patients improved, although many were agoraphobic. Thus 32% had zero panic attacks at endpoint, compared with 37% and 51% in the two drug groups. An even higher percentage (60%) in the placebo group experienced a reduction in panic attacks greater than 50%.

Clomipramine patients improved slowly with respect to panic attacks, and the drug was significantly better than placebo only at week 12. Paroxetine had a faster mode of action. (Figure 9.1).

When other outcome measures were considered (including anxiety, phobia and disability), the active drugs gave better improvement compared with placebo from week 9. There were no significant differences between the active components throughout the trial.

Forty-one patients discontinued because of adverse effects; of these, 15% were in the clomipramine group, 7% in the paroxetine group and 11% in the placebo group.

The results of this study are in accordance with the results from the meta-analysis of Boyer demonstrating the clinical efficacy of serotonin uptake inhibitors, even in a sample with a high frequency of placebo responders. Although the SSRIs are often claimed to be better tolerated than the TCAs, the differences in tolerability among panic patients were not impressive in this study.

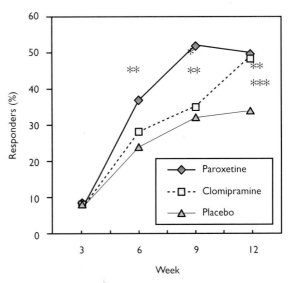

Figure 9.1 Reduction in number of panic attacks to zero in placebo, clomipramine and paroxetine-treated patients (modified after Ref 32). *$P < 0.05$, paroxetine vs clomipramine; **$P < 0.05$, paroxetine vs placebo; ***$P < 0.05$ clomipramine vs placebo.

Other studies

As mentioned, imipramine and clomipramine have been the most extensively studied among TCAs. Much less evidence is available for the clinical efficacy of other TCAs.

Fahy et al[49] compared clomipramine with lofepramine in a placebo-controlled trial where some behavioral counseling was also given. By the end of the acute phase at week 6, a pronounced placebo effect was seen. Forty-two percent had zero panic attacks, compared with 67% in the active drug groups. However, both drugs were superior to placebo on several other outcome measures.

Interestingly, no tendency to relapse was noted in the three months following taper-off of medication from week 12 to week 24. This is in contrast to a similar study of Clark et al.[11]

Studies applying a much less rigorous design suggest that desimipramine[50] and nortriptyline[51] are efficacious. There is a theoretically interesting double-blind study by Den Boer and Westenberg,[52] who compared fluvoxamine (an SSRI) and maprotiline (a specific noradrenergic uptake inhibitor). The former drug appears as a potent antipanic agent, while the latter had but slight effect on depressive symptoms (cf reference 39).

Tolerability and side-effects

The well-known spectrum of side-effects of TCAs (anticholinergic, cardiovascular, among others) may be a major hindrance for their wider applicability in panic patients, who are assumed to be very sensitive to any symptoms imitating anxiety attacks, such as palpitations and tremor. Thus high drop-out rates have often been noticed in controlled trials of TCAs. In the CNPCS, significantly more patients dropped out in the imipramine group (30%) compared with the alprazolam (a benzodiazepine) group (17%), but not compared with the placebo group (40%). Side-effects are frequently reported. Interestingly, clomipramine and paroxetine (an SSRI) did not differ widely in drop-out rates or reported side-effects.[32]

An initial exacerbation of anxiety symptoms has frequently been noticed,[51] and experts advise more gradual dose increases for panic patients than for depressed patients.[19]

The delay of onset of improvement may be troublesome to many patients seeking immediate relief for their suffering, but, considering the chronicity of the disorder, this is hardly a strong argument against the use of TCAs.

Discontinuation symptoms have also been described for antidepressants, but have not been observed as a major problem in controlled studies, in contrast to treatment with alprazolam. The major advantages of imipramine and other antidepressants with antipanic activity compared with alprazolam and other benzodiazepines are that physical dependence does not develop and that discontinuation can be instituted much more rapidly.

TCAs may be the drugs of choice for treating panic patients with current or previous alcohol or drug abuse.

Long-term treatment

Panic disorder is generally conceived as a chronic and recurrent disabling syndrome. Patients are often initially treated for 3 months, and those who respond continue treatment for 6–12 months, but some need even longer maintenance treatment.[53] The optimal time to treatment discontinuation has not been determined. In a comprehensive review of the course and outcome of panic patients by Roy-Burne and Cowley,[54] it is concluded that while most patients improve with modern treatment, few are cured. The presence of agoraphobia, depression and personality disorders indicate a poorer prognosis. Thus a majority of patients may require long-term treatment. This issue was reviewed in 1993 by Burrows et al.[55] They concluded that long-term treatment with TCAs did not lead to loss of efficacy. On drug withdrawal, high rates of relapse were observed.

Curtis et al[56] presented data from a systematic double-blind comparison of maintenance therapy for up to eight months in patients who participated in the CNCPS (phase II), i.e. who were treated with alprazolam, imipramine or placebo. One hundred and eighty-one patients participated, and the therapeutic gains obtained in the short-term trial persisted in all groups. However, fewer placebo patients remained throughout the whole study period. Tolerance to the antipanic efficacy of TCAs was not indicated and the drugs were well tolerated.

Similar conclusions were observed in a recently published study of long-term treatment (36 weeks) with clomipramine and paroxetine in panic patients.[53] This study is an extension of the short-term study of Lecrubier et al[32] previously mentioned. One hundred and seventy-six patients entered the 36-week extension study, and 66% completed the study. A higher percentage of patients withdrew from the placebo group (42%) than from the clomipramine (35%) and paroxetine (28%) groups. A similar distribution of percentages was obtained for patients who withdrew owing to lack of efficacy (9%, 3% and 3%). The active drugs were significantly more effective than placebo with respect to the reduction of full panic attacks from baseline. A surprising finding was that the large placebo response observed in the short-term study continued throughout the long-term extension phase.

Optimizing TCA treatment

Owing to their long elimination half-lives TCAs are often prescribed as single-dosage regimes in the treatment of depression, but in controlled trials in panic disorder imipramine has been administered in three or four doses for reasons of comparison with other drugs, especially alprazolam. Single-dose administration may be advantageous to minimize drug-intake-oriented behavior throughout daytime. Clinically, a dose of 150–200 mg of imipramine is assumed to be the most appropriate initial target dose, but, as in the treatment of depression, plasma monitoring of antidepressants should play a more prominent role in the future, considering the genetic polymorphism for cytochrome P450 isozymes.[57]

It has been suggested that some patients may improve with low-dose (10–50 mg) clomipramine treatment.[58,59] In a study by Modigh et al[36] comparing the efficacy of imipramine and clomipramine, the mean daily doses were 124 mg/24 h (range 50–250) for imipramine and 109 mg/24 h (range 25–200) for clomipramine. Further studies are needed to delineate a subgroup of patients in need of low-dose treatment (see also references 32 and 60).

The gradual increase in dose to improve tolerability to TCAs has been mentioned above.

Plasma levels

In the study by Modigh et al[36] comparing imipramine and clomipramine, no significant relations between plasma concentrations of imipramine or clomipramine or their metabolites and clinical response were observed.

Mavissakalian and Perel[61] have published an eight-week, double-blind, placebo-controlled dose-ranging trial in 80 panic patients with agoraphobia. They used weight-adjusted doses of imipramine: (low) 0.5 mg/kg per day, (medium) 1.5 mg/kg per day or (high) 3.0 mg/kg per day. Plasma levels of imipramine and N-methylimipramine and response to treatment were ascertained after four and eight weeks. There was a significant positive dose–response relationship. For phobias, the best total drug plasma levels were in the range 110–140 mg/ml. Higher doses had a detrimental effect. For panic, improvement was observed on increasing the dose, but with no improvement beyond 140 mg/ml.

A predictor analysis[62] of the data for the plasma concentrations of imipramine, desmethylimipramine and total drug concentration demonstrated that imipramine and total drug concentration were better predictors of most outcome measures considered than desmethylimipramine. As this major metabolite has higher noradrenergic affinity than imipramine, the authors suggest that the antipanic and antiphobic activity is predominantly mediated by serotonergic mechanisms (cf references 39 and 52).

An important clinical implication is that drug efficacy may decrease with increasing total plasma concentration, indicating the existence of a 'therapeutic window'. If replicated in future studies, this finding is further support for using therapeutic drug monitoring in optimizing TCA treatment of panic disorder.

Monoamine oxidase inhibitors (MAOIs)

See Table 9.5.

Irreversible MAOIs

The efficacy of monoamine oxidase inhibitors (MAOIs) against phobic anxiety symptoms was suggested by a series of early studies published before the appearance of DSM-III (cf references 2–4). Often a mixed group of phobic patients was included, and panic attacks were not always systematically evaluated. Thus Tyrer et al,[63] in a placebo-controlled double-blind study of 40 patients with agoraphobia and social phobia, found that the irreversible MAOI phenelzine (30–90 mg) was significantly superior to placebo with regard to overall improvement after eight weeks but not at four weeks.

The study by Sheehan et al[5] is widely cited as evidence for the efficacy of MAOIs in panic disorder, although strict DSM-III criteria were not applied. Seventy-seven patients with 'endogenous anxiety' (i.e. panic disorder with agoraphobia) were randomized to phenelzine (45 mg), imipramine (150 mg) and a placebo treatment. Several outcome measures were applied, but panic attacks were not analyzed. Both drugs gave superior improvement compared with placebo on most outcome measures at week 12. A trend for phenelzine to be superior to imipramine achieved significance on

scales measuring severity of symptoms, avoidance, and work and social disability. All patients received concomitant supportive group psychotherapy. The authors argue from clinical evidence based on the treatment of 300 patients that many patients need higher doses of phenelzine than those administered in the trial.

Buigues and Vallejo[64] presented an open dose-ranging trial over six months. Thirty-five of 40 completed the study. The drug blocked panic attacks completely in patients with uncomplicated panic disorder, and almost completely in patients with agoraphobia. Anticipatory anxiety and avoidant behavior improved markedly, although not statistically significantly, in 74% of patients with agoraphobia. The mean dose was 55 mg/day (range 45–75), but increasing the dose to 90 mg/day in four non-responders was followed by improvement. Thus some patients may require a high daily dose, as suggested by Sheehan et al.[5]

Considering that uncontrolled clinical experience has suggested phenelzine as a highly efficacious drug in the treatment of panic disorder,[3,65] it is surprising that phenelzine or other classical irreversible MAOIs (isocarboxazid or tranylcypromine) have not been subjected to rigorous controlled trials for panic disorder. However, this is probably due to the well-known spectrum of side-effects, especially the 'cheese' effect and the need to place patients on low-tyramine diets to avoid hypertensive crises, but other side-effects may also be troublesome. Thus Buigues and Vallejo[64] reported postural hypotension (64%), insomnia (40%), dry mouth (42%), sexual dysfunction (20%) and myoclonic jerks (23%). However, Sheehan et al[5] reported that phenelzine was better tolerated than imipramine.

The task force of the World Psychiatric

Table 9.5 Panic disorder: treatment with MAOIs

Study	Diagnosis[a]	MAOI[b], no. of drop-outs	Comparison drug, no. of drop-outs	Placebo, no. of drop-outs	Dose of MAOI	Duration (weeks)	Other therapy	Efficacy[b]	Comments[b]
Tyrer (1973)[63]	AG/SP	PHE, 20/6		20/2	45 mg	8		PHE > PLA	Overall improvement rated as significant by psychiatrist, but not by patient; panic attacks not evaluated
Sheehan (1980)[5]	AG[c]	PHE, 29/17	IMI, 28/18	30/22	45 mg	12	Supportive psychotherapy	PHE = IMI > PLA	Efficacy on several outcome measures, PHE > IMI on Work and Social Disability Scale at 12 weeks; panic attacks not evaluated
Buigues and Vallejo (1987)[64]	PD/AG	PHE, 40/5		No		24		PHE	Panic-attack block almost 100%; anticipatory anxiety and avoidant behavior improved markedly, but not significantly; open study
Bakish et al (1993)[70]	PD/AG	BRO, 47/27	CLO, 46/29		Maximum tolerable	8	Chloral hydrate p.n.	BRO = CLO	Efficacy toward several outcome measures
Van Vliet et al (1993)[4]	PD/AG	BRO, 15/15		15/14	150 mg	12 (+12)		BRO > PLA	Improvement in general anxiety and avoidance, but not in panic attacks
Van Vliet et al (1996)[71]	PD/AG	BRO, 15/?	FLU, 15/?		150 mg (both)	12 (+12)		BRO = FLU	No placebo control; outcome measures included panic attacks

[a] PD = panic disorder; AG = agoraphobia; SP = social phobia.
[b] PHE = phenelzine; BRO = brofaromine; IMI = imipramine; CLO = clomipramine; FLU = fluvoxamine; PLA = placebo.
[c] Nine patients with social phobia were analyzed separately.

Association[19] refers to clinical experience indicating that patients with refractory panic disorder may be the 'ideal candidates' for treatment with MAOIs. As underlined by Sheehan et al,[5] some patients may need as much as 90 mg/24 h of phenelzine to improve. Lydiard et al[66] suggest that patients with coexisting major depression may benefit more with MAOI treatment. This interesting possibility awaits further studies.

RIMAs

Reversible inhibitors of the monoamine oxidase type A (RIMAs) include several recently developed drugs (moclobemide, brofaromine, befloxatone, among others).[67] Moclobemide has been widely studied in the treatment of depression, and is indicated as an efficacious agent.[67,68] The drug has a very low incidence of side-effects. Thus safety data revealed only differences compared with placebo with respect to dizziness, nausea and insomnia.[67] Preliminary studies (reviewed by Buller[69]) suggest that the drug may have a role in the treatment of panic disorder. Unfortunately, an extremely large placebo response has invalidated the interpretation of results from a multicenter study of moclobemide in panic disorder (personal communication).

In a study by Bakish et al,[70] brofaromine was compared with clomipramine. Although efficacy was demonstrated in several outcome measures, neither drug was well tolerated (Table 9.5).

Van Vliet and co-workers[4,71] have presented the best studies on the efficacy of brofaromine in panic disorder. However, the drug is no longer developed for clinical purposes.

The first study[4] was placebo-controlled (Table 9.5), and brofaromine gave a marked reduction in general anxiety and avoidance behavior. No difference was seen regarding panic attacks, but the authors claim that often too much emphasis is laid on panic attacks in drug trials although they show large inter- and intraindividual variability. A remarkable finding compared with other recent studies is a very low placebo response. In fact, no significant improvement was observed on placebo.

This observation is important for the interpretation of the second brofaromine study by Van Vliet et al.[71] Brofaromine was compared with fluvoxamine (an SSRI), but without a placebo group. Again significant efficacy was found for brofaromine on most outcome measures, including panic attacks. Brofaromine was not significantly different from fluvoxamine. During a 12-week follow-up period, further improvements were observed in both groups. The most prominent side-effect was sleep disturbance and nausea, which was observed in the majority of patients.

In summary, the MAOIs are suggested as efficacious in the treatment of phobic anxiety symptoms in panic patients, and probably also of panic attacks, but it should be underlined that their efficacy on panic attacks has not been substantially documented in controlled trials. However, clinical experience suggests the drugs to be efficacious antipanic agents, especially for patients who are refractory to other drugs.

The classical irreversible MAOIs have had a more limited role than the TCAs because of their more troublesome side-effects. The RIMAs have a much better profile of side-effects, but the best documented compound, brofaromine, will probably not appear on the market in the near future. The RIMAs may especially benefit panic patients with phobic anxiety.

Conclusions

Among the TCAs, imipramine and clomipramine have been much studied. Despite some differences in research methodology across studies published in the last few decades, a consistent picture has emerged. Both drugs are efficacious in the treatment of panic disorder, and patients benefit with regard to most important clinical aspects, including panic attacks, anticipatory anxiety and phobic avoidance behavior. This improvement is not dependent on the treatment of concurrent affective symptoms. Interestingly, despite these repeat studies the tricyclics are not licensed for panic disorder in most countries. The exception is clomipramine which has this indication in a number of European states. The reasons for this are unclear.

A striking finding in recent multicenter studies following a rigorous research protocol is the very high proportion of patients responding to placebo. Some evidence has been obtained that more severe states as defined by the presence of agoraphobia benefit mostly from drug treatment.

Reviews of the literature applying meta-analytic techniques do generally demonstrate moderate but clinical meaningful effect sizes on major outcome measures.

Panic patients may be especially sensitive to the well-known spectrum of side-effects of the drugs, which may limit their role in the long-term treatment of a chronic disorder.

Clomipramine is suggested as more efficacious than imipramine in some studies, indicating that drugs with predominantly serotonergic affinity may be clinically more efficacious in the treatment of panic disorder.

Although MAOIs are widely claimed to be efficacious in the treatment of panic disorder much less evidence based on controlled trials is available for them – both the classical irreversible and modern reversible (RIMA) inhibitors. The main mode of action may be on phobic anxiety, an effect that was suggested several decades ago. As the RIMAs are very well tolerated, further controlled trials are warranted.

The future role of classical antidepressants such as the TCAs and the irreversible MAOIs awaits future studies after the appearance of the SSRIs and the RIMAs.

References

1. Klein DF, Delineation of two drug-responsive anxiety syndromes. *Psychopharmacologia* 1964; **5**: 397–408.
2. Roth M, Argyle N, Anxiety, panic and phobic disorders: an overview. *J Psychiatr Res* 1988; **22**(Suppl 1): 33–54.
3. Hollander E, Hatterer J, Klein DF, Antidepressants for the treatment of panic and agoraphobia. In: *Handbook of Anxiety* (Noyes R, Roth M, Burrows GD, eds). Amsterdam: Elsevier, 1990: 207–31.
4. Van Vliet IM, Westenberg HG, Den Boer JA, MAO inhibitors in panic disorder: clinical effects of treatment with brofaromine. A double blind placebo controlled study. *Psychopharmacology Berl* 1993; **112**: 483–9.
5. Sheehan DV, Ballenger JC, Jacobsen G, Treatment of endogenous anxiety with phobic, hysterical, and hypochondriacal symptoms. *Arch Gen Psychiatry* 1980; **37**: 51–9.
6. Johnson MR, Lydiard RB, Ballenger JC, Panic disorder: pathophysiology and drug treatment. *Drugs* 1995; **49**: 328–44.
7. Krystal JH, Deutsch DN, Charney DS, The biological basis of panic disorder. *J Clin Psychiatry* 1996; **57**(Suppl 10): 23–31; discussion 32–3.
8. Klein DF, Anxiety reconceptualized. In: *Anxiety: New Research and Changing Concepts* (Klein DF, Rabkin J, eds). New York: Raven Press, 1981: 235–63.
9. Rosenberg R, Ottosson JO, Bech P et al,

Validation criteria for panic disorder as a nosological entity. *Acta Psychiatr Scand* 1991; **83**(Suppl 365): 7–17.

10. Klein DF, Treatment of panic disorder, agoraphobia and social phobia. *Clin Neuropharmacol* 1995; **18**(Suppl 2): 45–51.

11. Clark DM, Salkovskis PM, Hackmann A et al, A comparison of cognitive therapy, applied relaxation and imipramine in the treatment of panic disorder. *Br J Psychiatry* 1994; **164**: 759–69.

12. Barlow DH, Lehman CL, Advances in the psychosocial treatment of anxiety disorders. Implications for national health care. *Arch Gen Psychiatry* 1996; **53**: 727–35.

13. Liebowitz MR, Fyer AJ, Gorman JM et al, Tricyclic therapy of the DSM-III anxiety disorders: a review with implications for further research. *J Psychiatr Res* 1988; **22**(Suppl 1): 7–32.

14. Balestrieri M, Ruggeri M, Bellantuono C, Drug treatment of panic disorder – a critical review of controlled clinical trials. *Psychiatr Devel* 1989; **4**: 337–50.

15. Matuzas W, Jack E, The drug treatment of panic disorder. *Psychiatr Med* 1991; **9**: 215–43.

16. Rosenberg R, Drug treatment of panic disorder. *Pharmacol Toxicol* 1993; **72**: 344–53.

17. Bandelow B, Sievert K, Rothemeyer M et al, Panic disorder and agoraphobia: What is effective? *Fortschr Neurol Psychiatr* 1995; **63**: 451–64.

18. Jefferson JW, Antidepressants in panic disorder. *J Clin Psychiatry* 1997; **58**(Suppl 2): 20–4; discussion 24–5.

19. Klerman GL, Hirschfeld RMA, Weissman MM et al (eds), *Panic Anxiety and its Treatments*. Washington, DC: American Psychiatric Press, 1993.

20. McNally RJ, *Panic Disorder. A Critical Analysis*. New York: The Guildford Press, 1994.

21. Breier A, Charney DS, Heninger GR, Agoraphobia with panic attacks: development, diagnostic stability, and course of illness. *Arch Gen Psychiatry* 1986; **43**: 1029–36.

22. Katschnig H, Amering M, Stolk JM et al, Long-term follow-up after a drug trial for panic disorder. *Br J Psychiatry* 1995; **167**: 487–94.

23. Zitrin CM, Klein DF, Woerner G, Treatment of agoraphobia with group exposure in vivo and imipramine. *Arch Gen Psychiatry* 1980; **37**: 63–72.

24. Marks IM, Gray S, Cohen D et al, Imipramine and brief therapist-aided exposure in agoraphobics having self-exposure homework. *Arch Gen Psychiatry* 1983; **40**: 153–62.

25. Zitrin CM, Klein DF, Woerner MG, Ross DC, Treatment of phobias. I. Comparison of imipramine hydrochloride and placebo. *Arch Gen Psychiatry* 1983; **40**: 125–38.

26. Evans L, Kenardy J, Schneider P, Hoey H, Effect of a selective serotonin uptake inhibitor in agoraphobia with panic attacks. A double-blind comparison of zimeldine, imipramine and placebo. *Acta Psychiatr Scand* 1986; **73**: 49–53.

27. Gould RA, Otto MW, Pollack MH, A meta-analysis of treatment outcome for panic disorder. *Clin Psychol Rev* 1995; **15**: 819–44.

28. American Psychiatric Association, *Diagnostic and Statistical Manual of Mental Disorders*, 3rd edn. Washington, DC: American Psychiatric Association, 1980.

29. World Health Organization, *The ICD-10 Classification of Mental and Behavioural Disorders. Diagnostic Criteria for Research*. Geneva: World Health Organization, 1993.

30. Shear MK, Maser JD, Standardized assessment for panic disorder research. A conference report. *Arch Gen Psychiatry* 1994; **51**: 346–54.

31. Cross-National Collaborative Panic Study SP, Drug treatment of panic disorder. Comparative efficacy of alprazolam, imipramine, and placebo. *Br J Psychiatry* 1992; **160**: 191–202.

32. Lecrubier Y, Bakker A, Dunbar G, Judge R, The Collaborative Paroxetine Panic Study Investigators, A comparison of paroxetine, clomipramine and placebo on the treatment of panic disorder. *Acta Psychiatr Scand* 1997; **95**: 145–52.

33. Pecknold JC, McClure DJ, Appeltauer L et al, Does tryptophan potentiate clomipramine in the treatment of agoraphobic and social phobic patients? *Br J Psychiatry* 1982; **140**: 484–90.

34. Charney DS, Woods SW, Goodman WK et al, Drug treatment of panic disorder: the comparative efficacy of imipramine, alprazolam, and trazodone. *J Clin Psychiatry* 1986; **47**: 580–6.

35. Andersch S, Ottosson J-O, Bech P et al, Efficacy

and safety of alprazolam, imipramine, and placebo in the treatment of panic disorder. *Acta Psychiatr Scand* 1991; **83**(Suppl 365): 18–27.

36. Modigh K, Westberg P, Eriksson E, Superiority of clomipramine over imipramine in the treatment of panic disorder: a placebo-controlled trial. *J Clin Psychopharmacol* 1992; **12**: 251–61.

37. Clum GA, Surls R, A meta-analysis of treatments for panic disorder. *J Consult Clin Psychol* 1993; **61**: 317–26.

38. Wilkinson G, Balestrieri M, Ruggeri M, Bellantuono C, Meta-analysis of double-blind placebo-controlled trials of antidepressants and benzodiazepines for patients with panic disorders. *Psychol Med* 1991; **21**: 991–8.

39. Boyer W, Serotonin uptake inhibitors are superior to imipramine and alprazolam in alleviating panic attacks: a meta-analysis. *Int Clin Psychopharmacol* 1995; **10**: 45–9.

40. Mattick RP, Andrews G, Hadzi Pavlovic D, Christensen H, Treatment of panic and agoraphobia. An integrative review. *J Nerv Ment Dis* 1990; **178**: 567–76.

41. Cox BJ, Endler NS, Lee PS, Swinson RP, A meta-analysis of treatments for panic disorder with agoraphobia: imipramine, alprazolam, and in vivo exposure. *J Behav Ther Exp Psychiatry* 1992; **23**: 175–82.

42. Klerman GL, Overview of the Cross-National Collaborative Panic Study. *Arch Gen Psychiatry* 1988; **45**: 407–12.

43. Marks I, Are there anticompulsive or antiphobic drugs? Review of the evidence. *Br J Psychiatry* 1983; **143**: 338–47.

44. Deltito JA, Argyle N, Klerman GL, Patients with panic disorder unaccompanied by depression improve with alprazolam and imipramine treatment. *J Clin Psychiatry* 1991; **52**: 121–7.

45. Maier W, Rosenberg R, Argyle N et al, Subtyping panic disorder by major depression and avoidance behaviour and the response to active treatment. *Eur Arch Psychiatry Clin Neurosci* 1991; **241**: 22–30.

46. Rosenberg R, Jensen PN, Treatment of panic disorder with alprazolam and imipramine: clinical relevance of DSM III dysthymia. *Eur Psychiatry* 1994; **9**: 27–32.

47. Maier W, Roth SM, Argyle N et al, Avoidance behaviour: a predictor of the efficacy of pharmacotherapy in panic disorder? *Eur Arch Psychiatry Clin Neurosci* 1991; **241**: 151–8.

48. Klein DF, Gorman JM, A model of panic and agoraphobic development. *Acta Psychiatr Scand* 1987; **335**(Suppl): 87–95.

49. Fahy TJ, O'Rourke D, Brophy J et al, The Galway Study of Panic Disorder. I: Clomipramine and lofepramine in DSM III-R panic disorder: a placebo controlled trial. *J Affect Disord* 1992; **25**: 63–75.

50. Kalus O, Asnis GM, Rubinson E et al, Desipramine treatment in panic disorder. *J Affective Disord* 1991; **21**: 239–44.

51. Munjack DJ, Usigli R, Zulueta A et al, Notriptyline in the treatment of panic disorder and agoraphobia with panic attacks. *J Clin Psychopharmacol* 1988; **8**: 204–7.

52. Den Boer JA, Westenberg HG, Effect of a serotonin and noradrenaline uptake inhibitor in panic disorder: a double-blind comparative study with fluvoxamine and maprotiline. *Int Clin Psychopharmacol* 1988; **3**: 59–74.

53. Lecrubier Y, Judge R, The Collaborative Paroxetine Panic Study Investigators, Long-term evaluation of paroxetine, clomipramine and placebo in panic disorder. *Acta Psychiatr Scand* 1997; **95**: 153–60.

54. Roy-Byrne PP, Cowley DS, Course and outcome in panic disorder: a review of recent follow-up studies. *Anxiety* 1994; **1**: 151–60.

55. Burrows GD, Judd FK, Norman TR, Long-term drug treatment of panic disorder. *J Psychiatr Res* 1993; **27**(Suppl 1): 111–25.

56. Curtis GC, Massana J, Udina C et al, Maintenance drug therapy of panic disorder. *J Psychiatr Res* 1993; **27**(Suppl 1): 127–42.

57. Meyer UA, Amrein R, Balant LP et al, Antidepressants and drug-metabolizing enzymes – expert group report. *Acta Psychiatr Scand* 1996; **93**: 71–9.

58. Modigh K, Antidepressant drugs in anxiety disorders. *Acta Psychiatr Scand* 1989; **76**(Suppl 335): 57–71.

59. Gloger S, Grunhaus L, Gladic D et al, Panic attacks and agoraphobia: low dose clomipramine treatment. *J Clin Psychopharmacol* 1989; **9**: 28–32.

60. Gentile V, Lotufo-Neto F, Andrade L et al, Clomipramine, a better reference drug for panic/agoraphobia. 1. Effectiveness comparison

with imipramine. *J Psychopharmacol* 1993; **7**: 316–24.

61. Mavissakalian MR, Perel JM, Imipramine treatment of panic disorder with agoraphobia: dose ranging and plasma level–response relationships. *Am J Psychiatry* 1995; **152**: 673–82.

62. Mavissakalian MR, Perel JM, The relationship of plasma imipramine and *N*-desmethylimipramine to response in panic disorder. *Psychopharmacol Bull* 1996; **32**: 143–7.

63. Tyrer P, Candy J, Kelly D, A study of the clinical effects of phenelzine and placebo in the treatment of phobic anxiety. *Psychopharmacologia* 1973; **32**: 237–54.

64. Buigues J, Vallejo J, Therapeutic response to phenelzine in patients with panic disorder and agoraphobia with panic attacks. *J Clin Psychiatry* 1987; **48**: 55–9.

65. Michelson LK, Marchione K, Behavioral, cognitive and pharmacological treatment of panic disorder with agoraphobia: critique and synthesis. *J Consult Clin Psychol* 1991; **59**: 100–14.

66. Lydiard RB, Brawman-Mintzer O, Ballenger JC, Recent developments in the psychopharmacology of anxiety disorders. *J Consult Clin Psychol* 1996; **64**: 660–8.

67. Priest RG, Gimbrett R, Roberts M, Steinert J, Reversible and selective inhibitors of monoamine oxidase A in mental and other disorders. *Acta Psychiatr Scand* 1995; **386**(Suppl): 40–3.

68. Angst J, Stabel M, Efficacy of moclobemide in different patients groups: a meta-analysis of studies. *Psychopharmacology* 1992; **106**: 109–13.

69. Buller R, Reversible inhibitors of monoamine oxidase A in anxiety disorders. *Clin Neuropharmacol* 1995; **18**(Suppl 2): 38–44.

70. Bakish D, Saxena BM, Bowen R, D'Souza JD, Reversible monoamine oxidase-A inhibitors in panic disorder. *Clin Neuropharmacol* 1993; **16**(Suppl 2): S77–82.

71. Van Vliet IM, Den Boer JA, Westenberg HG, Slaap BR, A double-blind comparative study of brofaromine and fluvoxamine in outpatients with panic disorder. *J Clin Psychopharmacol* 1996; **16**: 299–306.

72. Pohl R, Balon R, Yeragani VK et al, Serotonergic anxiolytics in the treatment of panic disorder: a controlled study with busiprione. *Psychopathology* 1989; **22**(Suppl 1): 60–7.

73. Robinson DS, Shrotriya RC, Alms DR et al, Treatment of panic disorder: nonbenzodiazepine anxiolytics, including buspirone. *Psychopharmacol Bull* 1989; **25**: 21–6.

74. Taylor CB, Hayward C, King R et al, Cardiovascular and symptomatic reduction effects of alprazolam and imipramine in patients with panic disorder: results of a double-blind, placebo-controlled trial. *J Clin Psychopharmacol* 1990; **10**: 112–8.

75. Uhlenhuth EH, Matuzas W, Glass RM et al, Response of panic disorder to fixed doses of alprazolam or imipramine. *J Affect Disord* 1989; **17**: 261–70.

10

The treatment of panic disorder with benzodiazepines

Graham D Burrows and Trevor R Norman

Treatment of panic disorder

Guidelines for the pharmacological management of panic disorder have been developed into a decision tree (Figure 10.1). Clearly the decision to implement pharmacological management must be based on an accurate history, on any associated co-morbid diagnoses and whether the panic disorder is primary or secondary. It is essential to treat the primary disorder first.[1] For example, panic attacks are frequently associated with alcoholism or major depression. While the pharmacotherapy for both conditions may be the same, other requirements, such as hospitalization and psychotherapy, may not. The decision to implement pharmacotherapy will clearly depend on the severity and frequency of panic attacks in the current episode and the degree to which these limit the capacity of the patient to function normally (e.g. at work or socially). The presence of associated morbidity with the disorder, such as alcohol abuse, development of secondary demoralization or suicidal ideation, suggests that treatment should be instituted. A significant family history of suicide or alcohol abuse has been argued as another indicator for instituting pharmacotherapy.[2] In milder forms of panic disorder with no other complications, pharmacotherapy can be postponed, while presenting complaints are dealt with by other therapies (e.g. cognitive–behavioural therapy).

Benzodiazepines in panic disorder

Efficacy in the treatment of panic disorder has been established for the tricyclic antidepressants, monoamine oxidase inhibitors, specific serotonin reuptake inhibitors and benzodiazepines.[3] Comparative studies suggest that there is little to choose between drugs in each of these classes with respect to their efficacy. Differences are apparent with respect to speed of onset, side-effect profiles, safety and complications of longer-term therapy, such as the ease of withdrawal of medication. The latter consideration is particularly important, since it appears that, for the majority of patients, panic

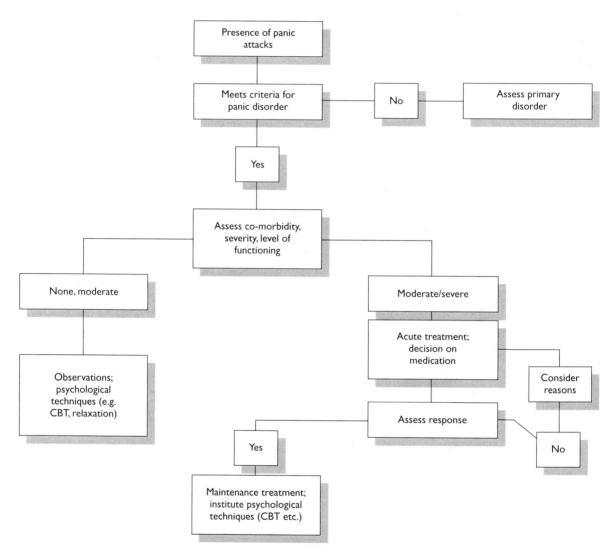

Figure 10.1 Treatment guidelines for the management of panic disorder. (Adapted from Ballenger[1])

disorder is a continuous, chronic disorder requiring treatment for at least 6–8 months, and longer in some cases.[1]

Benzodiazepines were once generally regarded as ineffective in the treatment of panic disorder, their main role being confined to the alleviation of anticipatory anxiety accompanying the attacks. However, studies with relatively high doses of diazepam (up to 50 mg/day) and early results with alprazolam challenged that view.[4-7] The benzodiazepine for which most evidence of efficacy in the treatment of panic disorder has since been gathered is alprazolam.

Alprazolam

Structurally, alprazolam, a triazolobenzodiazepine, is distinguished from other benzodiazepines by the presence of a triazole ring (Figure 10.2). The first controlled study suggesting antipanic efficacy for this agent was published in 1982.[8] A summary of some clinical trials of alprazolam in panic disorder is presented in Table 10.1. The efficacy of alprazolam in panic has been confirmed by these studies, where it has been demonstrated

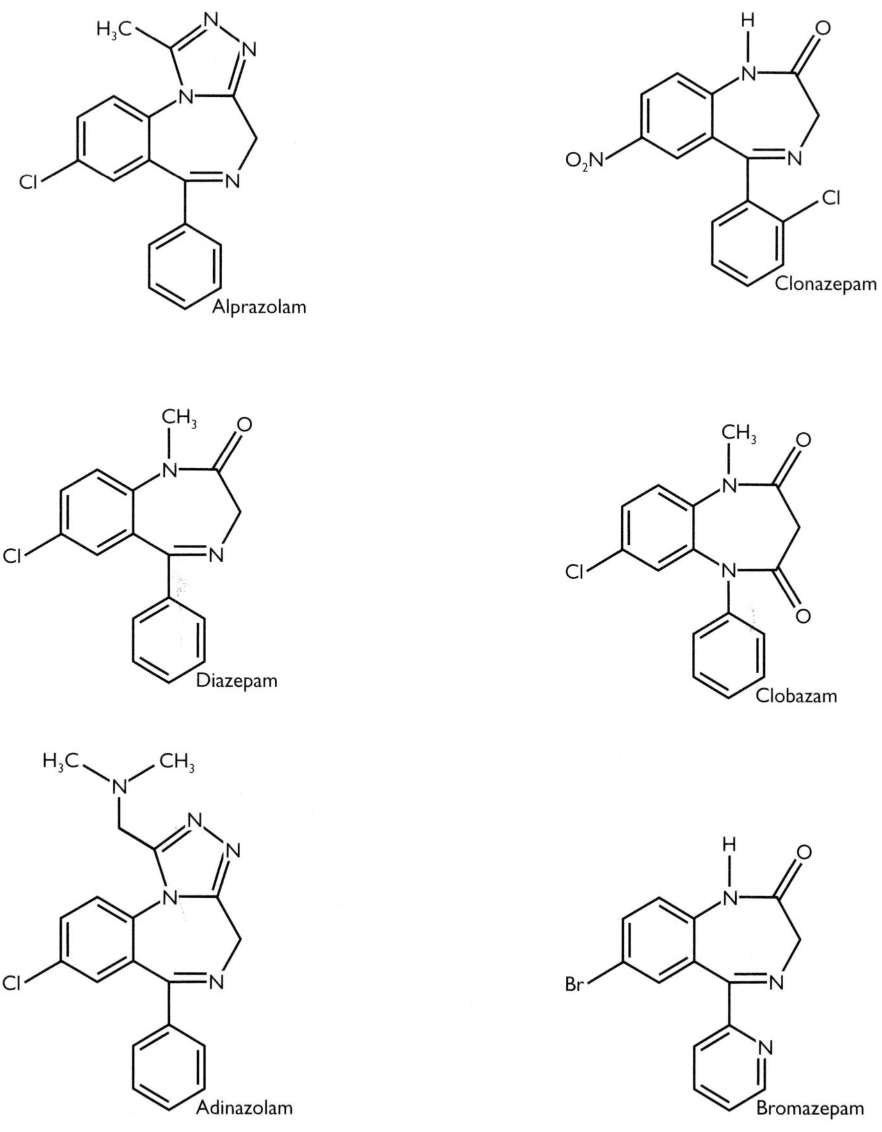

Figure 10.2 Chemical structures of some benzodiazepines used in the treatment of panic disorder.

Table 10.1 Some evaluations of alprazolam in the treatment of panic disorder

Design of study	Drugs,[a] dosage (mg)	N	Results	Ref
Single blind, randomized; 2 weeks placebo, 8 weeks drug	ALP, 5.4 IBU, 2130	16 16	ALP > IBU for panic attacks; onset of action ALP within 1 week	54
Double-blind, randomized, placebo-controlled 6-week study	ALP, 4 DIA, 44 PBO	16 16 16	ALP = DIA > PBO	6
Open label, 3-week fixed-dose study	ALP, 1 DIA, 10	10 8	ALP, DIA reduced anxiety; ALP more effective for panic	55
Non-random, flexible-dose study; behaviour therapy weekly; 3 weeks placebo, 8 weeks drug	ALP, 3.1 IMI, 141 TRZ, 250	23 24 27	ALP = IMI > TRZ using anxiety scales, panic attack frequency; ALP faster onset	56
Double-blind, randomized, flexible dose; 12-week study	ALP, 2.8 IMI, 132.5	22 22	ALP = IMI; ALP faster onset	57
Double-blind, randomized crossover study; 4 weeks per drug; flexible dose	ALP, 3.1 ADN, 95.5	14	ALP = ADN for panic attacks	25
Double-blind, randomized, 6 weeks; flexible dose	ALP, 1 ETZ, 1	15 15	ALP = ETZ; onset of action same for both drugs	58
Double-blind, randomized, placebo controlled, 8-week fixed-dose study	ALP, 2 ALP, 6 IMI, 225 PBO	20 21 20 20	ALP6 = IMI > ALP2 = PBO	59
Double-blind, randomized, flexible-dose study; 3 weeks placebo, 6 weeks drug; behaviour therapy weekly	ALP, 2.7 LRZ, 6.0	27 21	ALP = LRZ panic attacks, phobic anxiety	60
Double-blind, randomized, placebo-controlled, flexible-dose study; 5 weeks drug	ALP, 3.62 PRO, 184.6 PBO	20 19 16	ALP > PRO = PRO; similar rank order on other anxiety scales	61
Double-blind, randomized, placebo-controlled, flexible-dose study; 9 weeks drug	ALP, 3.7 IMI, 147 PBO	26 27 26	ALP = IMI > PBO for panic attacks	62

Table 10.1 Continued				
Design of Study	Drugs,[a] dosage (mg)	N	Results	Ref
Double-blind, randomized, flexible-dose study; 9 weeks drug	ALP, 4.9 IMI, 130	27 28	ALP = IMI; ALP faster onset	63
Double-blind, randomized, flexible: dose study; 6 weeks drug	ALP, 3.0 LRZ, 7.0	34 33	ALP = LRZ on panic attacks, relief of anxiety	64
Double-blind, randomized, placebo-controlled, flexible-dose study; 6 weeks drug	ALP, 5.2 CLN, 2.4 PBO	24 26 22	ALP = CLN > PBO	65
Double-blind, randomized, flexible-dose study; 6 weeks drug	ALP, 5 PRO, 182	14 15	ALP = PRO; ALP rapid onset	66
Double-blind, randomized, placebo-controlled, flexible-dose study; 8 weeks drug	ALP, 5.7 IMI, 155 PBO	386 391 391	ALP = IMI > PBO; ALP rapid onset	67
Double-blind, randomized, placebo-controlled, flexible-dose study; 8 weeks drug	ALP and exposure ALP and relaxation PBO and exposure PBO and relaxation	40 38 37 39	All treatments equally effective; longer-lasting gains with exposure alone than with ALP following withdrawal of treatment	68
Double-blind, randomized, placebo-controlled, flexible-dose study; 8 weeks drug	ALP, 4.9 DIA, 43 PBO	80 82 80	ALP = DIA > PBO for panic attacks; other anxiety measures	7

[a] ADN = adinazolam; ALP = alprazolam; CLN = clonazepam; DIA = diazepam; ETZ = etizolam; IBU = ibuprofen; IMI = imipramine; LRZ = lorazepam; PBO = placebo; PRO = propranolol; TRZ = trazodone.

that alprazolam is superior to placebo and comparable to a number of other agents, notably the tricyclic antidepressants. Other open evaluations of alprazolam confirm its efficacy as an antipanic drug.

The effective doses of alprazolam in clinical studies have varied widely, with up to 10 mg/day being necessary in some patients and as low as 0.5 mg/day in others. An average dose of 4–6 mg/day is generally regarded as effective in the majority of patients.[9] Alprazolam acts rapidly in alleviating panic attacks. For example, in the Cross National Panic Disorder Study,[10] half of the eventual improvement observed in the frequency of panic attacks was noted after the first week of treatment. Further slower improvements were noted with continued treatment. This is in contrast to studies with imipramine or phenelzine, where 3–6 weeks are necessary for marked improvement to occur.[11] A further advantage of alprazolam is that it is better tolerated than the antidepressants because it has fewer side-effects.

Alprazolam is not without side-effects or adverse reactions, and these are well documented for the Cross National Study.[12] The major side-effects that became worse with alprazolam to a greater degree than with placebo were sedation, ataxia, fatigue, slurred speech, amnesia, change in libido, constipation and incontinence. Only sedation, ataxia and fatigue were worse with alprazolam than placebo throughout the eight weeks of treatment. In addition to these side-effects, several potentially serious adverse events occurred during treatment. Severe intoxication occurred in three subjects receiving 1–2 mg/day of alprazolam, amnesia in another subject receiving 6 mg/day, and aggressive behaviour in another subject on 4 mg/day; two subjects developed hepatitis probably related to alprazolam; two subjects became hypomanic and another experienced an episode of major depression while receiving alprazolam. However, the very large size of this trial (over 1100 patients) means that the incidence of these adverse events was less than 4%, while most patients who received alprazolam experienced some side-effects.

Clonazepam

Clonazepam is a 1,4-benzodiazepine derivative (Figure 10.2) that is most often used for the treatment of certain types of seizures.[13] Like alprazolam, it has a high affinity for the benzodiazepine-binding site, but its half-life of elimination is much longer (20–80 hours compared with 10–14 hours). This latter property makes the drug suitable for once-daily dosing, while its potency at benzodiazepine receptors suggests that it may have antipanic efficacy equal to that of alprazolam.

The antipanic efficacy of clonazepam was first suggested by Fontaine and Chouinard.[14] At doses of 6–9 mg/day, clonazepam produced marked improvement in 10 of 12 patients with panic disorder. Clonazepam, because of its pharmacokinetic properties, was regarded as easier to use than alprazolam, which requires three-times-a-day dosage. A more extensive evaluation was conducted by Herman et al.[15] From patients treated for panic disorder with alprazolam, 48 who were experiencing inter-dose anxiety symptoms were switched to clonazepam. Clinical responses to clonazepam were rated better by 82% of patients. The average dose of clonazepam was 1.5 mg/day and was well tolerated. Although this was an open evaluation, it suggests the efficacy of clonazepam for panic attacks, which has been confirmed in subsequent studies. In these later studies, lower doses than that originally reported[14] have also been confirmed.

The side-effects reported with clonazepam treatment were typically sedation and ataxia. Most often, these were of mild to moderate severity, and usually diminished on continued treatment.[16] Follow-up of patients treated for a year with clonazepam has been reported.[17] Of 50 patients studied initially in an acute phase, 20 remained on clonazepam for one year and 18 had a positive response to the drug. The average dose required for these patients was 2.3 ± 1.6 mg/day, which was not significantly different from the dose requirement at the end of the acute phase (1.9 mg/day). Tolerance was not a significant problem in this group of patients. The main reasons for discontinuing clonazepam were lack of efficacy and side-effects – most often sedation, irritability and depression.

Diazepam

As noted previously, some studies suggest that diazepam has an antipanic effect, albeit at higher doses than those normally prescribed for generalized anxiety disorder. Noyes and colleagues[5] first challenged the notion of the ineffectiveness of benzodiazepines in the treatment of panic disorder in a two-week, double-blind, crossover study comparing diazepam and propranolol. Diazepam moderately improved 86% of patients compared with 33% receiving propranolol. There was no effect of propranolol on panic attacks, whereas it was reported that diazepam substantially reduced them. More convincing evidence for the efficacy of diazepam in panic disorder was provided in a three-way, double-blind comparison with alprazolam and placebo.[6] Both diazepam and alprazolam were more effective than placebo in blocking panic attacks, but at relatively high doses: 44 mg/day and 4 mg/day respectively. Similar findings were reported by Roy-Byrne and colleagues[18] in a three-way, double-blind comparison of diazepam, alprazolam and placebo. Diazepam at an average dose of 56 mg/day and alprazolam at an average dose of 4.3 mg/day were equally effective against panic attacks and more effective than placebo. Recently, a two-site, three-way, comparative study of diazepam, alprazolam and placebo in DSM-III panic disorder was reported.[7] Subjects were randomly allocated to one of the three treatment arms and the dose of drug adjusted according to individual response. Ratings of panic attacks, based on patient diaries, as well as anxiety, agoraphobic symptoms and depression were performed through the eight-week study period. A total of 241 subjects were enrolled in the study, with approximately 80 subjects in each group. At both weeks 4 and 8 of treatment, subjects on both active drugs experienced fewer panic attacks than those on placebo. The proportion of patients free of panic attacks at the end of the trial was 62.8% on diazepam, 71.4% on alprazolam and 37.5% on placebo, a highly statistically significant difference between active groups and placebo. No significant differences were noted between diazepam and alprazolam (Figure 10.3). At week 8, the mean dose of diazepam was 43 mg/day and that of alprazolam 4.9 mg/day, while an average of 7.4 capsules of placebo were taken. The data from this study confirm the efficacy of relatively high doses of diazepam for the treatment of panic attacks.

Other benzodiazepines

Limited clinical trials suggest that other high-potency benzodiazepines may also be effective in treating panic disorder. Clobazam, a 1,5-benzodiazepine (see Figure 10.1) has been evaluated in the treatment of panic attacks. An open evaluation noted the marked effects of clobazam in 11 patients with 'raptus' anxiety, which may have been panic attacks.[19] The effect of clobazam in 10 patients with DSM-III panic disorder or agoraphobia with panic attacks was evaluated over eight weeks of treatment.[20] Response, defined as a 75% reduction in the number of panic attacks from baseline, was observed in 6 of the 10 subjects, partial response in 2 subjects and no response in 2. Responders to medication achieved an average dose of 50 ± 17 mg/day of clobazam, which was well tolerated, with mild to moderate side-effects. The main emergent side-effects were sedation, lightheadedness, fatigue, weakness and headache. In this short evaluation, tolerance to the effects of clobazam did not

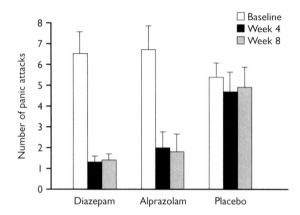

Figure 10.3 Comparative efficacies of alprazolam, diazepam and placebo in the treatment of panic attacks. Data are mean (±SEM) numbers of panic attacks in the past week. Results are taken from reference 7.

develop, while on withdrawal of the drug, by gradual dose tapering, there was no evidence of a withdrawal syndrome. Two cases of withdrawal syndrome have been described in which the patients were using clobazam for six months or more.[21] The syndrome was characterized by sleep disturbance, increased tension and anxiety, and perceptual disturbances (e.g. intolerance to light and sound). This report suggests that, on long-term administration, clobazam may prove difficult to withdraw.

There have also been three positive studies with the commonly used benzodiazepine lorazepam. The first of these[22] compared lorazepam with phenelzine, in a flexible-dose open trial with random patient allocation. Twenty-two patients were treated for three months with each drug and all patients also received group behavioural therapy. Both drugs appeared to be equally effective. However, the clinical effects began in the first 1–2 weeks with

lorazepam, whereas they were delayed for 4–6 weeks with phenelzine. The average doses of the drugs were 3.8 ± 1.3 mg/day lorazepam and 53 ± 12 mg/day phenelzine.

Subsequently, Charney and colleagues[23,24] conducted two studies comparing lorazepam and alprazolam. The first, on 48 patients, showed relatively equivalent efficacy of alprazolam and lorazepam in a double-blind study for six weeks. The later study was a six-week, multicentre, double-blind study of 102 patients treated for eight weeks (two weeks placebo washout and six weeks active treatment). Again, both drug groups showed a similar and significant decrease in anxiety symptoms. In both, the improvement began early in treatment (the first week). Spontaneous panic attack frequencies were reduced by both drugs, with lorazepam producing a 90% reduction and alprazolam an 83% reduction by the sixth week.

The dimethylamino derivative of alprazolam, adinazolam (see Figure 10.2) has been examined as an antipanic agent. In a double-blind, placebo-controlled, crossover study adinazolam 10–120 mg/day was compared with alprazolam 0.5–6 mg/day over a four-week period.[25] Both drugs were equally effective in the alleviation of panic attacks. Given the lack of a placebo control group and the relatively small number of patients involved, the data suggested further evaluation of the compound. Recent studies have focused on the use of a sustained-release formulation of the drug. Davidson and colleagues[26] treated 202 patients with panic disorder and agoraphobia for four weeks with either adinazolam sustained release or placebo. At the end of the study, 57.1% of adinazolam-treated compared with 39.2% of placebo-treated patients were free of panic attacks – a statistically significant difference. The relationship of dose of adinazolam sustained release to efficacy in panic disorder with agoraphobia was investigated in a double-blind, placebo-controlled, fixed-dose study.[27] Approximately 80 patients per group were randomized to receive placebo, 30, 60 or 90 mg/day administered as a divided dose for four weeks. Both the 60 and 90 mg/day groups were superior to the placebo and 30 mg/day groups for all clinical measures of anxiety and total number of panic attacks. Adinazolam is an alternative benzodiazepine for the treatment of panic disorder, although it is not yet available for this purpose.

The possible efficacy of another high potency 1,4-benzodiazepine, bromazepam (Figure 10.2), in the treatment of panic attacks has been suggested from a case report.[28] After four weeks of treatment with 18 mg/day bromazepam, a 28-year-old female patient with panic attacks improved markedly. Following withdrawal of bromazepam and substitution of placebo, she relapsed, and was later treated with a combination of imipramine and bromazepam with good response. Although by no means a definitive study, the data suggest that further evaluation of bromazepam in panic disorder would be worthwhile. As noted in Table 10.1, lorazepam has also been used as a comparative agent in clinical trials in panic disorder, and is an effective agent in this condition.

It can be concluded from this brief overview that, contrary to early clinical opinion, benzodiazepines are effective drugs in the treatment of panic disorder. Commonly, a marked reduction in the number of panic attacks is seen within the first week of treatment, while there is also a reduction of anticipatory anxiety. Benzodiazepines tend to be well tolerated, with oversedation being the major side-effect during treatment. Against their perceived advantages are the risks of dependence and withdrawal, which appear to be greater in patients with a history of personality disorder or substance abuse.[29] In such patients, the use of antidepressants may be more appropriate.

Duration of treatment

For the majority of patients presenting for treatment, panic disorder is usually a chronic illness, often for a period of a decade or more.[1] Usually, despite its chronic nature, panic disorder has a fluctuating course, and in all likelihood will require long-term therapy. Despite the lack of a substantial body of controlled trials to support the long-term use of benzodiazepines in panic disorder[30] and the recommendations of some authorities to the contrary,[31,32] this is often clinical practice. In generalized anxiety disorder, limited data suggest that benzodiazepines are effective in the longer term.[33,34] Panic disorder is another condition where long-term therapy has been recommended.[35]

As part of the Cross National Panic Disorders Study, a subgroup of 85 patients with panic disorder (69 receiving alprazolam and 16 on placebo) were followed up for 24 weeks after their initial 8 weeks of treatment.[30] Double-blind treatment was maintained throughout the follow-up period, and regular ratings of panic attacks, anxiety and side-effects were completed. Throughout this period, alprazolam maintained its efficacy in blocking panic attacks without an increase in dose, suggesting that tolerance to the therapeutic effects did not develop. The average dose of alprazolam at week 8 was 5.3 ± 2.3 mg/day, which had decreased to 4.7 ± 2.1 mg/day at week 32. Other rating scales used also suggested a lack of therapeutic tolerance to the drug. On the other hand, the well-recognized tolerance to the side-effects of benzodiazepines did develop, as assessed by comparing the rate of appearance of side-effects during the acute and chronic phases.

In a similar study, the efficacies of alprazolam, imipramine and placebo were compared in 181 patients treated double-blind for up to

32 weeks.[1] Therapeutic gains following acute dosing were maintained for both drugs in the longer term without the necessity to increase the dose of either agent. This again supports the contention that therapeutic tolerance to benzodiazepines does not develop at least out to eight months and possibly beyond.

Evidence for the continued efficacy of alprazolam up to and beyond one year of treatment was found in two naturalistic follow-ups of patients with panic disorder. After one year of treatment, patients who continued on alprazolam, either alone or in combination with various behavioural therapies, had significantly decreased panic attack frequency compared with baseline.[36] More than half of the patients were panic-free. Similar results were observed for a group of patients treated with alprazolam and behavioural therapy for four months and followed up by interview two to four years later.[37] No tolerance to the antipanic effect of alprazolam was observed, while the dose of drug was the same or lower in 65% of patients, higher in 5% and discontinued in 30%. Remission was achieved by about 40% of patients.

A group of 50 patients treated initially with clonazepam was followed up over one year.[17] A positive response to treatment was maintained by 62% of subjects, while clonazepam dosage increased slightly from 1.9 mg/day at four months to 2.3 mg/day at one year. Tolerance to the therapeutic effects of clonazepam was not a significant problem.

Efficacy after drug withdrawal

One of the important issues concerning the use of medications in the treatment of panic disorder is whether or not short- or long-term therapy with these agents provides lasting gains once they are withdrawn. Additionally for the benzodiazepines, the optimal strategies to adopt to avoid the withdrawal syndrome need to be considered as well; for instance, Otto et al[38] have shown that cognitive–behavioural therapy is effective.

Evidence suggests that relapse is frequent once medications are withdrawn. In 18 patients treated for 12–47 weeks with alprazolam for panic disorder, a rapid recurrence of panic attacks was noted, including 14 patients who were previously panic-free.[39] Despite a slow tapered medication withdrawal schedule in this study, the majority of patients experienced a withdrawal syndrome characterized by the appearance of new symptoms. This contrasts with the 30 day taper from the phase I alprazolam/placebo trial that found 35% withdrawal rate and 35% rebound rate.[40] Nevertheless, about a third of patients were experiencing few or no panic attacks 1–5 months after completing drug withdrawal. For these patients, recurrence of panic may be temporary – a finding supported by studies of alprazolam after short-term administration.[41]

Withdrawal of alprazolam and diazepam compared with placebo was studied following short-term administration for the treatment of panic disorder.[18] A tapered withdrawal schedule was used for two days, then drugs were abruptly withdrawn when the dose was about half. When tapered to about half the dose, there were few differences between drugs and placebo. Abrupt withdrawal caused marked increases in anxiety, but not panic attacks, for alprazolam, and less effects for diazepam – but still more than placebo patients, who showed little or no effect. Rather than withdrawal, the effects recorded in this study may represent a rebound of the underlying anxiety state.

By contrast, severe difficulties were experienced by 20–30% of 88 patients with panic disorder treated for up to eight months with alprazolam, diazepam or placebo during tapered withdrawal over a 4–6-week period.[42] Significantly, 46 of the 88 subjects were not able to successfully complete the taper. For patients completing the taper, there was no difference with respect to difficulties encountered between active drugs and placebo. Somewhat different results were reported for 50 patients withdrawing from alprazolam, diazepam or placebo after eight months treatment.[43] Following a slow taper, alprazolam withdrawal was associated with more distress than discontinuation from diazepam. Following complete withdrawal from the drugs, a 70–80% relapse rate was noted. Relapse was more likely to occur in the more severely ill patients, while rebound and withdrawal syndrome were more closely allied to plasma elimination half-life.

Conclusions

It can be concluded from these studies that benzodiazepines maintain their efficacy as antipanic agents during chronic therapy. Significant tolerance to the therapeutic effects does not appear to occur, with lower doses often employed during maintenance treatment. Similar conclusions have been reached regarding chronic benzodiazepine therapy in generalized anxiety disorder.[34] Relapse rates are high when benzodiazepines are withdrawn, while many patients experience a withdrawal syndrome even during a slow tapering of the drug. In benzodiazepine-dependent patients, withdrawal reactions were observed in the majority of patients following abrupt discontinuation of the drug.[44] Peak severity occurred 2–7 days after discontinuation, but, for those patients able to remain drug-free, anxiety scores fell to below the levels before discontinuation. During tapered withdrawal, 90% of patients experienced a withdrawal reaction of mild to moderate severity.[45] About one-third of patients were not able to achieve drug-free status. Despite the pessimism of some workers associated with the results, it has been suggested that the risks of dependence on, and addiction to, benzodiazepines is low compared with their widespread use.[46] Furthermore, most long-term users can discontinue the drugs if required. This contention is supported by the observation that 73% of patients who were tapered off benzodiazepines were still drug-free after three years.[47] Benzodiazepine overuse may have been exaggerated, and some patients who would otherwise benefit from the drugs are being denied effective therapy.[46]

The effects of benzodiazepine withdrawal are well recognized.[48-52] While a high dose and long duration of benzodiazepine administration is most often associated with withdrawal syndromes, both short-term therapy[52] and normal or low doses[49] are also implicated in withdrawal phenomena. A practical approach to the withdrawal of benzodiazepines has been described.[53] Experiencing withdrawal effects of benzodiazepines could lead to reinstituting the drug and reinforcing psychological and physical dependence. Non-pharmacological management of anxiety states may be particularly beneficial, and should not be overlooked. Although most controlled trials are drug-only for panic attacks, in clinical practice it is common to use a combination of pharmacotherapy and behavioural therapy. Behavioural or cognitive therapy commenced during maintenance may help alleviate some of the problems associated with drug withdrawal and may prevent relapse. This assertion needs to be tested by appropriate studies.

Finally, although this chapter has focussed on the use of benzodiazepines as primary treatments for panic disorder they are often co-prescribed as adjunctive agents when other drug therapies are used. This is particularly common when the SSRIs are instigated in PD. They can cause an exacerbation of anxiety plus some worsening of sleep early in treatment. Many experts advise covering patients with a benzo-diazepine during this period and then taking it off after 2–4 weeks once the anti-panic benefits of the antidepressant have become established.[69]

References

1. Ballenger JC, Long-term pharmacologic treatment of panic disorder. *J Clin Psychiatry* 1991; **52**(Suppl 2): 18–23.

2. Weissman MM, Panic disorder: impact on quality of life. *J Clin Psychiatry* 1991; **52**(Suppl 2): 6–8.

3. Burrows GD, Norman TR, Judd FK, Panic disorder: a treatment update. *J Clin Psychiatry* 1991; **52**(Suppl 7): 24–6.

4. Judd FK, Norman TR, Burrows GD, Pharmacotherapy of panic disorder. *Int Rev Psychiatry* 1990; **2**: 399–410.

5. Noyes R, Anderson DJ, Clancy J et al, Diazepam and propranolol in panic disorder and agoraphobia. *Arch Gen Psychiatry* 1984; **41**: 287–92.

6. Dunner DL, Ishiki D, Avery DH et al, Effect of alprazolam and diazepam on anxiety and panic attacks in panic disorder: a controlled study. *J Clin Psychiatry* 1986; **47**: 458–60.

7. Noyes R, Burrows GD, Reich JH et al, Diazepam versus alprazolam for treatment of panic disorder. *J Clin Psychiatry* 1996; **57**: 349–55.

8. Chouinard G, Annable L, Fontaine R, Solyom L, Alprazolam in the treatment of generalised anxiety and panic disorders: a double-blind, placebo controlled study. *Psychopharmacology* 1982; **77**: 229–33.

9. Sheehan DV, Current perspectives in the treatment of panic and phobic disorders. *Drug Ther* 1982; **12**: 49–57.

10. Ballenger JC, Burrows GD, DuPont RL et al, Alprazolam in panic disorder and agoraphobia: results from a multicentre trial. I. Efficacy in short-term treatment. *Arch Gen Psychiatry* 1988; **45**: 413–22.

11. Levin AP, Liebowitz MR, Drug treatment of phobias: efficacy and optimum use. *Drugs* 1987; **34**: 504–14.

12. Noyes R, DuPont RL, Pecknold JC et al, Alprazolam in panic disorder and agoraphobia: results from a multicenter trial II. Patient acceptance, side effects, and safety. *Arch Gen Psychiatry* 1988; **45**: 423–8.

13. Browne TR, Drug therapy: clonazepam. *N Engl J Med* 1978; **299**: 812–16.

14. Fontaine R, Chouinard G, Antipanic effect of clonazepam. *Am J Psychiatry* 1984; **141**: 149.

15. Herman JB, Rosenbaum JF, Brotman AW, The alprazolam to clonazepam switch for the treatment of panic disorder. *J Clin Psychopharmacol* 1987; **7**: 175–8.

16. Svebak S, Cameron A, Levander S, Clonazepam and imipramine in the treatment of panic attacks: a double-blind comparison of efficacy and side effects. *J Clin Psychiatry* 1990; **51**(Suppl 5): 14–17.

17. Pollack MH, Tesar GE, Rosenbaum JF, Spier SC, Clonazepam in the treatment of panic disorder and agoraphobia: a one-year follow-up. *J Clin Psychopharmacol* 1986; **6**: 302–4.

18. Roy-Byrne P, Dagen SF, Cowley DS et al, Relapse and rebound following discontinuation of benzodiazepine treatment of panic attacks: alprazolam versus diazepam. *Am J Psychiatry* 1989; **146**: 860–5.

19. Gisselman A, Bouhey J, Mignot G, Marin A, Essai ouvert d'une nouvelle benzodiazepine: le clobazam. *Psychol Medicale* 1976; **8**: 1421–8.

20. Judd FK, Burrows GD, Marriott PF, Norman TR, A short term open clinical trial of clobazam in the treatment of patients with panic attacks. *Int Clin Psychopharmacol* 1989; **4**: 285–93.

21. Peturrson H, Lader MH, Withdrawal reaction from clobazam. *Br Med J* 1981; **282**: 1931–2.

22. Howell EF, Laraia M, Ballenger JC, Lydiard RB, Lorazepam treatment of panic disorder. In: *New Research Programs and Abstracts, 140th Annual Meeting of the American Psychiatric Association*, 1987: Abst NR 466, 111.

23. Charney DS, Woods SW, Goodman WK et al, The efficacy of lorazepam in panic disorders. In: *New Research Programs and Abstracts, 140th Annual Meeting of the American Psychiatric Association*, 1987: Abst NR 165, 119.

24. Charney DS, Woods SW, Benzodiazepine treatment of panic disorder. A comparison of alprazolam and lorazepam. *J Clin Psychiatry* 1989; **50:** 418–23.

25. Pyke RE, Greenberg HS, Double-blind comparison of alprazolam and adinazolam for panic and phobic disorders. *J Clin Psychopharmacol* 1989; **9:** 15–21.

26. Davidson JR, Beitman B, Greist JH et al, Adinazolam sustained-release treatment of panic disorder: a double-blind study. *J Clin Psychopharmacol* 1994; **14:** 255–63.

27. Carter CS, Fawcett J, Hertzman M et al, Adinazolam-SR in panic disorder with agoraphobia: relationship of daily dose to efficacy. *J Clin Psychiatry* 1995; **56:** 202–10.

28. Beaudry P, Fontaine R, Chouinard G, Bromazepam, another high potency benzodiazepine, for panic attacks. *Am J Psychiatry* 1984; **141:** 464–5.

29. Salzman C, Benzodiazepine treatment of panic and agoraphobic symptoms: use, dependence toxicity, abuse. *J Psychiat Res* 1992; **27**(Suppl 1): 97–110.

30. Burrows GD, Judd FK, Norman TR, Long term drug treatment of panic disorder. *J Psychiat Res* 1992; **27**(Suppl 1): 111–25.

31. Committee on the Review of Medicines, Systemic review of the benzodiazepines. *Br Med J* 1980; **i:** 910–12.

32. Greenblatt DJ, Shader RI, Abernethy DR, Current status of the benzodiazepines. *N Engl J Med* 1983; **309:** 410–16.

33. Fabre LF, McLendon DM, Stephens AG, Comparison of the therapeutic effect, tolerance and safety of ketazolam and diazepam administered for six months to outpatients with chronic anxiety neurosis. *J Int Med Res* 1981; **9:** 191–8.

34. Rickels K, Case G, Downing RG, Winokur A, Long-term diazepam therapy and clinical outcome. *J Am Med Assoc* 1983; **250:** 767–71.

35. Rickels K, Antianxiety therapy: potential value of long-term treatment. *J Clin Psychiatry* 1987; **48**(Suppl): 7–11.

36. Judd FK, Burrows GD, Norman TR, Follow-up study of patients with panic disorder. *Arch Gen Psychiatry* 1991; **48:** 860–2.

37. Nagy LM, Krystal JH, Woods SW, Charney DS, Clinical and medication outcome after short-term alprazolam and behavioral group treatment in panic disorder. *Arch Gen Psychiatry* 1989; **46:** 993–9.

38. Otto MW, Pollack MH, Sachs GS et al, Discontinuation of benzodiazepine treatment: efficacy of cognitive–behavioral therapy for patients with panic disorder. *Am J Psychiatry* 1993; **150:** 1485–90.

39. Fyer AJ, Liebowitz MR, Gorman JM et al, Discontinuation of alprazolam treatment in panic patients. *Am J Psychiatry* 1987; **144:** 303–8.

40. Howell SF, Laraia M, Ballenger JC, Lydiard RB, Lorazepam treatment of panic disorder. In: *New Research Programs and Abstracts, 140th Annual Meeting of the American Psychiatric Association*, 1987: Abst NR 166, 111.

41. DuPont RL, Pecknold JC, Alprazolam withdrawal in panic disorder patients. In: *New Research Abstracts of the 138th Annual Meeting of the American Psychiatric Association, Washington, DC*, 1985.

42. Burrows GD, Norman TR, Judd FK, Marriott PF, Short-acting versus long-acting benzodiazepines: discontinuation effects in panic disorders. *J Psychiat Res* 1990; **24**(Suppl 2): 65–72.

43. Noyes R, Garvey MJ, Cook B, Suelzer M, Controlled discontinuation of benzodiazepine treatment for patients with panic disorder. *Am J Psychiatry* 1991; **148:** 517–23.

44. Rickels K, Schweizer E, Case WG, Greenblatt DJ, Long-term therapeutic use of benzodiazepines I: Effects of abrupt discontinuation. *Arch Gen Psychiatry* 1990; **47:** 899–907.

45. Schweizer E, Rickels K, Case WG, Greenblatt DJ, Long-term therapeutic use of benzodiazepines II: Effects of gradual taper. *Arch Gen Psychiatry* 1990; **47:** 908–15.

46. Uhlenhuth EH, DeWit H, Balter M et al, Risks and benefits of long-term benzodiazepine use. *J Clin Psychopharmacol* 1988; **8:** 161–7.

47. Rickels K, Case WG, Schweizer E et al, Long-term benzodiazepine users 3 years after participation in a discontinuation program. *Am J Psychiatry* 1991; **148**: 757–61.

48. Greenblatt DJ, Shader RI, Dependence, tolerance and addiction to benzodiazepines: clinical and pharmacokinetic considerations. *Drug Metab Rev* 1978; **8**: 13–28.

49. Hallstrom C, Lader MH, Benzodiazepine withdrawal phenomenon. *Int Pharmacopsychiatry* 1981; **16**: 235–44.

50. Owen RT, Tyrer P, Benzodiazepine dependence: a review of the evidence. *Drugs* 1983; **25**: 385–98.

51. Browne JL, Hauge KJ, A review of alprazolam withdrawal. *Drug Intelligence Clin Pharmacy* 1986; **20**: 837–41.

52. Tyrer P, Murphy S, The place of benzodiazepines in psychiatric practice. *Br J Psychiatry* 1987; **151**: 719–23.

53. DuPont RL, A practical approach to benzodiazepine discontinuation. *J Psychiat Res* 1990; **24**(Suppl 2): 81–90.

54. Sheehan DV, Coleman JH, Greenblatt DJ et al, Some biochemical correlates of panic attacks with agoraphobia and their response to a new treatment. *J Clin Psychopharmacol* 1984; **4**: 66–75.

55. Wilcox JA, An open comparison of diazepam and alprazolam. *J Psychoactive Drugs* 1986; **18**: 159–60.

56. Charney DS, Woods SW, Goodman WK et al, Drug treatment of panic disorder: the comparative efficacy of imipramine, alprazolam and trazodone. *J Clin Psychiatry* 1986; **47**: 580–6.

57. Rizley R, Kahn RJ, McNair DM et al, A comparison of alprazolam and imipramine in the treatment of agoraphobia and panic disorder. *Psychopharmacol Bull* 1986; **22**: 167–72.

58. Meco G, Capriani C, Bonifati V et al, Etizolam: a new therapeutic possibility in the treatment of panic disorder. *Adv Ther* 1989; **6**: 196–206.

59. Uhlenhuth EH, Matuzas W, Glass RM et al, Response of panic disorder to fixed doses of alprazolam or imipramine. *J Affect Disord* 1989; **17**: 261–70.

60. Charney DS, Woods SW, Benzodiazepine treatment of panic disorder: a comparison of alprazolam and lorazepam. *J Clin Psychiatry* 1989; **50**: 418–23.

61. Munjack DJ, Crocker B, Cabe D et al, Alprazolam, propranolol and placebo in the treatment of panic disorder and agoraphobia with panic attacks. *J Clin Psychopharmacol* 1989; **9**: 22–7.

62. Taylor CB, Hayward C, King R et al, Cardiovascular and symptomatic reduction effects of alprazolam and imipramine in patients with panic disorder: results of a double-blind, placebo controlled trial. *J Clin Psychopharmacol* 1990; **10**: 112–18.

63. Lepola U, Heikkinen H, Rimon R et al, Clinical evaluation of alprazolam in patients with panic disorder: a double blind comparison with imipramine. *Hum Psychopharmacol* 1990; **5**: 159–64.

64. Schweizer E, Pohl R, Balon R et al, Lorazepam v alprazolam in the treatment of panic disorder. *Pharmacopsychiatry* 1990; **23**: 90–3.

65. Tesar GE, Rosenbaum JF, Pollack MH et al, Double-blind, placebo controlled comparison of clonazepam and alprazolam for panic disorder. *J Clin Psychiatry* 1991; **52**: 69–76.

66. Ravaris CL, Friedman MJ, Havri PJ et al, A controlled study of alprazolam and propranolol in panic-disordered and agoraphobic outpatients. *J Clin Psychopharmacol* 1991; **11**: 344–50.

67. Cross-National Collaborative Panic Study, Drug treatment of panic disorder. *Br J Psychiatry* 1992; **160**: 191–202.

68. Marks IM, Swinson RP, Basoglu M et al, Alprazolam and exposure alone and combined in panic disorder with agoraphobia. *Br J Psychiatry* 1993; **162**: 776–87.

69. Nutt DJ, The psychopharmacology of anxiety. *Br J Hosp Med* 1996; **55**: 187–91.

11

Selective serotonin reuptake inhibitors (SSRIs) in panic disorder

James C Ballenger

Introduction

Over the past 25 years, we have witnessed the development of multiple effective treatments for panic disorder (PD). Both psychological and pharmacological treatments have been shown to be effective in PD, including most of the tricyclic antidepressants (TCAs), the monoamine oxidase inhibitor (MAOI) antidepressants and high-potency benzodiazepines (BZs), particularly alprazolam and clonazepam. However, during a recent NIMH Algorithm Development Meeting, the expert panel reached the conclusion that the selective serotonin reuptake inhibitors (SSRIs) had in fact become the pharmacological treatment of choice for PD.[1] This was in spite of the fact that, except for clomipramine and fluvoxamine, there were almost no controlled data to support this conclusion. As this chapter will review, there is now a large body of evidence documenting that the SSRIs are effective and probably deserve to be the pharmacological treatment of first choice in PD for many patients.

Preclinical animal studies of the role of 5-HT in panic disorder

Although the role of serotonin (5-hydroxytryptamine, 5-HT) in PD is controversial, there is considerable evidence that it is, in fact, involved.[2–4] The 5-HT inhibitor, *p*-chlorophenylalanine (PCPA) has been shown to reduce anxiety in multiple paradigms in animals.[4] The 5-HT precursor 5-hydroxytryptophan reverses the anxiety reducing effects of PCPA.[5,6] When the 5-HT-rich median raphe nucleus is simulated, behavioral inhibition is produced and is thought to be an anxiety equivalent. These effects are reversed by the injection of 5-HT into the raphe[7] or when PCPA is administered.[8] Other investigators utilizing similar techniques have been less supportive of the role of 5-HT in anxiety.[9,10]

Other studies suggest that reduced 5-HT activity is anxiolytic. Serotonin antagonists and 5-HT lesions both decrease suppressed behavior,[11] and electrical stimulation increases behavioral suppression.[6,8]

In the model of separation-induced distress cries, there are seemingly contradictory observations. The separation-induced vocalizations are thought to represent a good animal model of panic/agoraphobic anxiety; these separation vocalizations are increased following 5-HT blockade with methysergide,[12] and clomipramine and paroxetine reduce these vocalizations.[13]

It is difficult to reach a clear-cut conclusion based on preclinical animal studies because of the observations that both increasing and decreasing 5-HT function are associated with reduction in anxiety. This leaves open the possibility that both increases and decreases in 5-HT function, perhaps in different parts of the brain, may be helpful in panic anxiety (see below).

Human studies of 5-HT function in panic anxiety
Challenge studies

If panic patients have abnormal serotonin function, one might reason that the 5-HT agonist *m*-chlorophenylpiperazine (mCPP) might have a different response in panic patients versus controls, although mCPP did induce anxiety in both groups. Charney and colleagues[15] observed no differences between PD patients and controls. In a subsequent study with lower doses, they were able to demonstrate increased effects in PD patients.[14] Consistent with this latter study, Kahn and colleagues[16] observed increased anxiety and panic attacks in 60% of PD patients, which they interrupted as reflecting hypersensitive post-synaptic 5-HT receptors.

Fenfluramine

In a similar fashion, Targum and colleagues[17] demonstrated an enhanced response to fenflu-

ramine, which is thought to release 5-HT and to have direct postsynaptic agonist effects.

The ability of lactate infusion and CO_2 inhalations to stimulate panic attacks in PD subjects but rarely in normals has also been linked to the 5-HT system.[18–20] Both have been demonstrated to increase brain 5-HT reuptake.[21,22]

Chemical studies in humans

Although contradictory, some studies do suggest abnormalities in 5-HT function in human patients. The growth hormone response to clonidine infusion is thought to reflect serotonin activity[23] and has been demonstrated to be blunted in PD patients.[24] Cerebrospinal fluid (CSF) concentration of 5-hydroxyindoleacetic acid (5-HIAA), the principal serotonin metabolite, has been shown to correlate with anxiety in depressed individuals.[3] Platelet imipramine binding sites and 5-HT platelet transporter sites are both thought to reflect brain 5-HT functioning, and have been shown to be decreased in panic patients.[25–27] This was not replicated in a subsequent study.[28] However, in a similar fashion, Schneider and colleagues[29] observed low plasma serotonin levels in agoraphobic individuals.

Summary of studies of the role of 5-HT

The preclinical animal work and biological investigations in PD humans remain contradictory.[30,31] There are studies that suggest decreased 5-HT function in PD, and others that suggest increases. The suggestions of decreased 5-HT function in PD are consistent with the bulk of evidence that suggests that the SSRIs ameliorate PD by having a net increased effect on 5-HT neurotransmission in the brain by desensitization of somatodendritic autoreceptors.[32-35] Klein[36] has suggested that SSRIs may normalize abnormal internal controls to regulate perturbations in either direction, and Grove and colleagues[37] that they may regulate fluctuations in the dorsal raphe nucleus.

Serotonin reuptake inhibitors in panic disorder

The SSRI medications became available for use in Europe 25 years ago with the introduction of clomipramine. Zimelidine was available in the early 1980s in Europe, and was shown to be effective in PD before it was taken off the market because of adverse events. The remaining SSRIs have been available for less than a decade, and include fluvoxamine, fluoxetine, paroxetine, sertraline and citalopran.

Clomipramine

Although clomipramine is a TCA, it is included in this chapter for several reasons. It is an SSRI, but its actions are not as specific to serotonin neurons as the remaining SSRI agents discussed below. It has also been extensively studied, and for varying reasons (discussed below) has become the agent considered the 'gold standard' for treatment of PD in Europe. However, it was not widely available in the USA during much of this period of time, and has therefore occupied a less central position in the psychopharmacological treatment of PD in the USA.

The first study by Gloger and colleagues[38] in a small sample (N = 20) demonstrated that clomipramine was effective in 75% of these patients with PD or agoraphobia with panic attacks, and this study was one of the first to show a direct reduction in panic attack frequency. The medication was begun at 25 mg/day, and 40% of patients had an initial increase in the frequency and severity of panic attacks, thought to represent the 'hyperstimulation' excitatory effects of TCAs in PD patients. Beneficial effects began to appear toward the end of the second week. Although patients could reach a maximum of 75–100 mg/day, fully 45% of patients did not need more than 50 mg/day. Also, 85% of these patients improved to the point where they had only mild symptoms or none at all.

In a follow-up study by the same group,[39] even lower doses of clomipramine were effective. The average daily dose was 40 mg/day, with almost half of the patients receiving less than 25 mg/day. However, even with these low doses, 13 out of 17 patients became completely panic-free and the remaining four showed improvement in panic attack frequency. It was observed that higher doses were needed when agoraphobia was present – a finding also found with alprazolam[40] and with imipramine.[41]

After positive open trials by Pecknold and associates[42] and Caetano,[43] Johnston and colleagues[44] designed a large and methodologically rigorous trial with a sample of 108 agoraphobic women, who were studied in an eight-week, placebo-controlled, double-blind study. This was one of the first studies to investigate a diagnostically homogenous PD group with a placebo control. This study provided unequivocal controlled data documenting the clinical effectiveness of clomipramine in reducing not only panic attacks, but agoraphobic and depressive symptomatology as well.

Fahy and colleagues[45] compared clomipramine, placebo and lofepramine, a TCA with reduced anticholinergic side-effects. They studied 79 outpatients, who were treated initially with 50 mg/day, with increases to 100 mg, compared with 70 mg of lofepramine, which could be increased to a maximum of 140 mg/day over a two-week period. Clomipramine was more effective than both lofepramine and placebo, although 67% of patients in both active groups had resolution of their panic attacks, compared with only 42% of the placebo group. Interestingly, clomipramine's effects began in the second week. These patients could continue for a total of 24 weeks, and, at that point, 93% of the clomipramine patients were panic-free, compared with 64% of the lofepramine and 60% of the placebo group. Interestingly, there was little to no relapse from either drug following gradual taper of medication from week 12 on.

Hoffart and colleagues[46] studied a group of 18 patients with PD and agoraphobia who had failed to respond to inpatient behavioral treatment. They studied them in a 12-week placebo-controlled, double-blind, crossover study with a maximum dose of 150 mg clomipramine. The 17 of 18 patients who completed the trial did have significant reduction in their symptom scores while on clomipramine compared with placebo, demonstrating efficacy even in this very treatment-resistant group.

One study by Feet and colleagues[47] suggests a method to increase the response to clomipramine. They observed that dixtyrazine combined with imipramine had a greater anti-depressant effect, and reasoned that it could have similar results with clomipramine in PD. The patients treated with dixtyrazine and clomipramine did, in fact, experience significantly greater improvement than those treated with clomipramine alone.[48] This was one of the first studies to document that daily functioning was also significantly improved, especially in the dixtyrazine + clomipramine group. Not only was this combination treatment more effective, but side-effects were also found to be lower in that group.

These studies provide some confirmatory evidence suggesting serotonergic abnormalities in PD. In the Feet and Gotestan[48] study mentioned above, there was a positive correlation between the serum concentration of clomipramine, similar to the observation of Mavissakalian and Michelson that the anti-panic effect of imipramine was related to the imipramine and not desipramine metabolite levels (see Chapter 9).[49] Because imipramine and clomipramine are both more serotonergic than noradrenergic, this is supportive of a serotonin role in PD.

There were two studies that suggested that clomipramine was in fact the best of the available agents prior to the development of the SSRI class. In a study by Cassano and colleagues,[50] clomipramine was compared with imipramine (thought to be the best treatment at the time) in 59 PD patients. Both drugs were approximately equally effective, but clomipramine was more effective on some outcome measures and its effect was earlier, becoming evident at the end of the second week. In a subsequent trial, Modigh and colleagues[51] again compared imipramine and clomipramine with placebo in 57 PD patients. In this 12-week trial, both medications could be raised to a maximum of 250 mg/day, with mean doses of 124 ± 9 mg/day of imipramine and 109 ± 8 mg/day of clomipramine. Despite the lower doses of clomipramine, the effects on all major outcome measures (panic attacks, anticipatory anxiety, etc.) were significantly greater in the clomipramine group. The significant effects of clomipramine were observed by the end of the fourth week, in contrast to after eight weeks with imipramine patients. It was largely the two studies by Cassano[50] and Modigh[51] that established clomipramine as the so-called 'gold standard' of the antidepressant treatments of PD in Europe.

Den Boer and colleagues[52] compared clomipramine and a more modern SSRI, fluvoxamine, in a six-week trial of 58 mixed anxiety patients, 38 of who had agoraphobia with panic attacks. Doses were increased gradually over two weeks to a maximum dosage of 150 mg/day of clomipramine or 100 mg/day of fluvoxamine. Both drugs were felt to be about equal in efficacy, with approximately 60% of both patient groups experiencing almost complete amelioration of symptoms. There was some suggestion on the Symptom Checklist (SCL-90) that clomipramine's effects were superior to fluvoxamine, although this may have been related to the fact that doses of clomipramine were higher than that of fluvoxamine (150 mg/day versus 100 mg/day).

Clomipramine has recently been compared with paroxetine, the first of the more modern SSRIs released after fluvoxamine and citalopram (see below).

Fluvoxamine

A series of eight-week placebo-controlled trials have demonstrated that fluvoxamine is superior to placebo in the treatment of PD. The study of Asnis and colleagues[53] in 188 PD patients demonstrated significantly greater improvement with fluvoxamine than placebo in a well-controlled trial. Fluvoxamine was administered up to 300 mg/day. This was followed by a trial by Hoehn-Saric and colleagues[54] in 50 PD patients. The mean daily dose of fluvoxamine was 206.8 mg/day. Patients began to improve as early as the third week in terms of panic attacks, but improvement in anticipatory/general anxiety and depression did not occur until week six. However, by week eight, 61% of the fluvoxamine patients were panic-free (versus 22% of placebo).

This same group[55] reported another eight-week multicenter trial with 117 patients, again demonstrating reductions in panic attacks and the remaining other domains of PD symptomatology, including phobic avoidance and anticipatory anxiety. Woods and colleagues[56] studied 189 PD patients, with 58 fluvoxamine and 63 placebo patients completing the trial. Panic attacks began improving even in the first and second weeks of treatment, and, by study end, 64% of the fluvoxamine patients (versus 40% of placebo) were panic-free.

This is in contrast to the study by Nair and colleagues[57] comparing fluvoxamine, imipramine and placebo in 148 outpatients with PD. Despite treatment with 171.4 mg/day of fluvoxamine, compared with 164.4 mg/day of imipramine, the study failed to demonstrate efficacy for fluvoxamine, although significant differences were observed for imipramine. There was also a high drop-out rate of patients on fluvoxamine (62% compared with 32% on imipramine and 58% on placebo). Given the relatively large number of positive trials described above, it is difficult to know whether this trial failed to show a positive effect because of the high drop-out rate or because of differences in baseline panic attack frequency.

Holland and colleagues[58] studied 73 PD patients in a maintenance trial for a year after the patients completed the two double-blind, eight-week studies referred to above.[54,55] As has been found with other medications, treatment gains in the initial few months were maintained for a full year on fluvoxamine. There was also a high rate of tolerability of treatment with fluvoxamine for this year. Interestingly, the placebo patients in the short-term trials were switched to fluvoxamine and had similar positive responses over the long-term maintenance trial. Improvement was excellent in 82–100% of these patients over the long-term 12-month maintenance trial.

Fluvoxamine has been compared with cognitive therapy in two eight-week trials. Black and colleagues[59] studied 55 patients treated with a mean daily dose of 230 mg/day. In this trial, fluvoxamine was superior to both cognitive therapy and placebo, with 90% of the fluvoxamine group attaining moderate to marked improvement (versus 50% with cognitive therapy and 39% on placebo). Also, 81% of the fluvoxamine patients were free of panic attacks (53% in cognitive therapy and 29% of the placebo group). In this study, fluvoxamine also had earlier efficacy than cognitive therapy.

The findings of Black and colleagues are in contrast to those of Sharp and colleagues.[60] In their study of 190 patients with PD and agoraphobia, fluvoxamine and cognitive behavioral therapy (CBT) were much more comparable. Doses of fluvoxamine in this trial were only 150 mg/day, which may or may not have made a difference, since most of the previous trials, including the Black trial, used doses up to a maximum of 300 mg/day.

Black and colleagues[61] utilized their study comparing fluvoxamine with cognitive therapy and placebo to investigate potential predictors of response to fluvoxamine. They observed that a low panic attack severity score and absence of a comorbid personality disorder was predictive of a positive response to fluvoxamine in this trial.

In a similar study of predictors of positive response, Dewulf and colleagues[62] studied the treatment of 229 patients in a 12-week treatment trial with fluvoxamine. Similar to the findings of Black and colleagues,[61] baseline severity of illness, psychiatric antecedents, and duration of PD were all negative predictors of response. In this study, fluvoxamine was clearly an effective treatment in the outpatient setting.

Spiegel has recently performed an open trial for a year of PD complicated by depression. This is a very pertinent trial, because 80% of PD patients develop depression some time in their life.[63] In the Spiegel trial, 17 patients with a prior diagnosis of PD but with comorbid depression were treated with fluvoxamine averaging 213 mg/day. Patients improved greatly on all measures of PD, including panic attacks, anticipatory anxiety, depression and disability, but failed to improve in agoraphobic avoidance. This is consistent with the many other studies indicating that depressed PD patients do less well.[64]

There are several studies comparing the efficacy of fluvoxamine with other agents that are worth mentioning. As mentioned earlier, in a study of 50 PD patients, fluvoxamine was compared with clomipramine. Although both drugs were effective, the positive effects of clomipramine occurred earlier and were somewhat superior to those of fluvoxamine.[52] The van Vliet group[65] compared fluvoxamine and brofaramine, a reversible MAOI. Both groups responded quite well, with 93% of the brofaramine group and 87% of the fluvoxamine group rating themselves as much or very much improved after 12 weeks. There were no significant differences between the treatment groups.

Den Boer and colleagues[66,67] have conducted two studies that are pertinent to the potential mechanism of the SSRI efficacy in PD. In the first, they compared fluvoxamine with maprotiline, a specific norepinephrine (noradrenaline) reuptake blocker. Both drugs were given at doses averaging 150 mg/day, with 20 patients on fluvoxamine and 20 patients on maprotiline. The patients on fluvoxamine experienced significant decreases in panic attacks, as well as the other symptoms of PD, but significant improvement was not seen in the maprotiline patients. When maprotiline patients were switched to fluvoxamine, most responded well. This is one of the clearest studies suggesting that a serotonin medication is more efficacious than a noradrenergic one.

If there were postsynaptic hyperactivity in PD, as some preclinical studies suggest,

Ritanserin, a 5-HT$_2$ postsynaptic blocker, should have a more rapid action. In a further study by den Boer and colleagues, 20 patients on Ritanserin were compared with 20 on fluvoxamine. There were striking differences in clinical efficacy. Although 75% of the fluvoxamine patients improved, only 10% of the Ritanserin group and 5% of the placebo group showed significant improvement. These studies would suggest that 5-HT$_2$ postsynaptic hyperactivity is not a part of PD.

Citalopram

Although citalopram was introduced some time ago in Europe, there have been relatively few studies of its efficacy in PD.[68] In the largest published trial, Humble et al studied 20 patients with PD with and without agoraphobia in an open trial with citalopram. After eight weeks, 13 out of 17 patients had responded in terms of an antipanic effect, and there were decreases in anticipatory anxiety, agoraphobia and the somatic symptomatology of PD. Doses ranged from 30 to 60 mg/day. After this trial, 16 of the patients continued in a 15-month long-term maintenance trial, with 11 of these patients completing this portion of the study. Initial gains were maintained throughout this longer period, with further improvement in some patients, including two patients who had failed to respond in the initial eight-week trial. As in other trials, there was no tolerance to early positive effects. The mean dose of citalopram fell from 41 mg/day after eight weeks to 38 mg/day at the end of the 15-month trial. Bertani and colleagues[69] reported a positive response in 4 of 5 patients on 20–40 mg/day.

Wade and colleagues[70] and Lepola[71] recently reported results of an eight-week, double-blind, placebo-controlled, fixed-dose multicenter trial of citalopram and clomipramine in 475 PD patients. Although not effective in doses of 10–15 mg/day, citalopram in higher doses (20–60 mg/day) was significantly better than placebo in reducing panic attacks, as was clomipramine. The 20–30 mg/day dose range for citalopram appeared to be the most effective dose. Interestingly, positive effects of citalopram were not observed until week 12. It remains to be seen if citalopram's antipanic effects take longer to be manifest.

Longer-term follow-up studies of citalopram in PD are underway following the large trial described above, and preliminary results suggest maintenance of positive acute effects for over a year.[71]

Lepola and colleagues[72] studied the treatment of early onset of PD and school phobia utilizing citalopram in three young patients. Panic attacks decreased, as did the school phobia thought to be secondary to PD. The children responded to low doses of citalopram, generally administered in the morning, and had few to no side-effects.

Paroxetine

This was the first SSRI to obtain a licensed indication for panic (1995), and has been the most extensively studied of the SSRIs in panic disorder.

The first publication of a placebo-controlled randomized trial of a true SSRI other than with fluvoxamine was a study by Oehrberg and colleagues.[73] They treated 60 patients with paroxetine and 60 with placebo in seven Danish centers. All patients also received standard cognitive behavioral treatment in this 12-week trial. Many of the patients were agoraphobic, with moderate or severe avoidance behavior. There was a high completion rate, with 92% of paroxetine patients and 87% of placebo patients finishing the 12-week trial. There were a significantly greater number of patients who had at least a 50% reduction in the number of panic attacks at weeks 6, 9 and 12 of the trial, with 82% of the paroxetine group and 50% of the placebo reaching this criterion. At week 12, there was a significant difference favoring paroxetine in the number of patients who had none or only one panic attack in the final three weeks of the trial, with 36% of the paroxetine patients and 16% of placebo patients meeting this criteria. The mean number of panic attacks in the paroxetine group fell from 21.2 to 5.2, compared with the placebo group, which decreased from 26.4 to 16.6 over the final three weeks of the study (not statistically significant).

Improvements in the secondary measures of outcome, which include the Hamilton-Anxiety ratings (HAM-A) and the Clinical Global Response (CGR), were all significantly greater in the paroxetine group. Response began in the first three weeks, and was statistically significant in some measures by week 6 and then throughout the remainder of the trial. Although the majority of patients had agoraphobia, the authors do not mention the effects of paroxetine on agoraphobia avoidance in this trial.

Although this study was not designed to determine the effective dose, 75% of patients were treated with either 40 or 60 mg and 47% received 60 mg during the trial.

Paroxetine was well tolerated, with a low drop-out rate. Side-effects observed were those expected of an SSRI, and included nausea, sweating, headache, dizziness, asthenia, decreased libido and dry mouth. The so-called 'jitteriness syndrome' was not observed in this trial, and there were no drop-outs during the first week. This may relate to the slow increase in dose, which began at 10 mg, increasing to 20 mg over the first two weeks of the trial.

Even more definitive evidence was provided by the large trial carried in 39 centers in 13 countries, mainly in Europe.[73] This trial involved 367 patients randomized to paroxe-

tine ($N = 123$), clomipramine ($N = 121$) and placebo ($N = 123$). Again, the majority of patients (<80%) had significant agoraphobia avoidance. Patients from this study could choose at the end of the 12-week trial whether they wanted to enter a long-term extension of the study for nine months or be titrated off over a three-week period. Patients were abruptly discontinued from paroxetine; however, there was no evidence of a withdrawal syndrome.

Paroxetine and clomipramine were begun at 10 mg for three days, with increases to 20 mg of paroxetine and 50 mg of clomipramine at the end of the first week. Dosages ultimately ranged between 20 and 60 mg for paroxetine and between 50 and 150 mg for clomipramine.

Again, no patients from either the paroxetine or the clomipramine groups discontinued during the first week, suggesting the absence of the 'jitteriness syndrome', perhaps because they were both begun at a low dose of 10 mg. Dropouts for adverse effects were lower in the paroxetine group (4.1%) compared with the clomipramine (8.3%) and placebo (8.95%) groups.

Paroxetine was again more effective than placebo in reducing the total number of panic attacks to zero at weeks 6, 9 and 12. At week 12, a higher percentage of patients (50.9%) in the paroxetine group had no panic attacks, compared with 36.7% of the clomipramine group and 31.6% of the placebo group. Clomipramine was significantly better than placebo only at week 12. In reduction in mean number of panic attacks, paroxetine was actually more effective than placebo at week 12 and more effective than clomipramine at week 6.

A significantly greater percentage of patients on paroxetine than placebo experienced a greater than 50% reduction in panic attacks at weeks 9 and 12. At week 12, 76.1% of the paroxetine, 64.5% of the clomipramine and 60.0% of the placebo group had a greater than 50% reduction in panic attacks. Paroxetine was significantly greater than clomipromine at week 6.

In addition, the other measures of anxiety (HAM-A, CGI-S and PGE) agoraphobia (MSPS), and measures of interference with work, social and family life (SDS) were all reduced to a greater extent by paroxetine and clomipramine than placebo. There were no significant differences between the two active agents in these secondary variables.

In terms of side-effects, there were no statistically significant differences between the paroxetine and placebo groups in the number of patients who had adverse effects. However, there were more patients with adverse effects in the clomipramine group compared with the paroxetine group. In particular, symptoms referable to the nervous system and digestive system were greater in the clomipramine group. Drop-outs from the paroxetine (7.3%), the clomipramine (14.9%) and the placebo (11.4%) groups were not significantly different. Nausea was the most common side-effect for the paroxetine group, and dizziness, dry mouth, nausea, somnolence and tremor in the clomipramine group.

Similar to the Oehrberg study, improvement was observed in the second and third weeks. In this study, the comparator drug of clomipramine allowed comparisons in both efficacy and side-effects between the previous 'gold standard' and a competitor for that designation. Paroxetine actually showed significant improvement 4–6 weeks faster than clomipramine, and was better tolerated. Both paroxetine and clomipramine reduced the other symptoms and functional disability of PD. Importantly, both drugs reduced agoraphobia avoidance.

Controlled, long-term data on psychophar-macological treatment of PD is very limited. An extension of the study mentioned above allowed the collection of data for a total of one year of treatment.[74]

This study was a double-blind continuation of patients from the 32 centers in 11 European countries described above. The patients continued on the same medication at the same dosage for the entire time without interruption. The study population included 176 patients who chose to continue treatment after the initial 12-week study. Sixty-six percent (116 patients) completed the study and 34% (60 patients) withdrew. The largest percentage of patients discontinuing the study was from the placebo group (42%), compared with clomipramine (35%) and paroxetine (28%). For both drugs, the most common reason for withdrawal was side-effects, which was highest in the clomipramine group (19%) versus the other two treatment groups (paroxetine 7.4% and 6.7% for placebo). As seen in Table 11.1, the mean number of panic attacks in the paroxetine group continued to decrease throughout the study, and the paroxetine group decreased further than the placebo group by weeks 24 and 36. After 36 weeks of treatment, almost 85% of the paroxetine group were free of panic attacks (Table 11.1), which was significantly greater than the 59% on placebo, but not significantly different from the clomipramine group (72.4%).

The global measures and measures of anxiety and agoraphobia also improved in a similar fashion for both active treatment groups. The most common side-effects were dizziness (approximately 11% with both medications) and headache (approximately 10–13% in all three groups). There was a higher percentage of patients experiencing sweating and dry mouth on clomipramine than on paroxetine. Discontinuation because of side-effects was most frequent in the clomipramine group

Table 11.1 Reduction in panic attacks (PAs) over 48 weeks of treatment with paroxetine, clomipramine (CLO) and placebo (PBO) (adapted from LeCrubier et al[75])

	Mean number of PAs			Percentage free of PAs		
	Paroxetine	CLO	PBO	Paroxetine	CLO	PBO
Baseline	17.5	16.0	14.3	0	0	0
Week 12	2.2	3.9	4.1	55.2	65.1	46.5
Week 24	1.1[a]	1.4	3.8	73.8	77.6	65.1
Week 36	0.9[a]	2.2	4.0	84.6[b]	72.4	59.1

[a] $p < 0.049$ versus PBO.
[b] $p = 0.004$ versus PBO.

(19%), and lower in the paroxetine (7.4%) and placebo (6.7%) groups. Although there were more side-effects in the higher doses of both medications, there was, in fact, no significant evidence of a dose–response relationship to side effects.

This is a valuable study in that it documented that with both paroxetine and clomipramine patients continued to improve in both panic attacks, anxiety, agoraphobia and functional disability for the entire year of treatment. Although both medications were effective, paroxetine was more effective in terms of some secondary measures of efficacy, and was clearly better tolerated.

A fixed-dose, 10-week, double-blind comparison of 10, 20 or 40 mg/day compared with placebo allowed determination of the target dose of paroxetine in PD.[76] Approximately 70 patients were randomized to each group, and 68% completed the 10-week trial. The most common reasons for discontinuation were for adverse effects, and ranged from 6% to 13.9% for the three paroxetine groups, but was 13.0% in the placebo group. Withdrawal secondary to a lack of efficacy was lower for the higher doses of paroxetine (6–1.4%) and highest for placebo (8.7%).

Patients treated with 40 mg/day of paroxetine had significantly greater improvements compared with placebo on three out of the four primary outcomes measures, including reduction to zero (or one) panic attacks, reduction in number of full panic attacks, and improvement in global severity (not in 50% reduction in panic attacks). This was apparent by week 4. During the final two weeks of the study, the highest percentage of patients free of panic attacks were on 40 mg (86%) compared with 20 mg (65.2%), 10 mg (67.4%) and placebo (50.0%). On the CGI, 81.2% of the 40 mg, 75.4% of 20 mg, 57.8% of 10 mg and 51.5%

of placebo patients were much or very much improved. Avoidance also declined in all groups (nonsignificantly). Agoraphobic fear scores were significantly lower at weeks 4 (40 mg) and 10 (20 and 40 mg), when compared with placebo. Improvements in anxiety and depression ratings were also significantly greater in the 40 mg group.

Side-effects were greater than placebo on relatively few measures (asthenia, diarrhea, dry mouth, dyspepsia, tremor and sexual side-effects). Again, in this trial there were no increases in drop-outs in the first two weeks because of increases in anxiety.

Although this trial did not show decreases in agoraphobia avoidance, agoraphobia fears did decrease significantly. As mentioned, agoraphobia avoidance was reduced in other trials with paroxetine.[73–75] Like the other trials, this trial showed paroxetine to be effective and well tolerated, and established a target dose as 40 mg.

A final controlled trial with paroxetine has provided further unique data in providing an estimated relapse rate after discontinuation from effective treatment in a controlled study.[77] Patients in the fixed-dose study described above who responded to treatment were invited to enter a treatment re-randomization study. They were re-randomized in a double-blind fashion to either the treatment and dose they had been on before, or to placebo for three months of further treatment. This was the first and most controlled trial to date to study relapse after rotation onto placebo, and certainly the first with an SSRI. Of paroxetine patients randomized to placebo, 30% (11/37) relapsed, but only 5% (2/43) relapsed if they continued on paroxetine – a statistically significant difference. In the 30% of placebo patients who relapsed, relapse occurred over 30 days, with relapses occurring in each of the first four weeks.

Sertraline

Two large, identical, double-blind, placebo-controlled, flexible-dose trials have been completed with sertraline,[78,79] and will be discussed as one trial.[80,81] A total of 342 patients from 20 US and Canadian centers were randomized to either sertraline or placebo. Dosages began at 25 mg/day for one week, and were then flexibly increased to between 50 and 200 mg/day based on tolerability and clinical response over the 10-week trial.

Panic-attack frequency was reduced significantly more in the sertraline group beginning at week 2 and was sustained throughout each week of the trial. This trial employed a new measure entitled Panic Attack Burden (PAB), which was the frequency of panic attacks multiplied by their severity. Significant differences between sertraline and placebo emerged at week 1 on this measure. The percentage of patients who reached zero panic attacks (59.3%) was higher than the percentage on placebo (46.3%). The reductions in panic attacks were greater than for placebo as early as weeks 2 and 4.

This pattern of improvement was seen across the other measures as well, including the CGI, which favored sertraline from week 2, and the patient globals from week 4 to the end of the trial. Phobic avoidance was also significantly reduced on sertraline over placebo by week 10 and anticipatory anxiety at week 4.

This study also had a rich battery of quality-of-life outcome measures, which demonstrated significantly greater improvement on sertraline than placebo. The sertraline patients had a higher overall improvement in quality of life, with specific significant improvements in mood, work and household activities, as well as social, family and leisure activities. Similar improvements were seen in occupational/economic issues, as well as in physical mobility, ability to work on hobbies, and an overall sense of satisfaction and wellness. There was also significantly greater improvement on measures of satisfaction with medication and overall satisfaction with life. These outcome measures represent significant improvement over previously available measures for this type of outcome.

Sertraline treatment was well tolerated, with 8.3% discontinuation for adverse events (2.3% placebo). The side-effects significantly greater for sertraline than placebo were diarrhea (25.6% versus 10.8%), nausea (15.5% versus 8.5%), dry mouth (8.9% versus 4.9%) and ejaculation failure (5.4% versus 0.0%).

Again, there were only 6% of patients who discontinued sertraline in the first week, compared with 2.3% on placebo. The low rate of discontinuation suggests again that a low starting dose (25 mg/day) reduces the rate of occurrence of the 'jitteriness syndrome'. The higher discontinuation rate early in treatment (10.5% for sertraline, 0% for placebo) suggests that doses even lower than 25 mg might be indicated to initiate treatment.

The remaining completed sertraline trial is a multicenter, placebo-controlled, fixed-dose study in 177 patients.[78,82] In this 12-week trial at seven US centers, approximately 45 patients were randomly assigned to placebo, and equal numbers to 50, 100 and 200 mg/day. Again, sertraline patients experienced a 65% decrease in panic attack frequency, compared with 39% of placebo patients. There were also greater reductions on sertraline in anticipatory anxiety and HAM-A anxiety scores.

Side-effects that were greater in the sertraline group included nausea (33% versus 20%), diarrhea (15% versus 9%), dry mouth (14% versus 2%) and fatigue (13% versus 4%). There were significant differences in only two adverse experiences: dry mouth and increased latency to ejaculation.

Although all three dosage groups had significantly greater reductions in panic attacks relative to placebo, they were not significantly different from each other. The 100 mg group had the greatest reduction in full panic attacks, limited symptom panic attacks and anticipatory anxiety. Unlike other SSRIs, these results do not provide evidence for a dose–response relationship in the 50–200 mg range for sertraline.

Fluoxetine

Although controlled trials are underway for fluoxetine in PD, these have not yet been presented or published. However, fluoxetine was the first of the SSRIs beyond fluvoxamine to be investigated in PD. Gorman and colleagues[83] studied 16 patients in an 18-week open trial, beginning treatment at 10 mg/day and increasing by 10 mg/week to a maximum dose of 80 mg/day. Most patients had a significant reduction in their panic attacks in about six weeks, and 7 of the 16 subjects were considered responders, with no panic attacks for at least four weeks in a row. On the other hand, of the nine who did not respond, eight actually discontinued the medication because of side-effects. Seven of the terminators discontinued because of what we now understand as the hyperstimulation or 'jitteriness syndrome' characterized by increased anxiety, sleep disturbances, jitteriness, GI symptoms and panic attacks.

The group involved in the initial fluoxetine trial went on to study 25 more PD patients, hoping they could decrease the drop-out rate by beginning at lower doses. Fluoxetine was generally begun at 5 mg/day and gradually increased every week. In this trial, 76% of 25 patients had a moderate to marked reduction in panic symptomatology, despite the fact that most of these patients previously had had a poor response to other anti-anxiety agents or had negative side-effects. Almost all of the patients (12/13) who had previously responded to other medications but had experienced adverse side-effects had a marked response to fluoxetine. Of the other nine patients who had previously been nonresponsive, four of these had a moderate or marked response.

Pecknold and colleagues[84] had 28 patients begin an eight-week open trial, but 36% dropped out of treatment, primarily because of increased anxiety or lack of efficacy. However, 32% of the patients had no panic attacks by week 3. At the end of the eight-week trial, 48% of the patients had resolution of their panic attacks. There was also significant reduction in anxiety and phobic avoidance, but almost 20% of the patients failed to respond.

Solyom and colleagues[85] reported two remarkable responses to fluoxetine in very treatment-unresponsive patients. One patient had three hospitalizations and two years of psychoanalytical therapy, behavior therapy, imipramine up to 300 mg/day, alprazolam up to 4 mg/day and clonazepam up to 8 mg/day. Phenelzine was effective, but a 50 lb (23 kg) weight loss led her to discontinue this. She had approximately 100 panic attacks per day in multiple situations, and was depressed much of the time. She began fluoxetine at 20 mg/day, which was increased to 80 mg/day. Her panic attacks began responding in the first week, and by the end of the second week were significantly improved. By nine weeks, she was considerably improved, and maintained this improvement over a two-year period while she remained on fluoxetine. She was unable to discontinue fluoxetine without a marked increase in symptomatology.

The second patient had also been unsuccessfully treated with behavior therapy, psychotherapy, imipramine to 400 mg/day, phenelzine to 90 mg/day and alprazolam to 7 mg/day. She was treated with fluoxetine to 80 mg/day, and by the third week there was a marked reduction in her symptomatology. She relapsed when fluoxetine was discontinued, but recovered when it was reinstituted and maintained that improvement for $2\frac{1}{2}$ years on 80 mg/day.

Louie and colleagues[86] studied a large group ($N = 133$) of depressed patients, some of whom also had PD ($N = 27$). Of the 13 PD patients who were able to reach 20 mg/day, nine discontinued fluoxetine because of side-effects. When compared with the noncomorbid depressed patients, this level of intolerance of side-effects was much higher.

Interestingly, a recent open trial studied fluoxetine treatment in children and adolescents (9–18 years old) with mixed anxiety disorders.[87] Each of these patients was nonresponsive to psychotherapy, and fluoxetine was instituted at 5 mg/day and increased to a maximum of 40 mg in children and 80 mg in adolescents. A significant improvement was observed in all 10 patients with concurrent separation anxiety, and in 8/10 with social phobia, 4/6 with specific phobia, 3/5 with panic disorder and 1/7 who had generalized anxiety disorder. The average doses were 24 mg/day for children and 40 mg/day for adolescents, with a mean time for improvement of approximately five weeks. This is a unique study, given the age group of the patients studied.

In a small open study in adults, 10 of 12 PD patients attained at least moderate improvement.[88] Patients were treated with a mean of 17.9 (±16.7 mg/day). In another trial, Veria and Donnelly[89] attempted to reduce the side-effects related to TCAs by utilizing fluoxetine as adjunctive treatment. Patients received 20 mg of fluoxetine and 25–50 mg TCAs. Interestingly, 14/16 patients did improve, with relatively few side-effects.

Dosage

The only SSRI that has a clear target dose is paroxetine. As described, a careful fixed-dose study has demonstrated that 40 mg is the target dose, although some patients do respond at lower and higher doses. The available literature suggests that there is no clear cut difference between 50, 100 and 200 mg of sertraline in the treatment of PD. However, there is some suggestion that 100–150 mg might be the recommended dosage range. Fluoxetine in the range between 20 and 80 mg has been associated with response.

As described in this chapter, fluvoxamine has been demonstrated to be effective at 50–150 mg, with somewhat increased side-effects at higher doses. Clomipramine has been utilized in studies with doses ranging from 25 to 300 mg/day, and some patients have responded to doses as low as 10–30 mg/day.[90] In two studies by Gloger and colleagues,[38,39] approximately half of their patients responded to less than 50 mg/day, and in the subsequent study, about half responded to 25 mg/day. However, most clinicians have been treating patients using the 100–150 mg/day range.

The other important issue with dosing is the clear evidence that patients should begin treatment with as low a dose of the medication as can be practically arranged. There has been the most evidence that fluoxetine needs to be started in the dosage range of 2.5–5 mg/day with slow increases of 5 mg every 4–14 days after that. Roy-Byrne and Wingerson[91] found that beginning with 2 mg/day of fluoxetine enabled a group who had previously been unable to successfully start fluoxetine to initiate treatment without difficulty. It is also true that paroxetine should probably be started with 10 mg and clomipramine, fluvoxamine and sertraline at no more than 25 mg/day, and perhaps lower if practical.

Comparisons between SSRIs

To date, there have been very few trials comparing SSRI-type drugs in PD patients. As mentioned, paroxetine and clomipramine have been compared directly, in both short-term and long-term maintenance treatment over a year.[74,75] Although both were effective, there was some evidence that paroxetine's action was somewhat more rapid, and there was reduction of more of the ancillary symptoms of PD (anxiety, depression, functional disability) in the long-term maintenance trial on paroxetine. The other major difference was in side-effects, again with paroxetine having significantly fewer side-effects than clomipramine.

As mentioned, den Boer and colleagues[52] compared clomipramine and fluvoxamine, and although both drugs were approximately equal, clomipramine was more effective than fluvoxamine in terms of reducing anxiety symptoms and depression. Other studies have suggested the two agents are approximately equal.[92] In the trial comparing citalopram and clomipramine, both drugs were effective, with little reported differences.[71,93]

In the absence of adequate direct comparisons, it would be difficult to compare these agents in terms of side-effects. While it seems clear that clomipramine probably has more side-effects than the traditional SSRIs, the remaining SSRIs seem to share a cluster of side-effects (nausea, asthenia, etc.). Whether there are lower rates of these various symptoms with one agent or another will have to wait for trials on direct comparisons.

There are three trials in the depression literature comparing the SSRIs on these issues.[94–96] In 78 depressed outpatients, the effects of fluoxetine (40 mg/day) and paroxetine (30 mg/day) were compared. In parallel to the paroxetine and clomipramine trial described above, both drugs had equal efficacy, but there was a statistically significant decline in depression earlier with paroxetine. In a subsequent trial comparing these two medications, Tignol[95] failed to observe any significant differences in efficacy, side-effects or onset of action.

A third eight-week trial compared sertraline and fluoxetine, and found approximately equal efficacy for these two drugs.[96] Although there were no apparent differences in the incidence of adverse effects, the authors felt that the severity of the adverse effects was greater with fluoxetine, particularly in the elderly. Whereas all of the elderly patients on sertraline completed the study, approximately 20% of fluoxetine patients dropped out of the trial.

Certainly, the most important clinical comparison has been that between the SSRIs and the TCAs. As a class, the SSRIs cause less weight gain, anticholinergic side-effects, sedation and dangerous interactions with the cardiovascular system. Overall, the frequency of side-effects with the SSRIs is probably as high as with the TCAs. However, it seems clear from years of use that these side-effects are milder, briefer and cause less difficulty for patients. Nausea is the most common side-effect, as mentioned above. Diarrhea and insomnia, agitation and headache are probably the next most common side-effects. Almost all SSRI-type agents are best administered in a single daily dose with breakfast. Fluvoxamine is generally administered at bedtime, with a maximum individual dose of 150 mg. The other SSRIs, if not well tolerated with breakfast, are often switched to bedtime with good results.

Most clinicians feel that interference with sexual function is the most important of the side-effects of the SSRIs. This is primarily related to delayed ejaculation or orgasm, and is probably more common in men. Another important issue in both depression and PD is that the SSRIs are clearly safer in overdose.

Withdrawal syndrome

Black and colleagues[59] have studied 14 PD patients who abruptly withdrew from fluvoxamine doses of up to 300 mg/day for eight months (mean 236 mg). One of the 14 patients had a full relapse five days after discontinuation, and had to be retreated. The remaining patients developed a cluster of symptoms unlike PD. In general, within 24 hours of discontinuation, they developed dizziness, nausea, incoordination, irritability and headache. Symptoms peaked on the fifth day after discontinuation, and were considered withdrawal symptoms.

In direct contrast to these findings, Holland and colleagues[58] in their study failed to observe symptoms of relapse or withdrawal-type symptoms in fluvoxamine patients compared with placebo patients.

As mentioned above, Oehrberg and colleagues[73] observed minor symptoms in a few patients after discontinuation. In this trial, more than three-quarters of the patients had been taking 40 mg or more, and yet did not evidence a withdrawal syndrome. It remains an open research issue as to whether there is a withdrawal syndrome with SSRIs in PD, but titration over several weeks would seem wise.

Emergence of depression

Despite the obvious efficacy of the SSRIs as antidepressants and anti-anxiety agents, there are reports that they appear to induce depressive symptoms in some patients. Fux and colleagues[96] reported that 7 out of 80 patients treated with fluvoxamine for PD (doses 50–200 mg/day) developed symptoms of depression during treatment, despite a positive response in terms of their anxiety symptoms. Five of these patients were treated with 20 mg of fluoxetine, and experienced continued depression, which actually worsened in four patients. Because depression is very common in PD, it is unclear whether the depression observed in this single study was related to the SSRI. However, it does appear that patients on SSRIs should be monitored closely for this possibility.

Pharmacodynamic/pharmacokinetic differences

There is little difference in absorption rates between the SSRIs, with peak levels for all of them occurring approximately 4–6 hours after ingestion. Plasma-protein binding varies widely, and is above 95% for fluoxetine, paroxetine and sertraline, but is actually low for fluvoxamine and citalopram. Whether or not this is clinically important is unclear. Since SSRIs are metabolized in the liver and then excreted in urine and feces, impaired liver and/or renal function lead to increased plasma concentrations.

One of the bigger differences between SSRIs is certainly the oxidation metabolism differences in the cytochrome P450 enzymes of the liver which metabolize the SSRIs and drugs used with the SSRIs. Important interactions that have been observed include fluoxetine raising serum levels of TCAs, BZs, carbamazepine, valproate, alprazolam and haloperidol. Fluvoxamine increases the levels of propranolol, warfarin, coumadin, theophylline, carbamazepine and the TCAs.

Paroxetine has been observed to increase levels of digoxin and the TCAs, and sertraline to elevate warfarin and to a lesser extent some of the antidepressants, particularly desipramine.

Citalopram has been observed to increase the levels of phenothiazines, but does not appear to affect TCA levels.

Although most SSRIs have elimination half lives of about 24 hours that for fluoxetine is very much longer (7–10 days if one includes the active metabolites). This can present management problems if patients are intolerant of the drug or have adverse reactions.

Conclusions

In conclusion, this review has shown there is now a large body of evidence documenting that the SSRIs are effective and probably deserve to be the pharmacological treatment of first choice in PD for many patients.

References

1. Jobson KO, Potter WZ, International Psychopharmacology Algorithm Project report. *Psychopharmacol Bull* 1995; **31**: 457–507.
2. Humble M, Wistedt B, Serotonin, panic disorder and agoraphobia: short-term and long-term efficacy of citalopram in panic disorders. *Int Clin Psychopharmacol* 1992; **6**(Suppl 5): 21–39.
3. Banki CM, Correlation of anxiety and related symptoms with cerebrospinal fluid 5-hydroxyindoleacetic acid in depressed women. *J Neural Transm* 1977; **41**: 135–43.
4. Pecknold JC, Serotonin abnormalities in panic disorder. In: *Neurobiology of Panic Disorder* (Ballenger JC, ed.). New York: Wiley-Liss, 1990: 121–42.
5. File SE, Hyde JRG, The effects of *p*-chlorophenylalanine and ethanolamine-O-

sulphate in an animal test of anxiety. *J Pharmacol* 1977; **29**: 735–8.

6. Stein L, Wise CD, Berger BD, Antianxiety action of benzodiazepines: decrease in activity of serotonin neurons in the punishment systems. In: *The Benzodiazepines* (Garrattini S, Mussini E, Randall LO, eds). New York: Raven Press, 1973: 299–326.

7. Thiebot MH, Hamon M, Soubrie P, Attenuation of induced anxiety in rats by chlordiazepoxide: role of raphe dorsalis benzodiazepine binding sites and serotonergic neurones. *Neuroscience* 1982; **7**: 2287–94.

8. Graeff NG, Filho NGS, Behavioural inhibition induced by electrical stimulation of the median raphe nucleus of the rat. *Physiol Behav* 1978; **21**: 477–84.

9. Blakey TA, Parker LF, Effects of parachlorophenylalanine on experimentally induced conflict behavior. *Pharmacol Biochem Behav* 1973; **1**: 600–13.

10. Cook L, Sepinwall J, Behaviour analysis of the effects of mechanisms of action of benzodiazepines. In: *Mechanism of Action of Benzodiazepines* (Costa E, Greengard P, eds). New York: Raven Press, 1975: 1–28.

11. Tye NC, Iversen SD, Green AR, The effects of benzodiazepines and serotonergic manipulations on punished responding. *Neuropharmacology* 1979; **18**: 689–95.

12. Panksepp J, Meeker R, Bean NJ, The neurochemical control of crying. *Pharmacol Biochem Behav* 1980; **12**: 437–43.

13. Winslow JT, Insel TR, Serotonergic and catecholaminergic reuptake inhibitors have opposite effects on the ultrasonic isolation calls of rat pups. *Neuropsychopharmacology* 1990; **3**: 51–9.

14. Germine M, Goddard AW, Sholomaskers DE et al, Response to metachlorphenylpiperazine in panic disorder and healthy subjects: influence of reduction in intravenous dosage. *Psychiatry Res* 1984; **54**: 115–33.

15. Charney DS, Woods SW, Goodman WK, Heninger GR, Serotonin function in anxiety. II. Effects of the serotonin agonist MCPP in panic disorder patients and health subjects. *Psychopharmacology* 1987; **92**: 14–24.

16. Kahn RS, Asnis GM, Wetzler S, van Praag HM, Neuroendocrine evidence for serotonin receptor hypersensitivity in panic disorder. *Psychopharmacology* 1988; **96**: 360–4.

17. Targum SD, Marshall LE, Fenfluramine provocation of anxiety in patients with panic disorder. *Psychiatry Res* 1989; **28**: 295–306.

18. Gorman JM, Askanazi J, Liebowitz MR et al, Response to hyperventilation in a group of patients with panic disorder. *Am J Psychiatry* 1984; **141**: 857–61.

19. Gorman JM, Liebowitz MR, Fyer AJ et al, Lacate infusions in obsessive–compulsive disorder. *Am J Psychiatry* 1985; **142**: 864–6.

20. Gorman JM, Liebowitz MR, Fyer AJ et al, A neuroanatomical hypothesis for panic disorder. *Am J Psychiatry* 1989; **146**: 148–61.

21. Lingjaerde O, Platelet update and storage of serotonin. In: *Serotonin in Health and Disease*, Vol IV (Essman EB, ed.). New York: Spectrum Publications, 1977: 139–99.

22. Lingjaerde O, Lactate-induced panic attacks: possible involvement of serotonin reuptake stimulation. *Acta Psychiatr Scand* 1985; **72**: 206–8.

23. Soderpalm B, Anderson L, Carlsson M et al, Serotonergic influences on the growth hormone response to clonidine in rats. *J Neural Transm* 1987; **41**: 135–43.

24. Roy-Byrne PP, Uhde TW, Panic disorder and major depression: biological relationships. *Psychopharmacol Bull* 1985; **21**: 551–4.

25. McIntyre IM, Judd FK, Burrows GD et al, Serotonin in panic disorder: platelet uptake and concentration. *Int Clin Psychopharmacol* 1989; **4**: 1–6.

26. Faludi G, Tekes K, Tothfalusi L, Comparative study of platelet 3H-paroxetine and 3H-imipramine binding in panic disorder patients and healthy controls. *J Psychiatry Neurosci* 1995; **20**: 193–8.

27. Lewis DA, Noyes R Jr, Coryell W et al, Tritiated imipramine binding to platelets is decreased in patients with agoraphobia. *Psychiatry Res* 1985; **16**: 1–9.

28. Innis RB, Charney DS, Heninger GR, Differential 3-H imipramine platelet binding in patients with panic disorder and depression. *Psychiatry Res* 1987; **21**: 33–4.

29. Schneider P, Evans L, Ross-Lee L et al, Plasma biogenic amine levels in agoraphobia with panic attacks. *Pharmacopsychiatry* 1987; **20**: 102–4.

30. Coplan JD, Gorman JM, Klein DF, Serotonin

related functions in panic-anxiety: a critical overview. *Neuropsychopharmacology* 1992; **6:** 189–200.

31. Grove G, Coplan JD, Hollander E, The neuroanatomy of 5-HT dysregulation and panic disorder. *J Neuropsychiatry* 1997; **9:** 198–207.

32. deMontigny C, Aghajanian GK, Tricyclic antidepressants: long-term treatment increases responsivity of rat forebrain neurons to serotonin. *Science* 1978; **202:** 1303–6.

33. Chaput Y, Blier P, deMontigny C, Acute and long-term effects of antidepressant serotonin (5-HT) reuptake blockers on the efficacy of 5-HT neurotransmission: electrophysiological studies in the rat central nervous system. *Adv Biol Psychiatry* 1988; **17:** 1–7.

34. Moret C, Briley M, Serotonin autoreceptor subsensitivity and antidepressant activity. *Eur Neuropsychopharmacol* 1990; **180:** 351–6.

35. Willner P, Antidepressants and serotonergic transmission: an integrative review. *Psychopharmacology* 1985; **85:** 387–404.

36. Klein DF, Gittelman R, Quitkin F, Rifkin A, *Diagnosis and Drug Treatment*, 2nd edn. Baltimore: Williams & Wilkins, 1980: 793–818.

37. Grove G, Coplan JD, Hollander E, The neuroanatomy of 5-HT dysregulation and panic disorder. *J Neuropsychiatry* 1997; **9:** 198–207.

38. Gloger S, Grunhaus L, Birmacher B, Troudarf T, Treatment of spontaneous panic attacks with clomipramine. *Am J Psychiatry* 1981; **138:** 1215–17.

39. Gloger S, Grunhaus L, Gladic et al, Panic attacks and agoraphobia: low dose clomipramine treatment. *J Clin Psychopharmacol* 1989; **9:** 28–32.

40. Lesser JM, Lydiard RB, Antel E et al, Alprazolma plasma concentrations and treatment response in panic disorder and agoraphobia. *Am J Psychiatry* 1992; **149:** 1556–62.

41. Mavissakalian MR, Perel JM, Imipramine treatment of panic disorder with agoraphobia: dose ranging and plasma level response relationships. *Am J Psychiatry* 1995; **152:** 673–82.

42. Pecknold JC, McClure DJ, Appeltauer L et al, Does tryptophan potentiate clomipramine in the treatment of agoraphobic and social phobic patients? *Br J Psychiatry* 1982; **140:** 484–90.

43. Caetano D, Treatment for panic disorder with clomipramine (Anafranil): an open study of 22 cases. *J Bras Psiquiatr* 1985; **34:** 123–32.

44. Johnston DG, Troyer IE, Whitsett SF, Clomipramine treatment of agoraphobic women. An eight week controlled trial. *Arch Gen Psychiatry* 1988; **45:** 453–9.

45. Fahy TJ, O'Rourke DO, Brophy J et al, The Galway study of panic disorder I. Clomipramine and lofepramine in DSM III-r panic disorder: a placebo controlled trial. *J Affect Disord* 1992; **25:** 63–76.

46. Hoffart A, Due-Madsen J, Lande B et al, Clomipramine in the treatment of agoraphobic inpatients resistant to behavioral therapy. *J Clin Psychiatry* 1993; **54:** 481–7.

47. Feet PO, Larsen S, Lillevold PD et al, Comparison of the serum levels in primary nonagitated depressed outpatients treated with imipramine in combination with placebo, diazepam or dixtyrazine. *Acta Psychiatr Scand* 1987; **75:** 435–40.

48. Feet PO, Gotestan KG, Increased antipanic efficacy in combined treatment with clomipramine and dixtyrazine. *Acta Psychiatr Scand* 1994; **89:** 230–4.

49. Mavissakalian M, Perel JM, Imipramine dose–response relationship in panic disorder with agoraphobia. *Arch Gen Psychiatry* 1989; **46:** 127–31.

50. Cassano GB, Petracca A, Perugi G et al, Clomipramine for panic disorder: I. The first 10 weeks of a long-term comparison with imipramine. *J Affect Disord* 1988; **14:** 123–7.

51. Modigh K, Westberg P, Eriksson E, Superiority of clomipramine over imipramine in the treatment of panic disorder: a placebo-controlled trial. *J Clin Psychopharmacol* 1992; **51(4S):** 53–8.

52. Den Boer JA, Westenberg HGM, Kamerbeek WDJ et al, Effect of serotonin uptake inhibitors in anxiety disorders; a double-blind comparison of clorimipramine and fluvoxamine. *Int Clin Psychopharmacol* 1987; **2:** 21–32.

53. Asnis GM, Effects of fluvoxamine on the treatment of panic disorder: a placebo-controlled trial. *An Psiquiatric (Madrid)* 1992; **8(Suppl 1):** 78.

54. Hoehn-Saric R, McLeod DR, Hipsley PA, Effect of fluvoxamine on panic disorder. *J Clin Psychopharmacol* 1993; **13:** 321–6.

55. Hoehn-Saric R, Fawcett J, Munjack DJ, Roy-

Byrne PP, A multicentre, double-blind, placebo-controlled study of fluvoxamine in the treatment of panic disorder. In: *Neuropsychopharmacology, Part 2, Oral Communications and Poster Abstracts of the XIXth Collegium International Neuropsychopharmacologicum Congress: 27 June–1 July, 1994, Washington, DC:* Abst P-58-33.

56. Woods S, Black D, Brown S et al, Fluvoxamine in the treatment of panic disorder in outpatients: A double-blind, placebo-controlled study. In: *Neuropsychopharmacology, Part 2, Oral Communications and Poster Abstracts of the XIXth Collegium International Neuropsychopharmacologicum Congress: 27 June–1 July, 1994, Washington, DC:* Abst P-58-37.

57. Nair NP, Bakish D, Saxena B et al, Comparison of fluvoxamine, imipramine, and placebo in the treatment of outpatients with panic disorder. *Anxiety* 1996; **2**: 192–8.

58. Holland RI, Fawcett J, Hoehn-Saric R et al, Long-term treatment of panic disorder with fluovoxamine in outpatients who had completed double-blind studies. *Neuropsychopharmacology* 1994; **10**(3S, Part 2): 102S.

59. Black DW, Wesner R, Bowers W, Gabel J, A comparison of fluvoxamine, cognitive therapy, and placebo in the treatment of panic disorder. *Arch Gen Psychiatry* 1993; **50**: 44–50.

60. Sharpe DM, Power KG, Simpson RJ et al, Fluvoxamine, placebo, and cognitive behavior therapy used alone and in combination in the treatment of panic disorder and agoraphobia. *J Anxiety Disord* 1996; **10**: 219–42.

61. Black DW, Wesner RB, Gabel J et al, Predictors of short-term treatment response in 66 patients with panic disorder. *J Affective Disord* 1994; **30**: 233–41.

62. Dewulf L, Hendrickx B, Lesaffre E, Epidemiological data of patients with fluvoxamine: results from a 12 week non-comparative multicentre study. *Int Clin Psychopharmacol* 1995; **9**(Suppl 4): 67–72.

63. Spiegel DA, Saeed SA, Bruce TJ, An open trial of fluvoxamine therapy for panic disorder complicated by depression. *J Clin Psychiatry* 1996; **57**(suppl 8): 37–40.

64. Ballenger JC, Comorbidity of panic and depression. *Int Clin Psychopharmacol* 1998; in press.

65. Van Vliet IM, den Boer JA, Westenberg HG et al, A double-blind comparative study of brofaromine and fluvoxamine in outpatients with panic disorder. *J Clin Psychopharmacol* 1996; **16**: 299–306.

66. Den Boer JA, Westenberg HG, Effect of a serotonin and noradrenaline uptake inhibitor in panic disorder: a double-blind comparative study with fluvoxamine and maprotiline. *Int Clin Psychopharmacol* 1988; **3**: 59–74.

67. Den Boer JA, Westenberg HGM, Serotonin function in panic disorder: a double blind placebo controlled study with fluvoxamine and ritanserin. *Psychopharmacology* 1990; **102**: 85–94.

68. Humble M, Koczkas C, Wistedt B, Serotonin and anxiety: an open study of citalopram in panic disorder. In: *Psychiatry Today: VIII World Congress of Psychiatry Abstracts* (Stefanis CN, Soldatos CR, Rabavilas AD, eds). New York: Elsevier, 1989: 151.

69. Bertaini A, Perna G, Politi E, Bellodi L, Citalopram and panic disorder. *Depression and Anxiety* 1996–1996; **4**: 253.

70. Wade AG, Lepola U, Koponen HJ et al, The effect of citalopram in panic disorder. *Br J Psychiatry* 1997; **170**: 549–53.

71. Lepola U, Long-term citalopram is effective in relieving panic disorder. Presented at the 17th Annual Meeting of the Anxiety Disorders Association of America, New Orleans, LA, March 1997.

72. Lepola U, Leinonen E, Koponen H, Citalopram in the treatment of early-onset panic disorder and school phobia. *Pharmacopsychiatry* 1996; **29**: 30–32.

73. Oehrberg S, Christiansen PE, Behnek K et al, Paroxetine in the treatment of panic disorder, a randomized double blind placebo controlled study. *Br J Psychiatry* 1995; **167**: 374–9.

74. LeCrubier Y, Bakker A, Judge R, and the Collaborative Paroxetine Study Investigators, A comparison of paroxetine, clomipramine and placebo in the treatment of panic disorder. *Acta Psychiatr Scand* 1997; **95**: 145–52.

75. LeCrubier Y, Judge R, and the Collaborative Paroxetine Study Investigators, Longterm evaluation of paroxetine, clomipramine and placebo in panic disorder. *Acta Psychiatr Scand* 1997; **95**: 153–60.

76. Ballenger JC, Steiner M, Bushnell W, Gergel I, Double-blind, fixed-dose, placebo-controlled study of paroxetine in the treatment of panic disorder. *Am J Psychiatry* 1998; **155**: 36–42.

77. Burnham DB, Steiner MX, Gergle IP et al, Paroxetine long-term safety and efficacy in panic disorder and prevention of relapse: a double-blind study. Presented in poster session at the American College of Neuropsychopharmacology, 1995, San Juan, Puerto Rico.

78. Baumel B, Bielski R, Carman J et al, Double-blind comparison of sertraline and placebo in patients with panic disorder. Presented at Collegium Internationale Neuro-Psychopharmacologicum, June 1996, Melbourne, Australia.

79. Wolkow R, Apter J, Clayton A et al, Double-blind flexible dose study of sertraline and placebo in patients with panic disorder, Presented at Collegium Internationale Neuro-Psychopharmacologicum, June 1996, Melbourne, Australia.

80. Pollack M, Wolkow R, Clary C, Sertraline treatment of panic disorder: combined results from two placebo-controlled trials. Presented at the annual meeting of the New Clinical Drug Evaluation Unit, May 1997.

81. Pohl RH, Clary C, Wolkow R, Sertraline treatment of panic disorder: combined results from two placebo-controlled trials. Presented at the Annual Meeting of the American Psychiatric Association, San Diego, May 1997.

82. DuBoff E, England D, Ferguson JM et al, Sertraline in the treatment of panic disorder. Presented at the VIII Annual European College of Neuropsychopharmacology, Venice, Italy, October 1995.

83. Gorman JM, Lieowitz MR, Fyer AJ et al, An open trial of fluoxetine in the treatment of panic attacks. *J Clin Psychopharmacol* 1987; **7**: 329–32.

84. Pecknold JC, Luthe L, Iny L, Ramdoyal D, Fluoxetine in panic disorder: pharmacological and tritiated platelet imipramine and paroxetine binding study. *J Psychiatry Neurosci* 1995; **20**: 193–8.

85. Solyom L, Solyom C, Ledwidge B, Fluoxetine in panic disorder. *Can J Psychiatry* 1991; **36**: 378–80.

86. Louie AK, Lewis TB, Lannon RA, Use of low-dose fluoxetine in major depression and panic disorder. *J Clin Psychiatry* 1993; **54**: 435–8.

87. Fairbanks JM, Pine DS, Tancer NK et al, Open fluoxetine treatment of mixed anxiety disorders in children and adolescents. *J Child Adolescents* 1997; **7**: 17–29.

88. Coplan JD, Papp LA, Pine D et al, Clinical improvement with fluoxetine therapy with noradrenergic function in patients with panic disorder. *Arch Gen Psychiatry* 1997; **54**: 643–8.

89. Varia IM, Donnelly DL, Fluoxetine augments tricyclics in panic disorder. In: *New Research Program and Abstracts*. Washington, DC: American Psychiatric Association, 1991: NR 368, 136.

90. Walker L, Ashcroft G, Pharmacological approaches to the treatment of panic. In: *Panic Disorder: Theory Research and Therapy* (Baker R, ed.). New York: Wiley, 1989: 301–14.

91. Roy-Byrne PP, Wingerson D, Pharmacotherapy of anxiety disorder. In: *Review of Psychiatry*, Vol 11 (Tasman A, Riba MB, eds). Washington, DC: American Psychiatric Press, 1992: 260–84.

92. Dick P, Ferrer E, A double-blind comparative study of the clinical efficacy of fluvoxamine and chlorimipramine. *Br J Clin Pharmacol* 1983; **15**(S3): 419S–25S.

93. Wade AG, The optimal therapeutical area for SSRIs: panic disorder. Presented at the VIII Annual European College of Neuropsychopharmacology, Venice, Italy, October 1995.

94. DeWilde J, Spiers R, Mertens C et al, A double-blind, comparative, multicentre study comparing paroxetine with fluoxetine in depressed outpatients. *Acta Psychiatr Scand* 1993; **87**: 141–5.

95. Tignol J, A double-blind, randomized, fluoxetine-controlled multicentre study of paroxetine in the treatment of depression. *J Clin Psychopharmacol* 1993; **13**(Suppl 2): 18–22.

96. Aguglia E, Casacchia M, Cassano GB et al, Double-blind study of the efficacy and safety of sertraline versus fluoxetine in major depression. *Int Clin Psychopharmacol* 1993; **8**: 197–202.

97. Fux M, Taub M, Zohar J, Emergence of depressive symptoms during treatment for panic disorder with specific 5-hydroxytryptophan reuptake inhibitors. *Acta Psychiatr Scand* 1993; **88**: 235–7.

12

Other drug treatments and augmentation therapies for panic disorder

Neil Laufer and Abraham Weizman

CONTENTS • Introduction • Other drug treatments • Augmentation therapy

Introduction

Treatment of panic disorder (PD) with tricyclic antidepressants (TCAs), monoamine oxidase inhibitors (MAOIs), benzodiazepines (BZs), and selective serotonin reuptake inhibitors (SSRIs) has been discussed in Chapters 9–11. In a review of the subject, Ballenger[1] suggested that about 75% of patients show good responses to these three classes of classical antipanic agents. However, treatment response is more limited when considering complete remission of multiple symptom domains, such as panic attacks (PAs), phobic anxiety and avoidance, generalized anxiety, depressive symptoms, functional impairment and global status (reviewed by Roy-Byrne and Cowley[2]). Further treatment is often limited by significant side-effects. Thus, although in various studies 70–90% patients treated with antipanic agents show marked or moderate improvement, half of the patients treated long-term with TCAs experienced significant side-effects, such as significant weight gain.[3] MAOIs may be limited by insomnia and weight gain,[4] and BZs may be problematic in patients with concomitant alcohol or substance abuse.[5] Further medical conditions or other comorbid psychiatric disorders may require alternative treatments.

Other drug treatments

There have been studies of other drug treatments (non-antidepressant and non-BZs) with limited controlled double-blind studies of efficacy. The reasons for limited study in these areas remain speculative, but might include the relatively good efficacy of standard agents (70–90%) in comparison with other psychiatric conditions, as well as the efficacy of cognitive–behavioral therapy (CBT) as a single treatment or recently, with increasing efficacy, combined with pharmacological treatment.[6,7]

Drug treatments that will be discussed include noradrenergic receptor agonists and antagonists, anticonvulsants, $GABA_B$ agonists, dopaminergic agents, calcium-channel blockers and drugs active at neuropeptide receptors, as well as strategies involving second-messenger systems. In general, despite encouraging results for many of these agents in case reports and open trials, efficacy has not been substantially established in double-blind controlled studies. For each agent, a rationale for use will be provided, including background preclinical and clinical evidence.

The results of the various pharmacological strategies are summarized in Tables 12.1–12.3.

Noradrenergic agents

A relationship between noradrenergic activity and anxiety was postulated when stimulation of the primate locus coeruleus (LC) caused anxiety reactions very similar to human panic attacks.[8] Further, abnormal β-adrenergic receptor function has been implicated in the pathophysiology of PD as shown by increased sensitivity to the anxiogenic effects of the selective β-adrenergic agonist isoprenaline,[9] although increased receptor sensitivity would seem unlikely from a report that panic patients showed blunted heart-rate response to isoprenaline, suggesting subsensitive peripheral β receptors.[10]

Challenge studies using the α_2 antagonist yohimbine have shown panic patients to possess enhanced sensitivity to the anxiogenic effects of this agent, as well as exaggerated blood pressure and 3-methoxy-4-hydroxy-phenylethylene glycol (MHPG) responses.[11–14] Some studies using the α_2 antagonist clonidine have suggested possible abnormal α_2 pre- as well as postsynaptic receptor function, although other studies have failed to replicate this finding.[15–20]

However, propranolol and clonidine, two agents that directly decrease noradrenergic neurotransmission, have generally not been found to be useful in the treatment of PD.

β-blockers

Use of β-adrenergic blocking agents in the treatment of anxiety began in 1966, when it was suggested that propranolol might be beneficial in managing the autonomic symptoms of anxiety, especially cardiovascular complaints.[21] Later, relief of psychic as well as somatic symptoms of anxiety disorders was also demonstrated.[22] However, a number of open trials, as well as the only placebo-controlled double-blind trial, have shown modest to no significant effect. An uncontrolled study by Heiser and Defrancisco[23] on the treatment of 10 patients with PAs (6 PD patients) with propranolol 20–80 mg daily demonstrated PA suppression in patients with a six-month history or less, but was ineffective in the three patients with a more chronic course with agoraphobia. It is of note that two patients demonstrated phobic response to first doses of propranolol and therefore did not undergo a treatment trial.

A double-blind placebo-controlled crossover study with propranolol resulted in reduction of both somatic and psychic symptoms in 17 of 26 patients with chronic anxiety disorders, including over 70% patients with PD and agoraphobia with panic attacks. It was noted that women and the presence of agoraphobia predicted better response, as opposed to men and patients with PD without agoraphobia.[22] In a double-blind crossover trial by Noyes et al[24] in 21 patients comparing two weeks diazepam with two weeks propranolol treatment, 18 patients showed moderate improvement with diazepam compared with 7 patients with propranolol. In a double-blind five-week trial by Munjack et al,[25] comparing propranolol with alprazolam and placebo, the 43% response rate in the propranolol group did not differ from placebo (40%) as measured by complete panic attack remission response. Further, acute blockade of β-adrenoreceptors with propranolol did not block lactate-induced panic attacks – a commonly used measure of drug response.[26] However, the effect of chronic propranolol treatment on lactate-induced PAs was not evaluated. In contrast, in an earlier six-week crossover trial by Mujack et al[27] comparing imipramine to propranolol treatment in 23 patients, approximately half of the PD patients achieved complete remission of PAs both on imipramine and on propranolol, with other patients partially responsive. Further, in a six-week double-blind comparison of propranolol ($n = 15$) and alprazolam ($n = 14$) by Ravaris et al,[28] both drugs were shown to be effective, with over 75% showing improvement. However, although a comparison was made with established antipanic treatment, no placebo group was studied.

Results of β-blocker studies in PD are summarized in Table 12.1.

Differences in the clinical characteristics of the population studied, study design, length of trial and dose/titration between the studies make comparison difficult. Thus, the different response rates in the studies by Munjack et al (1989)[25] and Ravaris et al (1991)[28] might be related to severity of PD, since the former study comprised primarily non-agoraphobic patients with a mean duration of illness of 6.4 years, in contrast to the latter study, with 65% patients showing moderate to severe agoraphobia and with a longer duration of illness. The two-week crossover trial of Noyes et al[24] with rapid dosage incrementation and subsequent significant side-effects contrasts with the maximal response to propranolol shown in other studies at two weeks, where no side-effects were reported due to gradual dosage increase.[28] Further, in view of demonstrated placebo response-rate variability, the lack of placebo washout or placebo control in several studies limits the conclusions that can be drawn.

Recommendations regarding the use of pro-

pranolol in PD remain somewhat tentative. It is noteworthy that, although not examined, propranolol has been considered the drug of choice for panic symptoms associated with mitral valve prolapse,[29] and may also represent a reasonable treatment in patients with other concomitant medical conditions where β blockers would be a recommended treatment, such as hypertension. However, it is important to remember that β blockers can be dangerous, especially in patients with medical illnesses such as asthma and diabetes.

Clonidine

Clonidine is an α_2-adrenergic receptor agonist that inhibits spontaneous firing of norepinephrine (noradrenaline) neurons in the locus coeruleus,[30] a site seemingly important in the mediation of anxiety.[31] Clonidine hydrochloride has been found to decrease acutely ratings of anxiety in patients with panic disorder in most,[16,17,32] although not all,[33] studies when administered intravenously in single doses of 1.5–2.0 µg/kg. Further, in the latter study,[33] assessing the ability of clonidine intravenous pretreatment to block lactate-induced panic, although clonidine significantly blocked lactate-induced panic in four out of ten subjects, over half still panicked in response to lactate despite clonidine at the dosages used. An eight-week open trial by Liebowitz et al[34] of 11 patients with panic disorder or agoraphobia with PAs, using clonidine to a maximal dose of 1 mg/day, showed four subjects to have a good antipanic response at dosages varying from 0.2 to 0.5 mg/day. Several subjects showed transient responses, although the beneficial effects could not be regained even with dosage increase to 0.7–1 mg/day. The remaining three were unable to tolerate increasing doses in attempts to achieve therapeutic benefit, and all subjects suffered bothersome side-effects,

Table 12.1 Beta-blocker treatment of panic disorder

Study	N	Design	Length of study	Mean dose[a] (range) (mg)	Results[b]	Limitations
Heiser and Defrancisco (1976)[23]	10[c]	Open	Variable	Pro (20–80)	Patients with recent panic states (less than 6 months); immediate ++/+++	Short trial, low doses
Kathol et al (1980)[22]	26[d]	Double-blind placebo cross-over	2 weeks × 2	Pro, 160	17/26 ++; psychic and cardiovascular symptoms, anxiety	Mixed diagnostic group
Noyes et al (1984)[24]	21	Double-blind crossover vs DZ	2 weeks × 2	Pro, 240 DZ, 30	DZ better than Pro 18/21 vs 7/21 ++	Short trial
Munjack et al (1985)[27]	38	Single-blind crossover vs Imi	7 weeks	Pro (<40–160) Imi (<50–300)	Imi = Pro, Pro 10/24 +++, 9/24 ++, Imi 13/25 +++, 5/25 ++	Only 23 completed both drug phases
Munjack et al (1989)[25]	55	Double-blind vs Alp and placebo	5 weeks	Pro, 184 Alp, 3.62	Pro = placebo, Alp better than placebo/Pro, Alp 15/20 +++, Pro 7/19 +++	
Ravaris et al (1991)[28]	29	Double-blind vs Alp	6 weeks	Pro, 182 Alp, 5.0	Pro = Alp, more rapid onset with Alp, both >79% ++/+++	

[a] Pro = propranolol; Imi = imipramine; DZ = diazepam; Alp = alprazolam.
[b] +, mild improvement; ++, moderate improvement; +++, marked improvement.
[c] Mixed patient sample: 6 PD.
[d] Chronic anxiety disorders: 70% PD.

including sedation, fatigue and loss of motivation. The authors concluded that the use of clonidine in PD should be restricted to patients with associated hypertension and those resistant or unable to tolerate standard therapies.

In a four-week double-blind placebo crossover study of 16 patients with panic or generalized anxiety disorder, clonidine in doses of 0.2–0.5 mg demonstrated only a modest clinical effect in PD.[35] Thus, although statistically significant improvement in psychic symptoms of anxiety was demonstrated, the decrease in somatic symptoms in the first week was not maintained. Further, 3 of the 14 PD patients worsened with treatment to the extent that therapy was discontinued, and although 8 patients found clonidine to be beneficial at reducing symptoms of anxiety relative to placebo, the effect was perceived as less so than conventional anxiolytic agents. Only the remaining 3 patients were nearly symptom-free and believed clonidine to be better than other medications. Also, undesirable side-effects were reported in the majority of subjects. This patient population had been previously treated for PD with medications not described, and might therefore represent a treatment refractory sample.

However, in a crossover study by Ko et al,[36] of six patients with PD who were treated for four weeks with placebo, clonidine hydrochloride (4–5 μg/kg/day) and a relatively low dose of imipramine hydrochloride (100 mg/day), clonidine was found to be more effective than imipramine in reducing anxiety stimulated by phobic exposure.

When oral clonidine was administered to 18 patients in a double-blind flexible-dose treatment trial lasting 10 weeks in duration,[32] although anxiolytic effects on several panic and anxiety measures were noticed in some patients, these effects did not emerge in the group as a whole. It is noteworthy that differ-ential responses of different aspects of each individual symptomatology, not evident on statistical analysis for the entire group, were found. The contrasting potential usefulness in short-term in contrast to long-term anxiolytic treatment might be explained by tolerance, which has also been reported for clonidine's sedative[37] and analgesic[38] properties. Tolerance to the anxiolytic effect of chronic clonidine treatment has been postulated to be due to desensitization of locus coeruleus α_2 autoreceptors.[39]

Results of studies of clonidine in PD are summarized in Table 12.2.

Anticonvulsants

A pathophysiological role of epileptiform activity in at least some PD patients has been raised by a number of lines of evidence.

(1) The phenomenology of PD including paroxysmal onset, short duration, psychosensory and dissociative symptoms, autonomic nervous system activation, and a chronic course resembles that of epilepsy – in particular, complex partial seizures.[40] Anxiety, particularly auras of fear or panic, is the most common mental system in temporal lobe epilepsy (TLE).[41] Further, stimulation of limbic and temporal lobe structures in humans produces fear and panic-like reactions.

(2) The co-occurrence of PD and epilepsy, especially temporal lobe epilepsy, has been reported, and sometimes presents problems of differential diagnosis.[42–45]

(3) The role of distinct brain structures (temporal/limbic) has been established for epilepsy. MRI studies have found brain abnormalities in these structures, suggesting that such dysfunctions may also be present in PD.[46,47] PET studies have found an abnormal interhemispheric asymmetry of

Table 12.2 Clonidine (α_2-agonist) treatment of panic disorder

Study	N	Design	Length of study	Mean dose (range) (mg/day)	Results
Liebowitz et al (1981)[34]	11	Open	8 weeks	Maximum 1	4/11 ++
Hoehn-Saric et al (1981)[35]	14[a]	Double-blind placebo crossover	4 weeks × 2	(0.2–0.5)	+, psychic symptoms > somatic symptoms
Ko et al (1983)[36]	6[b]	Double-blind crossover vs imipramine	6 weeks × 3	(4–5 µg/kg/day)	Clonidine more effective than imipramine in phobic anxiety reduction
Uhde et al (1989)[32]	18	Double-blind placebo crossover	10 weeks	0.6	No advantage over placebo

[a] Mixed sample: 8 generalized anxiety disorder (GAD); 6PD.
[b] Mixed sample: GAD and PD.
+, mild improvement; ++, moderate improvement; +++, marked improvement.

parahippocampal blood flow in PD.[47,48] Further, EEG abnormalities have been found in 14–60% of PD patients.[40,44,49,50] Although the majority of patients with PD have normal EEGs, this must be tempered by the failure of surface EEG studies to detect abnormal activity in deeper brain structures, such as the limbic system.[50]

(4) Some PD patients with concomitant or past evidence of a seizure disorder have been shown to improve with anticonvulsant therapy.[42,43,51] In fact, a subgroup of patients with atypical panic symptoms, such as hostility, irritability and social withdrawal, have been reported to display abnormal EEG findings and to show some response to carbamazepine or benzodiazepines, such as alprazolam or clonazepam.[52]

(5) Benzodiazepines, in particular high-potency anxiolytic and anticonvulsant agents such as alpazolam and clonazepam, enhancing GABA transmission, have been shown to be efficacious in the treatment of PD. However, limited controlled data exist for anticonvulsant treatment of PD.

Valproic acid (sodium valproate)

Data suggest that valproic acid may possess antipanic activity. Firstly, studies in animals and humans suggest that drugs enhancing GABA activity in the brain, such as benzodiazepines and valproic acid, exert anxiolytic effects.[53,54] Further, valproic acid seems to be unique among anticonvulsants in that it has been shown to possess properties comparable to those of benzodiazepines in animal models of anxiety.[55]

A small number of case reports have described antipanic effects of valproic acid.[56,57] In open trials, Primeau et al[58] reported moderate improvement in 6 out of 10 patients in panic attacks and diffuse anxiety, with less improvement in phobic anxiety measures. Although a rapid response was noticed during the first week of the treatment, additional improvement was seen in the six remaining weeks of the study. Woodman and Noyes[59] showed marked improvement in 9 out of 12 patients, with the remaining 3 showing moderate improvement in terms of panic attacks and phobic symptoms. Again, although some patients noted improvement in the first week of treatment, maximum effect was often not achieved until the second or third week. Further, the improvement was maintained at 6 months and 18 months follow-up. The medication was well tolerated, with patients experiencing few side-effects that limited treatment. Keck et al,[60] in a study of 16 patients, showed a 50% reduction in frequency of panic attacks in 10 out of 14 patients completing the trial, as well as a reduction in general anxiety, with 6 patients showing complete remission. Interestingly, valproic acid treatment blocked the reinduction of panic symptoms on lactate rechallenge in 10 of 12 patients who had initially experienced panic symptoms on initial infusion.

The only placebo-controlled double-blind crossover study showed a significant improvement in Clinical Global Impression severity and improvement, in length and intensity of panic attacks, and in psychic and somatic anxiety scores in PD patients withdrawn from BZs. This study included a seven-day placebo washout, following BZ use, and random assignment to two treatments of six weeks. Five patients reported valproic acid-related gastrointestinal dysfunction, dizziness and sleepiness. It should be noted that all patients were responders to BZ treatment. However, the relevance of this study to niaive or BZ non-responder PD patients remains to be determined.[61]

It is worth adding that valproic acid may have a role to play in patients with comorbid psychiatric disorders. Thus two patients with panic disorder and comorbid affective disorder (bipolar and organic affective disorder) and alcohol abuse were reported to respond to valproic acid treatment.[62] However, firm recommendations on the role of valproic acid as an anxiolytic and specifically antipanic agent will depend on results of rigorous controlled clinical trials that include comparisons with standard efficacious therapies and placebo.

Carbamazepine

Carbamazepine has been reported to be effective in ameliorating panic attacks in patients with EEG abnormalities.[43,51,52] In an open trial with 34 patients treated for a year with carbamazepine, good response was observed in 58.8% of the patients on the basis of the variation in the number of panic attacks, the degree of avoidance behavior and active functioning. Significant correlation between response and duration of treatment was found ($p < 0.02$). Good response was correlated with administration of carbamazepine for periods longer than an average of 7.2 months. Correlation was also noted between response and drug dose ($p < 0.05$; good response was correlated with doses ranging between 170 and 500 mg/day).[63] However, in 10 patients treated with carbamazepine, although decreases in help seeking and dysphoria were reported, no blockade of panic attacks was achieved.[64]

In the only controlled study, by Uhde et al,[65] carbamazepine was not found to be significantly superior to placebo in the patients with regard to outcome measures including frequency of panic attacks, global severity index, phobic anxiety, generalized anxiety, and panic anxiety and depression subscales, although statistically significant decreases in anxiety scores

were noted on several measures. All patients had a placebo period of at least two weeks before starting carbamazepine and at least three weeks carbamazepine treatment, with a mean ± SD duration of treatment 66 ± 43.4 days. The mean ± SD peak dose of carbamazepine was 679 ± 299 mg/day, with a mean blood level 8.4 ± 1.6 µg/ml (within the therapeutic range). Placebo–drug comparisons were between the week before initiation of carbamazepine treatment (while the patients were taking placebo) and the last week of treatment at the maximum dose of carbamazepine administered. Of note, 4 of the original 18 subjects recruited dropped out of the study. One patient became too 'agitated' while taking carbamazepine, one patient developed dizziness and blurred vision, and one patient developed a pruritic rash. The fourth patient showed a dramatic possibly placebo, response to carbamazepine and demanded treatment on an open basis. The presence of either EEG abnormalities or prominent psychosensory symptoms did not predict response to carbamazepine. Results from this study must be tempered with lack of placebo run-in and exclusion of placebo responders, as well as small numbers of patients. Furthermore, the possibly inadequate length of treatment may be relevant in view of the findings of the open study, where good response was correlated with administration of carbamazepine for periods longer than the average of 7.2 months – albeit a clinically questionable and very lengthy latency period. Carbamazepine, however, has been shown to be efficacious in assisting alprazolam withdrawal as measured by dropout rates from discontinuation in PD patients, who as a group are more vulnerable to alprazolam withdrawal.[66]

Differentiation of re-emergence of PD symptoms from BZ withdrawal symptoms is difficult to determine because of overlapping symptoms.

Further, PD symptoms were not measured, but it is noteworthy that, even with carbamazepine, 53% of patients ($n = 36$) dropped out of this benzodiazepine discontinuation study. This contrasts successful discontinuation of BZ (variety of BZs) treatment and PD symptom resolution in the 12 patients treated with valproic acid compared with placebo.[61] It is noteworthy that length of BZ treatment, prior experience to withdrawal, rate of dose reduction and pharmacokinetics of the specific BZ under investigation – factors also shown to play a significant role in determining the success of withdrawal – may have also contributed to the differential efficacy.[66,67]

The apparent differential efficacy of clonazepam and possible preliminary efficacy of valproic acid compared with carbamazepine, at least as shown in open trials, might allow speculation about mechanisms involved in the mediation of pathological anxiety and its treatment. Clonazepam, highly effective in the treatment of PD,[68,69] is active at the central benzodiazepine receptor.[70] Further, valproic acid enhances GABA activity within the brain by increasing synaptic levels of GABA and enhancing neuronal responsiveness to this inhibitory neurotransmitter, thereby increasing GABA activity at the $GABA_A$ and $GABA_B$ receptors. In contrast, carbamazepine has activity at the $GABA_B$ but weaker activity at the $GABA_A$ receptor complex and at the peripheral-type benzodiazepine receptor.[71,72] This would have virtually no effect on the GABA–BZ–chloride ionophore macromolecular complex.[73] Activity at the central rather than the peripheral BZ receptor might be crucial in treating panic attacks.

Other anticonvulsants

Phenobarbital and phenytoin have been reported to be effective in eliminating panic symptoms in single cases with concomitant EEG abnormalities.[51] However, the relevance of this observation to PD or even PD with historical or current epilepsy remains to be determined.

Results of anticonvulsant studies in PD are summarized in Table 12.3.

Other GABA-ergic agents: baclofen

Since several studies have suggested that antianxiety and antidepressant drugs that produce antipanic effects also augment GABA transmission,[74,75] a trial of baclofen, a selective $GABA_B$ agonist, in PD was carried out. Nine medication-free PD patients were treated with 30 mg/day of oral baclofen for four weeks in a double-blind placebo-controlled crossover trial. Baclofen was significantly more effective than placebo in reducing the number of panic attacks and scores on the Hamilton and Zung anxiety scales and Katz-R nervousness scales, with no effect on depressive symptoms. Few side-effects were reported. However, further studies are needed to support baclofen's efficacy in PD treatment.

CCK agents and other neuropeptides

As outlined in Chapter 5, an anxiogenic role of CCK was suggested by deMontigny,[76] who observed that intravenous injection of CCK in the tetrapeptide form (CCK-4) induced realistic panic-like attacks in healthy volunteers. Further, data suggested that patients with panic disorder seem to have an increased sensitivity to CCK-4.[77]

An exploratory double-blind placebo-controlled trial in patients with panic disorder showed that L-365,260, a compound with specific and high-affinity antagonist activity for the

Table 12.3 Reports of anticonvulsant treatment of panic disorder

Study	N	Design	Length of study	Mean dose (range) (mg)	Blood level	Results[a]	Comments
Carbamazepine							
Edlund et al (1987)[52]	6	Series	–	–	–	Decrease in help-seeking and dysphoria reported	5/6 had EEG abnormalities
Uhde et al (1988)[65]	14	Placebo-controlled	≥3 weeks	679	8.4 µg/µl	No significant reduction in care symptoms compared with placebo	12/14 totally normal EEG
Tondo et al (1989)[63]	34	Open-series	1 year	(170–500)	–	20/34 ++	EEG data not described
McNamara and Fogel (1990)[43]	1	Case	–	–	–	1 ++	EEG abnormal, left temporal lobe
Dantendorfer et al (1995)[51]	1	Case	12 months	–	20 µmol/l	1 +++	EEG abnormal, right temporal lobe
Valproic acid							
Roy-Byrne (1988)[56]	1	Case	1 year	–	–	1 ++	EEG abnormal, left temporal lobe
Primeau et al (1990)[58]	10	Open-series	7 weeks	Maximum 2250	Not stated	6 ++, panic attacks, diffuse anxiety, more improvement than phobic anxiety	–
Lum et al (1991)[61]	12	Double-blind placebo-controlled	6 weeks	Until maximum therapeutic dose (dose not stated)	–	12 ++/+++	Placebo washout post BZ discontinuation
Keck et al (1993)[60]	16	Open	4 weeks	1105	74 µg/ml	10/16 ++ 6/16 +++	10/12 blocked reinduction PAs on lactate rechallenge
Woodman and Noyes (1994)[59]	12	Open	6 weeks plus 6 and 18 months follow-up	1330	75 µg/ml	9/12 +++ 3/12 ++	–
Brady et al (1994)[62]	2	Series	6 months and 9 months	(1500–2000)	89.8 µg/ml and 74.6 µg/ml	2/2 +++	Concomitant mood disorder and alcohol abuse

Table 12.3 Reports of anticonvulsant treatment of panic disorder

Study	N	Design	Length of study	Mean dose (range) (mg)	Blood level	Results[a]	Comments
Phenytoin							
Dantendorfer et al (1995)[51]	1	Case	–	–	50 µmol/l	1 ++	EEG abnormal, left parietoccipital lobe
Phenobarbital							
Dantendorfer et al (1995)[51]	1	Case	–	–	75 µmol/l	1 ++	–

[a] +, mild improvement; ++, moderate improvement; +++, marked improvement.

CCKB receptor (subtype, primarily located in the brain), prevented CCK-4-induced panic attacks in a dose-related fashion. Thus pretreatment with the highest doses of L-365,260 (50 mg) prevented CCK-4-induced panic attacks in all PD patients ($n = 14$), in contrast to pretreatment with placebo, where panic attacks were observed in 85% of patients (12/14) when 20 µg of CCK-4 was administered 90 minutes later.[78]

In a multicenter placebo-controlled double-blind trial investigating the efficacy of L-365,260 in patients with PD with or without agoraphobia, 40 patients received L-365,260 (120 mg/day) and 43 placebo, following a one-week single-blind placebo period.[79] At the dose tested, there were no clinically significant differences between L-365,260 and placebo in global improvement ratings, Hamilton anxiety rating scale scores, panic attack frequency, intensity or disability measures. Although not statistically significant, there were numerical trends in favor of the drug at the end of the study in terms of higher response rate versus placebo (61% versus 48%), as measured by physicians' global improvement scale and mean change from baseline in number of weekly panic attacks and disability scores. The authors, however, suggested that the CCK hypothesis of PD could not be discarded on the basis of these results, since the potential site of action of L-365,260 is not known, and the drug may not have distributed to regions involved in the prevention of endogenous panic attacks. Secondly, although peak levels were constant, at values known to counteract the majority of CCK-4-induced panic attacks, trough levels may have been inadequate in blocking endogenous panic attacks.

It is noteworthy that, in a study of 24 patients, pretreatment with 50 mg L365,260, shown to prevent CCK-4-induced panic attacks in PD patients, did not block sodium lactate-induced panic attacks,[80] in contrast to clinically effective established antipanic agents.[33,81,82]

The role of other neuropeptides, such as corticotropin releasing factor (CRF) or neuropeptide Y (NPY), in PD is less clear. CRF seems to coordinate endocrine, physiologic and behavior responses to stressful stimuli,[83] and appears to be anxiogenic.[84] Interestingly, benzodiazepines would appear to reduce anxiogenic-like effects of CRF,[84] as well as to decrease CRF concentrations in the locus coeruleus.[85] Evidence from human and animal studies suggests that NPY may be a potent endogenous anxiolytic agent.[86] Further, the neuropeptide galanin, functionally related to NPY, has also been observed to possess specific anxiolytic-like actions similar to those of NPY.[87] However, drugs acting on receptors of these neuropeptides have yet to be investigated in PD.

Dopaminergic drugs

A small number of studies of dopamine function in PD have produced mixed results. An elevated growth hormone response to the dopamine agonist apomorphine was reported,[88] and although no difference was found in plasma homovanillic acid (HVA) values between PD patients and controls, a bimodal distribution was seen with patients in the high-HVA group being more symptomatic than patients in the low HVA group.[89] However, a study of plasma dopamine[90] and two studies of CSF HVA[91,92] failed to demonstrate abnormal dopamine metabolism in PD patients. It is of note that early trials of dopamine antagonists proved ineffective in PD.[93] However, a cross-sectional study of PD patients and treatments received showed that 29% of the patients received neuroleptic treatment.[94] Buproprion, a dopamine uptake inhibitor, has also been found in one study to be ineffective in treating panic attacks.[95]

As reported in previous chapters, MAOIs combining noradrenergic, serotonergic and dopaminergic activity have been established as effective antipanic agents, and clomipramine, a very effective antipanic agent, has some activity in the dopamine system in addition to its action in the serotonin system. Lastly, roxindole, a dopamine autoreceptor agonist and serotonin reuptake inhibitor, has been demonstrated in an open trial to have antipanic effects in five out of eight patients after four weeks of treatment.[96] However, the relevance of dopamine activity in the antipanic effect of this drug has yet to be determined.

Barbiturates

Trials of barbiturates were predominantly as adjuvant to exposure therapy, with intravenous administration of single doses. Out of five studies, two showed no or a negative effect,[97,98] with three studies showing some positive effect.[99,101] However, in these studies, no injection control was given and follow-up was inconclusive.

Side-effects of these agents, with very significant toxicity, have resulted in a marked decline in their use in clinical practice and there would be no indication for their use in the long-term treatment of PD. Further, recent evidence seems to suggest that sedative therapy prior to exposure in behavior therapies might impede efficacy.[102]

Second-messenger agents: inositol

Inositol is an isomer of glucose that is a key metabolic precursor in the phosphatidylinositol (PI) cycle. It is a precursor of an intracellular second-messenger system for numerous neurotransmitters.[103] Markedly reduced levels of inositol in CSF were reported in depressed patients,[104] and inositol was shown in both open and double-blind studies to cause significant improvements in depression.[105,106] Although no disturbance of inositol levels has yet been reported in PD, a double-blind random placebo-controlled crossover trial in 21 patients was studied, since some antidepressants are also effective in PD.[107]

Treatment phases lasted four weeks, consisting of 12 g inositol or placebo. Number of panic attacks, panic scores and phobia scores improved significantly more on inositol than on placebo, although Hamilton anxiety and depression scores did not show significantly more improvement. The patient population comprised predominantly mixed PD and agoraphobia patients (16/21), as well as those with PD without agoraphobia. However, 1 mg p.r.n. lorazepam was allowed, although use of this benzodiazepine did not differ between phases, nor did lorazepam use appear to interact with inositol's beneficial effect on panic attacks.

The efficacy of inositol administration alone in PD merits further investigation.

Verapamil

Calcium plays a central role in a variety of neurobiological processes, such as neurotransmitter release, postsynaptic effects, electrical activation of excitable cells and hormone release.[108-111] Calcium-channel blockers such as verapamil inhibit depolarization-induced calcium influxes into cells,[112] and can inhibit neurotransmitter (e.g. norepinephric) release from brain synaptosomal preparations.[113,114] They can also increase cerebral blood flow, which is possibly relevant since reductions in cerebral blood flow or brain hypoxia have been suggested in anxiety states.[115,116] Further, their negative chonotropic and inotropic effects[112,117] might improve panic-related cardiovascular manifestations, namely tachycardia, palpitations and increased blood pressure.

An open study of verapamil, 240 mg/day in which four of seven patients with PD had a favorable response suggested that verapamil treatment might reduce pathological anxiety and block panic attacks.[118] A 16-week double-blind crossover study in 11 patients with PD was carried out,[119] where patients received four weeks placebo followed by verapamil at a slowly increasing dose up to a maximum maintenance dose of 480 mg/day for five weeks, followed by placebo substitution for an additional four weeks. A statistically significant, although clinically modest, reduction in the number of panic attacks and Zung anxiety rating scores was observed, along with the expected hypotensive effect of this drug. Despite a significant decrease in the number of panic attacks, there was no significant improvement in agoraphobia over the relatively brief time course of the study. Four patients rated themselves as having markedly benefitted from the drug, three had a marginal response, and four were complete non-responders.

It is noteworthy that verapamil's anxiolytic action is unlikely to be mediated by its effects on cardiac and brain vascular systems, since nifedipine, which shares similar properties in these domains, would seem to be ineffective in the treatment of phobic anxiety (as cited in reference 119). As verapamil has been shown to be more potent than nifedipine in inhibiting noradrenergic release from synaptic vesicles,[113,114] this mechanism might be relevant to the antipanic efficacy.

Summary

Although a number of other drug treatments (non-antidepressants and non-BZs) have been reported in the treatment of panic disorder, data are as yet lacking to establish unequivocal efficacy. Although placebo-controlled trials have established efficacy for verapamil and valproic acid (at least after BZ discontinuation) in the treatment of PD, the small numbers of patients and lack of replications limit conclusions. Although open trials and case reports have suggested the efficacy of a variety of other agents, the placebo response in PD is high and has been reported to vary between 25% and 40%, although this may be short-lived, and thus necessitates placebo control to establish efficacy. Despite the paucity of available data, other treatments discussed may have a role to play in the treatment of PD or panic attacks when comorbid with other conditions. Further, conditions such as substance abuse may limit use and efficacy of other agents, particularly benzodiazepines. Lastly, these agents may have a role in cases with limited response and intolerable side-effects to other agents. However, much work is needed to establish the efficacy and the role of other drug treatments in PD.

Augmentation therapy
Introduction

As mentioned at the beginning of this chapter, although in general roughly 75% of patients show good responses to three classes of classical antipanic medication, namely TCAs, MAOIs and BZs, 5–20% of patients fail to respond to conventional treatment or experience unacceptable side-effects,[1,2] with a higher proportion showing only partial response in symptom domains. For example, in a $2\frac{1}{2}$-year mean follow-up study of PD patients treated with TCAs, with two-thirds of the patients remaining on medication at follow-up, although three-quarters of the patients reported at least moderate improvement, only 14% were free of symptoms (note, however, the mean dose of 109 mg/day imipramine).[3]

Augmentation therapy involves the addition of a second medication to increase the response to a partially effective medication, and is therefore indicated in cases of treatment-resistant anxiety.

Before starting augmentation therapy, an evaluation must first be made of contributing factors to 'treatment resistance'. Factors contributing to a patient remaining symptomatic despite pharmacotherapy may be divided into patient-related and pharmacologic factors.[120]

Patient-related factors

Comorbid psychiatric disorders
Comorbid depression, agoraphobia, social phobia, personality disorders and family dysfunction may all interfere with response to treatment for PD. Recognition of comorbid disorders allows tailoring of interventions to maximize response. Thus panic patients with significant comorbid depression may respond better to an antidepressant than to a benzodiazepine. Alternatively, significant personality dysfunction or psychosocial disturbance may contribute to ongoing symptoms unless specifically addressed during treatment.[120,121]

Untreated cognitive factors and anxiety sensitivity
Studies examining factors associated with chronicity and recurrence found untreated phobic fear, avoidance and sensitivity to anxiety to be associated with persistent symptomatology,[122,123] consistent with greater agoraphobic avoidance and comorbid social phobia as predictors of poor outcome in a number of follow-up studies of treated patients.[124,125] This is supported by one study where 40% of medication-refractory patients entered remission after addition of cognitive–behavioral therapy (CBT).[7] Further data also suggest better response with the addition of CBT to medication.[6,7,126]

Comorbid medical conditions
Although not systematically studied, comorbid medical conditions may contribute to chronicity. Factors may include direct anxiogenic effects of certain medical conditions (e.g. chronic obstructive pulmonary disease) or medications used to treat them (e.g. bronchodilators).[127] Some conditions, such as ischemic heart disease, may trigger anxiety by potential life-threatening significance or by mimicking anxiety symptoms, making diagnosis and treatment difficult. Further, medically ill patients may be more sensitive to the side-effects of medication and unable to tolerate therapeutic levels of antipanic medication. Thus optimal treatment of underlying medical factors may in itself improve response.[120]

Pharmacologic factors

Inadequate dose
Although anxiety disorder patients seem to be more sensitive to the initial phase of medication than depressive patients, they frequently require similar dosing. Studies measuring plasma levels of imipramine[128,129] and alprazolam[130] have supported a clear dose–response relationship in PD and agoraphobia patients. Thus doses of imipramine up to 300 mg/day should be tried, failing adequate response, with subsequent plasma levels determined when response is limited in order to detect rapid metabolizers.[131] Similarly, target doses of BZs include 4–10 mg/day for alprazolam and 2–5 mg/day for clonazepam.[120,132]

Inadequate frequency of administration
Medications with short half-lives will need appropriate frequency of administration. Thus short-acting benzodiazepines, such as alprazolam, must be administered three times a day to prevent rebound withdrawal/anxiety symptoms.

Inadequate length of treatment

Although most patients will respond to anti-depressant medication within 3–4 weeks, some patients may take 12–24 weeks to respond.[133]

Adverse side-effects

These may limit a patient's willingness or ability to receive an adequate trial of pharmacotherapy. Thus, in studies of antidepressant treatment, one-quarter to one-third of patients have been reported to drop out owing to troublesome side-effects.[134] In a $2\frac{1}{2}$-year follow-up study of TCA treatment of PD patients, more than half who stopped therapy did so because of medication side-effects, including increased anxiety early in the course of treatment and weight gain over the long term.[3] The most troublesome side-effects of MAOIs include insomnia and weight gain, while benzodiazepines show problems of sedation, cognitive impairment, somnolence, tolerance, abuse and dependence. Efficient and careful management of treatment-emergent side-effects,[135] as well as addressing cognitive fears of addiction and dependence, in addition to the development and use of newer agents with more favorable side-effect profiles may facilitate compliance and outcome.

However, when all factors are considered, the management of patients who remain symptomatic despite an adequate trial of treatment has not been well studied. Although no controlled study of augmentation treatment has yet been published, and the existing data consist of case series and reports, there is a rationale to combine agents with different pharmacological activities in the treatment of PD that is intolerant or resistant to monotherapy. Combination treatments, distinct from augmentation strategies (as described in major depression), will also be discussed here. Further, the concept of drug resistance in panic disorder, although commonly used in daily practise, is not well established or well defined.

Strategies used can be divided into several categories.

Combined treatment with different classes of medication

Antidepressant and benzodiazepines

Initial alprazolam supplementation during imipramine treatment followed by a gradual taper has been suggested in view of the different mode and time course (late versus immediate) of action of antidepressants on panic symptomatology and the difficulties experienced by some patients in discontinuing long-term benzodiazepine treatment. In a controlled trial of alprazolam supplementation to imipramine treatment, patients in combined treatment improved more rapidly, although they had more difficulty following the taper schedule.[136] Further, although combination treatment has been described as often used, it is unclear whether the combination represents supplementation of response to one of the agents.

Propranolol and benzodiazepines

Hallstrom et al[137] described the use of the combination of diazepam and propranolol in the treatment of 24 'chronically anxious' (including PD) outpatients, and reported the combination to be superior to either drug used alone. Shehi and Patterson[138] described the successful open-label treatment of 16 patients with PD using 40–160 mg propranolol combined with 1.5–3 mg alprazolam, with reduction of panic attacks within two weeks in all PD patients (excluding one dropout), as well as improvement of the somatic and psychic anxiety manifestations. Combination permitted the use of lower doses of each drug, allowing reduction in one or both medications below the level of the standard effective dose, with two patients reported to have discontinued scheduled doses of alprazolam. The role of each agent as augmentor has yet to be studied.

It is noteworthy that pindolol, a β-blocker with additional antagonistic serotenergic properties (5-HT$_{1A}$ receptor blockade), has been shown in some studies to be efficacious in the augmentation of antidepressant response in major depression.[139] Preliminary data have also suggested the efficacy of pindolol in augmenting response in PD non-responders to 20 mg fluoxetine.[140]

Combined treatment within classes of medication
Combination benzodiazepines

Although in a case series of 10 treatment-resistant PD patients responding to clonazepam, two patients described further relief on adding alprazolam to clonazepam,[141] there are at present few data to suggest efficacy of treatment with more than one benzodiazepine. It is possible that this finding may be related to the BZ withdrawal symptoms, rather than to the PD itself.

Combination antidepressants

In a case series of seven patients with refractory or relapsing PD, the majority with agoraphobia who had failed treatment with a wide range of different agents and psychological approaches, full remission was obtained with combinations of fluoxetine and TCAs, often with the second agent at subtherapeutic doses, indicating augmentory activity.[142] This could be pharmacokinetic, as serum levels of TCAs were not measured – a factor relevant in view of reported three- to fourfold increases in TCA levels with fluoxetine treatment.[143] It is noteworthy that this combination has been reported efficacious in depression non-responders,[144] although the efficacy of this combination has yet to be determined in placebo-controlled trials.

A further case report has demonstrated the efficacy of combination treatment of moclobemide with imipramine, as well as with behavior therapy, in a treatment-resistant patient.[145]

Augmentation of antidepressant or benzodiazepine response
Lithium

Two case reports of patients with panic disorder responding to lithium augmentation of TCAs have been reported,[146,147] supporting the possibility of lithium augmentation in PD.

A case series of five patients showing minimum benefit with six weeks tricyclic treatment showed complete resolution (four patients) or marked improvement (one patient) when lithium was added; recurrence occurred on lithium discontinuation (two patients) and resolution with reinstitution.[148] As in depression, response occurred within 10 days, and it is of note that none of the patients had a previous history of mood disorder.

Valproate

A case series of four patients unresponsive to antidepressants and/or benzodiazepine treatment showed marked improvement with the addition of valproate to clonazepam within four weeks. Clonazepam decrease resulted in recurrence of panic attacks, and although in two cases valproate was gradually decreased and stopped without relapse, in the other two patients it was reduced to 500 mg, resulting in relapse. An increase in GABA transmission via different mechanisms of actions of the two agents was postulated to account for the beneficial effect of the combination.[149]

A single case report of full response of panic attacks with comorbid depression after the addition of valproate to fluoxetine treatment has also been described.[150]

Buspirone

The addition of buspirone to ongoing long-term benzodiazepine with or without antidepressant treatment in four cases of PD resulted in marked improvements in the domains of anticipatory and generalized anxiety, allowing reduction of benzodiazepine dose in three patients.[151] (However, the authors mentioned three additional similar cases: one with marked, one with equivocal and one with no improvement in symptomatology.) Further, in one of the four patients, buspirone augmentation improved social phobic symptoms in addition to previously remitted panic attacks. Buspirone may thus have a role to play in PD treatment in the light of the persisting generalized, anticipatory or social anxiety that is often present in PD patients.

Future directions and conclusions

Despite some limited efficacy of pharmacological treatments of PD, no controlled data are available on augmentation treatments. Although combined treatments are often used, the rationale may be related to side-effects, time course or dose response of one medication. A number of authors have suggested similarities between PD and mood disorders with respect to course and treatment.[152] Much more data are available on the study of augmentation treatments in major depressive disorders, which may be relevant and applicable in the treatment of PD. The role of combined pharmacological and psychological treatments, as well as issues of length and doses of long-term treatments, have been studied and are continuing to be elucidated.

References

1. Ballenger JC, Panic disorder: efficacy of current treatments. *Psychopharmacol Bull* 1993; **29**: 477–86.
2. Roy-Byrne PF, Cowley DS, Course and outcome in panic disorder: a review of recent follow-up studies. *Anxiety* 1995; **1**: 151–60.
3. Noyes R, Garvey MJ, Cook BL et al, Problems with tricyclic antidepressant use in patients with panic disorder or agoraphobia: results of a naturalistic follow-up study. *J Clin Psychiatry* 1989; **50**: 163–9.
4. Sheehan DV, Ballenger J, Jacobsen G, Treatment of endogenous anxiety with phobic, hysterical and hypochondriacal symptoms. *Arch Gen Psychiatry* 1980; **37**: 51–9.
5. Ciraulo DA, Sands BF, Shader RI, Critical review of liability for benzodiazepine abuse among alcoholics. *Am J Psychiatry* 1988; **145**: 1501–6.
6. Mavissakalian M, Sequential combination of imipramine and self-directed exposure in the treatment of panic disorder with agoraphobia. *J Clin Psychiatry* 1990; **51**: 184–8.
7. Pollack MH, Otto MW, Kaspi SP et al, Cognitive–behavioral therapy for medication refractory panic disorder. *J Clin Psychiatry* 1994; **55**: 200–5.
8. Redmond D, Huang Y, Current concepts. II. New evidence for a locus coeruleus-norepinephrine connection with anxiety. *Life Sci* 1979; **25**: 2149–62.
9. Pohl R, Yeragani V, Balon R et al, Isoproterenol-induced panic attacks. *Biol Psychiatry* 1988; **24**: 891–902.
10. Nesse R, Cameron O, Curtis GC et al, Adrenergic function in patients with panic anxiety. *Arch Gen Psychiatry* (1984) **41**: 771–6.

11. Charney D, Heninger G, Breier A, Noradrenergic function in panic anxiety: Effects of yohimbine in healthy subjects and patients with agoraphobia and panic disorder. *Arch Gen Psychiatry* 1984; **41**: 751–63.

12. Charney D, Woods S, Goodman W et al, Neurobiological mechanisms of panic anxiety: biochemical and behavioral correlates of yohimbine-induced panic attacks. *Am J Psychiatry* 1987; **144**: 1030–6.

13. Charney DS, Woods SW, Krystal JH et al, Noradrenergic neuronal dysregulation in panic disorder: the effects of intravenous yohimbine and clonidine in panic disorder patients. *Acta Psychiatr Scand* 1992; **86**: 273–82.

14. Gurguis G, Uhde T, Plasma 3-methoxy-4-hydroxyphenyl ethylene glycol (MHPG) and growth hormone responses to yohimbine in panic disorder patients and normal controls. *Psychoneuroendocrinology* 1990; **15**: 217–24.

15. Uhde T, Vittone B, Siever L et al, Blunted growth hormone response to clonidine in panic disorder patients. *Biol Psychiatry* 1986; **21**: 1081–5.

16. Charney DS, Heninger GR, Abnormal regulation of noradrenergic function in panic disorder: effects of clonidine in healthy subjects and patients with agoraphobia and panic disorder. *Arch Gen Psychiatry* 1986; **43**: 1042–55.

17. Nutt D, Altered central alpha-2-adrenoreceptor sensitivity in panic disorder. *Arch Gen Psychiatry* 1989; **46**: 165–9.

18. Abelson J, Glitz D, Cameron O et al, Endocrine, cardiovascular, and behavioral responses to clonidine in patients with panic disorder. *Biol Psychiatry* 1992; **32**: 18–25.

19. Tancer ME, Stein MB, Black B et al, Blunted growth hormone responses to growth hormone-releasing factor and to clonidine in panic disorder. *Am J Psychiatry* 1993; **150**: 336–7.

20. Schittecatte M, Charles G, Depauw Y et al, Growth hormone response to clonidine in panic disorder patients. *Psychiatry Res* 1988; **23**: 147–51.

21. Granville-Grossman KL, Turner P, The effect of propranolol on anxiety. *Lancet* 1966; **i**: 788–90.

22. Kathol R, Noyes R Jr, Slymen DJ et al, Propranolol in chronic anxiety disorders: a controlled study. *Arch Gen Psychiatry* 1980; **37**: 1361–5.

23. Heiser JF, Defrancisco D, The treatment of pathological panic states with propranolol. *Am J Psychiatry* 1976; **133**: 1389–94.

24. Noyes RJ, Anderson DJ, Clancy J et al, Diazepam and propranolol in panic disorder and agoraphobia. *Arch Gen Psychiatry* 1984; **41**: 287–92.

25. Munjack DJ, Crocker B, Cabe D et al, Alprazolam, propranolol, and placebo in the treatment of panic disorder and agoraphobia with panic attacks. *J Clin Psychopharmacol* 1989; **9**: 22–7.

26. Gorman JM, Levy GF, Liebowitz MR et al, Effect of acute beta-adrenergic blockade on lactate-induced panic. *Arch Gen Psychiatry* 1983; **40**: 1079–82.

27. Munjack DJ, Rebal R, Shaner R et al, Imipramine versus propranolol for the treatment of panic attacks: a pilot study. *Compr Psychiatry* 1985; **26**: 80–9.

28. Ravaris CI, Friedman MJ, Hauri PJ et al, A controlled study of alprazolam and propranolol in panic-disordered and agoraphobic outpatients. *J Clin Psychopharmacol* 1991; **11**: 344–50.

29. Venkatesh A, Pauls DL, Crowe RR et al, Mitral valve prolapse in anxiety neurosis (panic disorder). *Am Heart J* 1980; **100**: 302–5.

30. Svensson TH, Bunney BS, Aghajanian GK, Inhibition of both noradrenergic and serotonergic neurons in brain by the alpha adrenergic agonist clonidine. *Brain Res* 1975; **92**: 291–306.

31. Redmond DE, New and old evidence for the involvement of a brain norepinephrine system in anxiety. In: *Phenomenology and Treatment of Anxiety* (Fann WE, Karacan I, Pokorny AD et al, eds). New York: SP Medical & Scientific Books, 1979: 152–203.

32. Uhde TW, Stein MB, Vittone BJ et al, Behavioral and physiologic effects of short-term and long-term administration of clonidine in panic disorder. *Arch Gen Psychiatry* 1989; **46**: 170–7.

33. Coplan JD, Liebowitz MR, Gorman JM et al,

Noradrenergic function in panic disorder: effects of intravenous clonidine pretreatment on lactate-induced panic. *Biol Psychiatry* 1992; **31**: 135–46.

34. Liebowitz MR, Fyer AJ, McGrath P et al, Clonidine treatment of panic disorder. *Psychopharmacol Bull* 1981; **17**: 122–3.

35. Hoehn-Saric R, Merchant AF, Keyser ML et al, Effects of clonidine on anxiety disorders. *Arch Gen Psychiatry* 1981; **38**: 1273–8.

36. Ko GN, Elsworth JD, Roth RH et al, Panic-induced elevation of plasma MHPG levels in phobic-anxious patients: effects of clonidine and imipramine. *Arch Gen Psychiatry* 1983; **40**: 425–30.

37. Drew GM, Gower AJ, Marriott AS, Alpha$_2$-adrenoreceptors mediate clonidine-induced sedation in the rat. *Br J Pharmacol* 1979; **67**: 133–41.

38. Paalzow G, Development of tolerance to the analgesic effect of clonidine in rats: cross-tolerance to morphine. *Naunyn Schmiedebergs Arch Pharmacol* 1978; **304**: 1–4.

39. Hsiao JK, Potter WZ, Mechanisms of action of antipanic drugs. In: *Clinical Aspects of Panic Disorder* (Ballenger JC, ed.). New York: Liss, 1990: 297–317.

40. Roth M, Harper M, Temporal lobe epilepsy and the phobic-anxiety depersonalization syndrome, Parts I and II. *Compr Psychiatry* 1962; **3**: 129–51, 215–26.

41. Gloor P, Olivier A, Quesney LF et al, The role of the limbic system in experiential phenomena of temporal lobe epilepsy. *Ann Neurol* 1982; **12**: 129–44.

42. Weilburg JB, Bear DM, Sachs G, Three patients with concomitant panic attacks and seizure disorder: possible clues to the neurology of anxiety. *Am J Psychiatry* 1987; **144**: 1053–6.

43. McNamara ME, Fogel BS, Anticonvulsant-responsive panic attacks with temporal lobe EEG abnormalities. *J Neuropsychiatry Clin Neurosci* 1990; **2**: 193–6.

44. Lepola U, Nousiainen U, Puranen M et al, EEG and CT findings in patients with panic disorder. *Biol Psychiatry* 1990; **28**: 721–7.

45. Spitz MC, Panic disorder in seizure patients: a diagnostic pitfall. *Epilepsia* 1991; **32**: 33–8.

46. Fontaine R, Breton G, Déry R et al, Temporal lobe abnormalities in panic disorder: an MRI study. *Biol Psychiatry* 1990; **27**: 304–10.

47. Reiman EM, Raichle ME, Butler FK et al, A focal brain abnormality in panic disorder, a severe form of anxiety. *Nature* 1984; **310**: 683–5.

48. Nordahl TE, Semple WE, Gross M et al, Cerebral glucose metabolic differences in patients with panic disorder. *Neuropsychopharmacology* 1990; **3**: 261–72.

49. Jabourian AP, Erlich M, Desvignes C et al, Attaques de panique et EEG ambulatoire de 24 heures. *Ann Med Psychol* 1992; **150**: 240–5.

50. Stein MB, Uhde TW, Infrequent occurrence of EEG abnormalities in panic disorder. *Am J Psychiatry* 1989; **146**: 517–20.

51. Dantendorfer K, Amering M, Baischer W et al, Is there a pathophysiological and therapeutic link between panic disorder and epilepsy. *Acta Psychiatr Scand* 1995; **91**: 430–2.

52. Edlund MJ, Swann AC, Clothier J, Patients with panic attacks and abnormal EEG results. *Am J Psychiatry* 1987; **144**: 508–9.

53. Rimmer EM, Richens A, An update on sodium valproate. *Pharmacotherapy* 1985; **5**: 171–84.

54. Sanger DJ, Minireview: GABA and the behavioral effects of anxiolytic drugs. *Life Sci* 1985; **36**: 1503–13.

55. Liljequist S, Engel JA, Reversal of the anti-conflict action of valproate by various GABA and benzodiazepine antagonists. *Life Sci* 1984; **34**: 2525–33.

56. Roy-Byrne PP, Anticonvulsants in anxiety and withdrawal syndromes: Hypotheses for future research. In: *Use of Anticonvulsants in Psychiatry: Recent Advances* (McElroy SL, Pope HG, eds). Clifton, NJ: Oxford Health Care, 1988: 155–68.

57. McElroy SL, Keck PE, Lawrence JL, Treatment of panic disorder and benzodiazepine withdrawal with valproate. *J Neuropsychiatry Clin Neurosci* 1991; **2**: 232–3.

58. Primeau F, Fontaine R, Beauclair L, Valproic acid and panic disorder. *Can J Psychiatry* 1990; **35**: 248–50.

59. Woodman CL, Noyes R, Panic disorder: treatment with valproate. *J Clin Psychiatry* 1994; **55**:134–6.

60. Keck PE, Taylor VE, Tugrul KC et al, Valproate treatment of panic disorder and lactate-induced panic attacks. *Biol Psychiatry* 1993; **33**: 542–6.

61. Lum M, Fontaine R, Elie R et al, Probable interaction of sodium divalproate with benzodiazepines. *Prog Neuropsychopharmacol Biol Psychiatry* 1991; **15**: 269–73.

62. Brady KT, Sonne S, Lydiard B, Valproate treatment of comorbid panic disorder and affective disorders in two alcoholic patients. *J Clin Psychopharmacol* 1994; **14**: 81–2.

63. Tondo L, Burrai C, Scamonatti L et al, Carbamazepine in panic disorder. *Am J Psychiatry* 1989; **146**: 558–9.

64. Klein E, Uhde TW, Post RM, Reply to a letter – Carbamazepine, alprazolam withdrawal and panic disorder. *Am J Psychiatry* 1982; **144**: 266.

65. Uhde TW, Stein MB, Post RM, Lack of efficacy of carbamazepine in the treatment of panic disorder. *Am J Psychiatry* 1988; **145**: 1104–9.

66. Klein E, Colin V, Sholk J et al, Alprazolam withdrawal in patients with panic disorder and generalized anxiety disorder. Vulnerability and effect of carbamazepine. *Am J Psychiatry* 1994; **151**: 1760–6.

67. Burrows GD, Norman TR, Judd FK et al, Short acting versus long acting benzodiazepines: discontinuation effects in panic disorders. *J Psychiatr Res* 1990; **26**(Suppl 2): 65–72.

68. Spier SA, Tesar GE, Rosenbaum JF, Treatment of panic disorder and agoraphobia with clonazepam. *J Clin Psychiatry* 1986; **47**: 238–42.

69. Tesar GE, Rosenbaum JF, Pollack MH et al, Double blind, placebo controlled comparison of clonazepam and alprazolam for panic disorder. *J Clin Psychiatry* 1991; **52**: 69–76.

70. Potter WF, Rudorfer MV, Manji HK, Potential new pharmacotherapies for refractory depression. In: *American Psychiatric Association Annual Review*, Vol 9 (Tasman A, Goldfinger SM, Kaufmann CA, eds). Washington, DC: American Psychiatric Press, 1990: 145–69.

71. Nutt DJ, Little KJ, Taylor SC et al, Investigating benzodiazepine receptor function in vivo using an intravenous infusion of DMCM. *Eur J Pharmacol* 1984; **103**: 359–62.

72. Skerritt JA, Johnston GAR, Chow SC, Interaction of carbamazepine with benzodiazepine receptors. *J Pharm Pharmacol* 1983; **35**: 464–8.

73. Post RM, Mechanisms of action of carbamazepine and related anticonvulsants in affective illness. In: *Psychopharmacology: The Third Generation of Progress* (Meltzer HY, ed.). New York: Raven Press, 1987: 567–76.

74. Lloyd KG, Pile A, Chronic antidepressants and GABA synapses. *Neuropharmacology* 1984; **23**: 841–2.

75. Breslow MF, Fankhauser MP, Potter RL et al, Role of GABA in antipanic drug efficacy. *Am J Psychiatry* 1989; **146**: 353–6.

76. deMontigny C, Cholecystokinin tetrapeptide induces panic-like attacks in healthy volunteers. *Arch Gen Psychiatry* 1989; **46**: 511–17.

77. Bradwejn J, Koszycki D, Shriqui C, Enhanced sensitivity to cholecystokinin tetrapeptide in panic disorder. *Arch Gen Psychiatry* 1991; **48**: 603–10.

78. Bradwejn J, Koszycki D, Couetoux-du Terte et al, L-365,260, a CCK_B antagonist, blocks CCK-4 panic. *Soc Neurosci Abstr* 1992; **18**: 763.

79. Kramer MS, Cutler NR, Ballenger JC et al, A placebo controlled trial of L-365,260, a CCK_B antagonist in panic disorder. *Biol Psychiatry* 1995; **37**: 462–6.

80. Van Megen HJ, Westenberg HG, den Boer JA, Effect of the cholecystokinin B receptor antagonist L-365,260 on lactate-induced panic attacks in panic disorder patients. *Biol Psychiatry* 1996; **40**: 804–6.

81. Cowley DS, Dager SR, Roy-Byrne PP et al, Lactate vulnerability after alprazolan versus placebo treatment of panic disorder. *Biol Psychiatry* 1991; **30**: 49–56.

82. Rifkin A, Klein DF, Dillon D, Blockade by imipramine or desipramine of panic induced by sodium lactate. *Am J Psychiatry* 1981; **138**: 676–7.

83. Vale W, Vaughan J, Smith M et al, Effects of synthetic ovine corticotropin releasing factor, glucocorticoids, catecholamines, neurohypophysial peptides, and other substances on cultured corticotropic cells. *Endocrinology* 1983; **113**: 1121–31.

84. Britton KT, Morgan J, Rivier J et al, Chlordiazepoxide attenuates response suppression induced by corticotropin-releasing factor in the conflict test. *Psychopharmacology* 1985; **86**: 170–4.

85. Owens MJ, Vargas AM, Nemeroff CB, The effects of alprazolam on corticotropin-releasing factor neurons in the rat brain: implications for a role for CRF in the pathogenesis of anxiety disorder. *J Psychiatr Res* 1993; **27**(Suppl 1): 209–20.

86. Heilig M, McLeod S, Brot M et al, Anxiolytic-like action of neuropeptide Y: mediation by Y1 receptors in amygdala, and dissociation from food intake effects. *Neuropsychopharmacology* 1993; **8**: 357–63.

87. Bing O, Moller C, Engel JA et al, Anxiolytic-like action of centrally administered galanin. *Neurosci Lett* 1993; **164**: 17–20.

88. Pitchot W, Ansseau M, Gonzalez MA et al, Dopaminergic function in panic disorder: comparison with major and minor depression. *Biol Psychiatry* 1992; **32**: 1004–11.

89. Roy-Byrne P, Uhde T, Sack D et al, Plasma HVA and anxiety in patients with panic disorder. *Biol Psychiatry* 1986; **21**: 847–9.

90. Schneider P, Evans L, Ross LL et al, Plasma biogenic amine levels in agoraphobia with panic attacks. *Pharmacopsychiatry* 1987; **29**: 102–4.

91. Eriksson E, Westberg P, Alling C et al, Cerebrospinal fluid levels of monoamine metabolites in panic disorder. *Psychiatry Res* 1991; **36**: 243–51.

92. Lydiard R, Ballenger J, Laraia M et al, Noradrenergic dysregulations in panic disorder: new CSF findings. Presented at the American College of Neuropsychopharmacology, Maui, HI, 10–15 December 1989: Abst. 181.

93. Johnson MR, Lydiard B, Ballenger JC, Panic disorder: pathophysiology and drug treatment. *Drugs* 1995; **69**: 328–44.

94. Bandelow B, Sieverk K, Rothemeger M et al, What treatment do patients with panic disorder and agoraphobia get? *Eur Arch Psychiatry Clin Neurosci* 1995; **245**: 165–71.

95. Sheehan D, Davidson J, Manshreck T, Lack of efficacy of a new antidepressant (bupropion) in the treatment of panic disorder with phobias. *J Clin Psychopharmacol* 1983; **3**: 28–31.

96. Kellner M, Wiedermann K, Krieg JC et al, Effects of the dopamine autoreceptor agonist roxindole in patients with depression and panic disorder. *Neuropsychopharmacology* 1994; **110**: 101S.

97. Husain MZ, Desensitization and flooding (implosion) in the treatment of phobias. *Am J Psychiatry* 1971; **127**: 1509–14.

98. Yorkston N, Sergeant H, Rachman S, Methohexitone relaxation for desensitising agoraphobics. *Lancet* 1968; **ii**: 651–3.

99. Lipsedge M et al, Iproniazid and systemic desensitization for severe agoraphobia. *Psychopharmacologica* 1973; **32**: 67–80.

100. Mawson AN, Methohexitone assisted desensitization for phobias. *Lancet* 1970; **i**: 1084–6.

101. Razari J, Treatment of phobias by systemic desensitization. *Arch Gen Psychiatry* 1974; **30**: 291–6.

102. Chambless DL, Foa EB, Groves G et al, Flooding with methohexitone in the treatment of agoraphobia. *Behav Res Ther* 1979; **17**: 243–51.

103. Holub BJ, Metabolism and function of myo-inositol and inositol phospholipid. *Am Rev Nut* 1986; **6**: 563–97.

104. Barkai A, Dunner DL, Gross HA et al, Reduced myo-inositol levels in cerebrospinal fluid from patients with affective disorder. *Biol Psychiatry* 1978; **13**: 65–72.

105. Levine J, Gonzalves M, Baber I et al, Inositol 6 gm daily may be effective in depression but not in schizophrenia. *Hum Psychopharmacol* 1993; **8**: 49–53.

106. Levine J, Barak Y, Gonzalves M et al, Double-blind controlled trial of inositol treatment of depression. *Am J Psychiatry* 1995; **152**: 792–4.

107. Benjamin J, Levine J, Fux M et al, Double blind, placebo controlled, crossover trial of inositol treatment for panic disorder. *Am J Psychiatry* 1995; **152**: 1004–6.

108. Blaustein MP, Effects of potassium, veratridine, and scorpion venom on calcium accumulation and transmitter release by nerve terminals in vitro. *J Physiol (Lond)* 1975; **247**: 617–55.

109. Eto S, Wood JM, Hutchins M et al, Pituitary

45 Ca ion uptake and release of ACTH, GH, and TSH: effect of verapamil. *Am J Physiol* 1974; **226**: 1315–20.

110. Katz B, Miledi R, Further study of the role of calcium in synaptic transmission. *J Physiol (Lond)* 1970; **207**: 787–801.

111. Russell JR, Thorn NA, Calcium and stimulus–secretion coupling in the neurohypophysis, II: Effects of lanthanum, a verapamil analogue (D600) and prenylamine on 45-calcium transport and vasopressin release in isolated rat neurohypophyses. *Acta Endocrinol (Copenh)* 1974; **76**: 471–87.

112. Antman EM, Stone PH, Muller JE et al, Calcium channel blocking agents in the treatment of cardiovascular disorders, Part 2: Hemodynamic effects and clinical applications. *Ann Intern Med* 1980; **93**: 886–904.

113. Ebstein RP, Daly JW, Release of norepinephrine and dopamine from brain vesicular preparations: effects of calcium antagonists. *Cell Mol Neurobiol* 1982; **2**: 205–13.

114. Callanan KM, Keenan AK, Differential effects of D600, nifedipine and dantrolene sodium on excitation–secretion coupling and presynaptic beta-adrenergic responses in rat atria. *Br J Pharmacol* 1983; **83**: 841–7.

115. Salaices M, Martin J, Rico ML et al, Effects of verapamil and manganese on the vasoconstrictor responses to noradrenaline, serotonin and potassium in human and goat cerebral arteries. *Biochem Pharmacol* 1983; **32**: 2711–14.

116. Reiman EM, Raichle ME, Robins E et al, The application of positron emission tomography to the study of panic disorder. *Am J Psychiatry* 1986; **143**: 469–77.

117. Antman EM, Stone PH, Muller JE et al, Calcium channel blocking agents in the treatment of cardiovascular disorders, Part 1: Basic and clinical electro-physiological effects. *Ann Intern Med* 1980; **93**: 875–85.

118. Goldstein JA, Calcium channel blockers in the treatment of panic disorder. *J Clin Psychiatry* 1985; **46**: 546.

119. Klein E, Uhde T, Controlled study of verapamil for treatment of panic disorder. *Am J Psychiatry* 1988; **145**: 431–44.

120. Pollack MH, Smoller JW, The longitudinal course and outcome of panic disorder. *Psychiatr Clin North Am* 1995; **18**: 785–801.

121. Coplan JD, Tiffon L, Gorman JM, Therapeutic strategies for the patient with treatment resistant anxiety. *J Clin Psychiatry* 1993; **54**(Suppl 5): 69–74.

122. Maier W, Buller R, One year follow up of panic disorder: outcome and prognostic factors. *Eur Arch Psychiatry Neurosci* 1988; **238**: 105–9.

123. Vollrath M, Angst J, Outcome of panic and depression in a seven-year follow-up; results of the Zurich study. *Acta Psychiatr Scand* 1989; **80**: 591–6.

124. Noyes R, Reich J, Christiansen J et al, Outcome of panic disorder: relationship to diagnostic subtypes and comorbidity. *Arch Gen Psychiatry* 1990; **47**: 809–18.

125. Pollack MH, Otto MW, Tesar GE et al, Long-term outcome after acute treatment with clonazepam and alprazolam for panic disorder. *J Clin Psychopharmacol* 1993; **13**: 257–63.

126. Otto MW, Gould R, Pollack MH, Cognitive–behavioral treatment of panic disorder: considerations or the treatment of patients over the long-term. *Psychiatr Ann* 1994; **24**: 299–306.

127. Rosenbaum JF, Pollack MH. Anxiety. In: *The Massachusetts General Handbook of General Hospital Psychiatry* (Cassem N, ed.). St Louis, MO: Mosby, 1991: 159–90.

128. Mavissakalian MR, Perel JM, Imipramine dose response relationship in panic disorder with agoraphobia. Preliminary findings. *Arch Gen Psychiatry* 1989; **46**: 127–31.

129. Mavissakalian MR, Perel JM, Michelson L, The relationship of plasma imipramine and N-desmethyl imipramine to improvement in agoraphobia. *Psychopharmacol Bull* 1984; **20**: 123–5.

130. Lesser IM, Lydiard RB, Antal E et al, Alprazolam plasma concentrations and treatment response in panic disorder and agoraphobia. *Am J Psychiatry* 1992; **149**: 1556–62.

131. Gorman JM, *The Essential Guide to Psychiatric Drugs*. New York: St Martin's Press, 1990.

132. Uhlenhuth EH, Matuzas W, Glass RM et al, Response of panic disorder to fixed dose of alprazolam or imipramine. *J Affect Disord* 1989; **17**: 261–70.

133. Muskin PR, Fyer AJ, Treatment of panic dis-

order. *J Clin Psychopharmacol* 1981; **1**: 81–90.

134. Fahy TJ, O'Rowhe DO, Brophy J et al, The Gateway study of panic disorder I: clomipramine and lofepramine in DSM III R panic disorder: a placebo controlled trial. *J Affect Disord* 1992; **25**: 63–75.

135. Pollack MH, Rosenbaum JF, The treatment of antidepressant induced side-effects. *J Clin Psychiatry* 1987; **43**: 3–8.

136. Woods SW, Nagy LM, Kolesgar A et al, Controlled trial of alprazolam supplementation during imipramine treatment of panic disorder. *J Clin Psychopharmacol* 1992; **12**: 32–8.

137. Hallstrom C, Treasden I, Guy Edwards J et al, Diazepam, propranolol and their combination in the management of chronic anxiety. *Br J Psychiatry* 1984; **139**: 418–21.

138. Shehi M, Patterson WM, Treatment of panic attacks with alprazolam and propranolol. *Am J Psychiatry* 1984; **141**: 900–1.

139. Blier P, Bergerson R, Effectiveness of pindolol with selected antidepressant drugs in the treatment of major depression. *J Clin Psychopharmacol* 1995; **15**: 217–22.

140. Danon P, Hirschmann S, Kindler S et al, Pindolol augmentation in the treatment of resistant panic disorder: a double blind placebo controlled trial. In: *Proceedings of the European College of Neuropsychopharmacology, Vienna, 15–19 September 1997*: Abst.

141. Tesar GE, Rosenbaum JF, Successful use of clonazepam in patients with treatment resistant panic disorder. *J Nerv Ment Dis* 1986; **174**: 477–82.

142. Tiffon L, Coplan J, Dapp LA et al, Augmentation strategies with tricyclic or fluoxetine treatment in seven partially responsive

panic disorder patients. *J Clin Psychiatry* 1994; **55**: 66–9.

143. Ciraulo DA, Shacher RI, Fluoxetine drug–drug interactions: I: Antidepressants and antipsychotics. *J Clin Psychopharmacol* 1990; **10**: 48–50.

144. Weilberg JB, Rosenbaum JF, Biederman J, Fluoxetine added to non MAOI antidepressants converts nonresponders to responders: a preliminary report. *J Clin Psychiatry* 1989; **50**: 447–9.

145. Boerner RJ, Treatment refractory panic disorder: success of a combined treatment with imipramine, moclobemide and behavior therapy. *Psychiatric Praxitum* 1995; **22**: 30–2.

146. Cournoyer J, Rapid response of a disorder to the addition of lithium carbonate: panic resistant to tricyclic antidepressants. *Can J Psychiatry* 1986; **31**: 335–8.

147. Feder R, Lithium augmentation of clomipramine. *J Clin Psychiatry* 1988; **49**: 458.

148. Carmara EG, Lithium potentiation of antidepressant treatment in panic disorder. *J Clin Psychopharmacol* 1990; **19**: 225–6.

149. Ontiveros A, Fontaine R, Sodium valproate and clonazepam for treatment resistant panic disorder. *J Psychiatry Neurosci* 1992; **17**: 78–80.

150. Corrigan FM, Sodium valproate augmentation of fluoxetine or fluoxamine effects. *Biol Psychiatry* 1992; **31**: 1178–9.

151. Gastfrend DR, Rosenbaum JF, Adjunctive buspirone in benzodiazepine treatment of four patients with panic disorder. *Am J Psychiatry* 1989; **146**: 914–16.

152. Kupfer DJ, Lessons to be learned from long-term treatment of affective disorders: potential utility in panic disorder. *J Clin Psychiatry* 1991; **52**(Suppl 2): 12–17.

13

Psychological treatment of panic disorder

Anne Chosak, Sandra L Baker, George R Thorn, David A Spiegel, David H Barlow

Introduction

Panic disorder takes a significant emotional toll on those who suffer from it, as well as contributing to lost productivity and increased health-care utilization.[1] Psychological treatment of panic disorder has been shown to be more effective than no treatment, psychosocial 'placebo' intervention, and even some psychopharmacological interventions.[2,3] In this chapter, we offer a brief review of the psychoanalytic/dynamic, behavioral and cognitive/cognitive–behavioral treatment of panic, as well as reviewing some current issues in the treatment of panic disorder.

Psychodynamic psychotherapy

The psychodynamic formulation of panic disorder continues to be primarily based on Freud's thinking about anxiety (see Chapters 1 and 8 in this volume). Although significant gains have been made in understanding the nature of panic disorder and in the development of effective therapeutic interventions, empirical research on psychodynamic interventions has lagged behind. Shear[4] reported that there is no formal body of prospective research data focusing on the psychodynamic treatment of panic disorder. This continues to be the case several years after Shear's review of the psychodynamic treatment literature. Coté and Barlow,[5] in their review of empirically validated treatment approaches for panic disorder, reported that there is no research demonstrating the efficacy of psychodynamic treatments by comparing these approaches with a waiting-list or credible placebo control, or with an empirically validated alternative psychotherapeutic intervention. Given the lack of empirical research supporting the efficacy of any psychodynamic treatments of panic disorder, in this chapter we shall present case study findings, one outcome study and two psychotherapy models that have been extensively described in the literature.

Several reasons are reported in the literature regarding why psychodynamic approaches to treating panic disorder should be explored.

Shear,[4] who has published extensively in this area, has suggested that psychodynamic perspectives on panic disorder can provide insight into questions that are presently unanswered. She has further stated that these treatments may be helpful in managing treatment-resistant patients or may provide protection against future panic vulnerability.

Like cognitive theories of panic disorder, psychodynamic theories predict that anxiety is generated when danger situations are activated. However, unlike cognitive theories that propose that these danger situations are due to cognitive misinterpretations of bodily sensations, dynamic theories propose that these danger situations are unconscious and include the threatened emergence of prohibited instinctual urges or the impending disruption of self or object representations.[4] Therefore psychodynamic treatments are focused primarily on the elucidation of underlying intrapsychic disturbances in treating symptoms and characterologically based maladaptive behaviors.[4] Generally, the curative interventions used in dynamic treatments of panic disorder involve the establishment of a transference relationship and the demonstration and acknowledgment of troublesome and angry feelings held by the patient that are connected with their panic attacks.[6] Dynamic treatments may also lessen repression of intense affects in general, thereby causing a decrease in panic symptoms.

Case studies

The literature on psychodynamic treatments of panic disorder is notable for the numerous case studies reporting the efficacy of these approaches.[7-13] These case reports are limited, however, because they lack appropriate experimental controls. There are no psychodynamic case reports utilizing a single subject experimental design.[5] The number of case reports in the literature suggests that psychodynamic treatments of panic disorder are quite popular and frequently used despite the lack of empirical support validating their efficacy. This assumption was supported by Goisman et al,[14] who reported, on a sample of 562 subjects with DSM-III-R diagnoses of panic disorder, panic disorder with agoraphobia (PDA) and agoraphobia without panic, that psychodynamic psychotherapy was the most frequently used psychosocial treatment.

Furthermore, Milrod and Shear[6] reviewed more than 100 case reports in the literature that used dynamic treatments of panic disorder. In 35 of these 100 cases, either the patients met strict DSM-III-R criteria for panic disorder or both authors agreed that the patients suffered from this disorder. Based on these 35 case studies where panic disorder diagnoses were confirmed, Milrod and Shear reported that all of the patients were considered improved by their therapist after being treated using dynamic interventions. Milrod and Shear provided some general information about dynamic treatments of panic disorder based on the cases reviewed. They reported that, during the initial phase of dynamic treatments, panic symptoms are managed through the establishment of a therapeutic relationship between the patient and the therapist. This phase of treatment also includes educating family members about panic disorder. The middle phase of treatment involves identifying and exploring patients' central conflicts and establishing links between precipitating events or fantasy and panic episodes. Although Milrod and Shear[6] reported that the termination phase of dynamic treatments in this literature was not regularly reported, ambivalent transference feelings were addressed, leading to greater overall psychological stability.

Comparative outcome study

A single study has evaluated the comparative efficacy of a psychodynamic treatment approach against another form of therapeutic intervention. Wiborg and Dahl[15] randomized 40 patients (17 males and 23 females), ranging in age from 18 to 50, with DSM-III-R diagnoses of panic disorder with or without agoraphobia, to either a clomipramine group (CG) or a clomipramine plus brief dynamic psychotherapy group (CPG). Subjects in the clomipramine group were treated with a maximum of 150 mg per day for nine months. All other subjects were treated with a maximum of 150 mg of clomipramine per day for nine months combined with 15 weekly sessions of brief dynamic psychotherapy (BDP). BDP included all of the main elements of dynamic psychotherapy, including clarification, confrontation, and interpretation of resistance, defensive styles and associated isolated affects.

Wiborg and Dahl[15] reported that all of the patients in the CPG were panic-free at the end of treatment, compared with 75% of the patients in the CG, using the Panic Attack and Anxiety Scale to monitor weekly panic attacks. All patients in both groups were panic-free at the 6-month follow-up. For the purposes of this study, relapse was defined as fulfilling DSM-III-R criteria for panic disorder after having been panic-free for at least eight weeks post-treatment. Using this criterion, Wiborg and Dahl found that 75% of the patients in the CG, in comparison with 20% of the patients in the CPG, relapsed during the nine months between the end of the clomipramine treatment and the 18-month follow-up. The authors reported that patients receiving BPD and clomipramine showed significantly greater global improvement on outcome measures than the patients treated with clomipramine alone.

Although a significant finding showing the effectiveness of a dynamic treatment of panic disorder in comparison to a pharmacological treatment, this study is limited because an adequate control group was not used.

Emotion-focused treatment for panic disorder

Shear and her colleagues[16,17] have developed an emotion focused treatment (EFT) for panic disorder that targets emotion regulation as it relates to interpersonal control and to fears of being abandoned or trapped. They state that EFT is not strictly a dynamic treatment in that it does not emphasize the interpretation of unconscious material or focus on linking early experiences with present symptoms. Instead, interventions used during EFT target fear and avoidance of negative affects and their triggers.

According to Shear and colleagues, there are two major components of EFT. The first component of treatment is psychoeducational, and involves providing information about panic disorder and explaining the hypothesized role of emotions. The second treatment component is the identification and clarification of emotional reactions and their consequences. Reflective listening is used by the therapist to identify and clarify emotional reactions of which the patient may not be aware.

EFT is conducted in 11 sessions of acute treatment, followed by 6 sessions of monthly maintenance. The acute phase is divided into initial, middle and termination subphases, with the goal of the initial phase being to provide information and the treatment rationale. During the middle phase of treatment, emotional reactivity is identified and the patient is encouraged to re-experience and think through specific problematic emotional reactions. The termination phase is used to discuss reactions to ending treatment, to review treatment progress and to help the patient consolidate therapeutic gains. Troubleshooting and a continuation of the work is the focus of the maintenance phase of treatment.

Shear et al[16] acknowledged that EFT has not been empirically validated, although they presented findings from case reports and studies comparing non-directive, empathic supportive therapy with traditional cognitive–behavioral treatments as preliminary support for their approach.[9,12,18–20] They compared treatment responses using cognitive–behavioral therapy and a non-prescriptive, empathic, reflective listening approach, and found that both treatments yielded similar results at post-treatment and 6-month follow-up.[20]

In a recent discussion of EFT, Shear and Weiner[17] noted several advantages to this approach. They hypothesized better treatment compliance with EFT in comparison with panic control therapy[21] – an empirically validated treatment approach – because less homework is used. This makes EFT a less time-consuming approach. Furthermore, EFT has an advantage over pharmacological treatment because of the avoidance of side-effects. Finally, EFT may have advantages in terms of quality of life, according to Shear.[4] Shear and her colleagues have reported that studies are underway to evaluate the efficacy of EFT.

Panic-focused psychodynamic psychotherapy

Panic-focused psychodynamic psychotherapy (PFPP)[22] is a brief form (approximately 3 months) of dynamic psychotherapy for panic disorder, focusing on rapid elimination of panic symptoms. PFPP can also be used as a longer-term treatment (9–12 months) aimed at decreasing vulnerability to panic relapse and functional impairment. PFPP is administered in three phases. During the first phase of treatment, interventions are aimed at exploring and relieving panic attacks. This phase focuses on the circumstances preceding panic onset, including the patient's thoughts and feelings during panic attacks, and the meanings of panic symptoms. The therapist then formulates psychological issues, including conflicts about separation, anger and sexuality that are involved in the genesis of the patient's panic episodes. Milrod and colleagues reported that panic symptoms are usually relieved in approximately 12–20 weeks using this approach.

The second phase of PFPP explores the patient's mental configurations and the characterological underpinnings to their symptoms that elicit panic. Furthermore, the working through of transference allows for increasing work on patterns in relationships, as they emerge in the relationship with the therapist.

Finally, the termination phase of treatment addresses the patient's difficulties with separation and independence. Addressing the patient's separation fears during the termination phase of treatment allows the patient to re-experience these conflicts directly with the therapist so that underlying fantasies can be worked through, thereby rendering them less frightening.

Milrod and colleagues[22] provide 32 cases that demonstrate each phase of intervention used in their treatment. They also note how PFPP can be used in conjunction with cognitive–behavioral therapy and pharmacotherapy. However, they have not undertaken any systematic research to ascertain the efficacy of this dynamic approach to panic disorder treatment. As with other psychodynamic psychotherapy models, until this approach can be empirically validated, its benefits remain conjectural.

Behavioral treatment of panic disorder

Behaviorally based treatments have had a central role in the treatment of panic disorder. The scope of this chapter permits a detailed review of only a few of the studies that are especially relevant in the history of behavioral treatments. The reader is referred to Barlow[23] and McNally[24] for more comprehensive reviews of behaviorally based treatments targeting panic disorder and PDA.

Exposure treatment

Behavioral treatments based on the technique of in vivo situational exposure have been well evaluated in the treatment of panic disorder and agoraphobic anxiety and avoidance. In vivo exposure involves having the patient enter a feared situation or confront a feared object. The rationale is that enduring the situational anxiety over time will promote habituation to the situation or object. This may be done at a graded, hierarchical pace or in an ungraded, massed fashion. Patients may also be taught strategies to help them control their anxiety before, during, and after exposure sessions.

In 1986, Telch et al[25] compared imipramine, imipramine plus exposure, and placebo plus exposure in the treatment of DSM-II-diagnosed agoraphobia with panic attacks. Participants in the imipramine-alone group were given specific anti-exposure instructions. Interestingly, those individuals who received imipramine alone experienced little to no improvement on measures of agoraphobic avoidance, panic or anxiety. That is, individuals who were specifically instructed not to engage in agoraphobic situations experienced little benefit. Overall, results favored the combination of imipramine plus

exposure, although both groups that included exposure treatment experienced significant improvements. However, on a composite index of treatment response, subjects who received cognitive therapy plus exposure evidenced the greatest improvement at post-treatment and 6-month follow-up.[25-27]

In a larger and more recent study, Marks et al[28] compared alprazolam plus exposure, alprazolam plus relaxation treatment, placebo plus exposure, and placebo plus relaxation treatment, in 154 individuals with panic disorder with agoraphobia. All treatments showed improvement on panic measures. However, on non-panic measures, the effect size of alprazolam was half the size of exposure. Additionally, following taper, all effects from the alprazolam were lost, in comparison with the effects of exposure, which endured. When interpreting these results, however, the reader should be cautious in drawing conclusions about the pure effects of exposure in both this study and that by Telch et al.[25] In both, participants actually received two treatments – exposure and placebo – despite the latter generally being considered a non-active treatment.

Several studies have compared pure exposure therapy to cognitive therapy or combinations of cognitive or relaxation therapies with exposure in patients with panic disorder with agoraphobia. In particular, in a study of 82 patients with panic disorder, Margraf and Schneider compared pure exposure therapy (in vivo and interoceptive), pure cognitive therapy (identification and restructuring of catastrophic misinterpretations and reattribution of anxiety symptomatology), a combination of exposure and cognitive therapy, and a wait-list control group.[29] Each of the treatments specifically targeted panic attacks or associated stimuli and thoughts. Few significant differences were found between the three active treatment conditions at post-treatment. At a one-month follow-up, 77–93% of patients remained panic-free, demonstrating that, despite different emphases, both exposure and cognitive therapy are efficacious in the treatment of panic disorder.

Recently, Michelson et al[30] examined the effectiveness of graded exposure alone (GE), cognitive therapy plus graded exposure (CT + GE), or relaxation training plus graded exposure (RT + GE), in a sample of 92 patients with moderate to severe PDA. All three treatments were found to be beneficial at post-treatment; however, CT + GE resulted in the greatest proportion with high end-state functioning at a one-year follow-up (71.4% versus 37.5% for GE and 33.0% for RT + GE). Furthermore, improvement in CT + GE was the most rapid and stable.

Bouchard and colleagues[31] examined differences in the rate of change between exposure therapy and cognitive restructuring to determine whether one treatment may be preferred over the other owing to its more rapid effect. In a sample of 28 individuals with PDA, behavioral, cognitive and clinical variables were assessed at pretreatment, weeks 6 and 12, post-treatment (week 18), and a 6-month follow-up. Both treatments were found to be equally effective and appeared to progress at the same rate of improvement. In addition, although exposure did not directly target panic-related cognitions, it appeared to be an effective means of changing beliefs about the harmfulness of panic symptoms as well as agoraphobic concerns.

Finally, exposure treatment also appears to have long-term benefits.[28,29,32] For example, Fava et al[32] treated 110 individuals with PDA using an exposure-based behavioral treatment program. Following 12 weeks of treatment, 81 individuals (74%) achieved panic-free status, and were followed for 2–9 years. Results indicated that an overwhelming 96.1% of these initial treatment responders remained panic-free after 2 years, 77.6% at a minimum of 5 years and 67.4% after 7 years. Further, relapse was higher among patients with co-morbid personality disorders and those with residual agoraphobia at post-treatment.

In summary, there is substantial research to support the utility of exposure treatment for panic and agoraphobia. However, behavioral treatment by itself is no panacea, with a large number of individuals remaining symptomatic at post-treatment and follow-up.[2] In addition, perhaps because of the anxiety-provoking nature of exposure treatment, difficulties with drop-out rates have been noted.

Relaxation treatments

In parallel with the development of cognitive and cognitive–behavioral treatment for panic disorder, other investigators have explored the utility of techniques based on behavioral relaxation strategies. Behaviorists who theorized that panic attacks were related to hyperventilation experimented with respiratory control strategies (e.g. deep diaphragmatic breathing) to help combat the physical symptoms of panic.[33,34] In uncontrolled studies, Clark, Salkovskis and their colleagues found that respiratory control strategies along with education about hyperventilatory sensations led to an abatement in panic attack frequency. However, other studies produced mixed results.[35,36] For instance, de Ruiter, Rijken and their colleagues found that supplementing in vivo exposure with respiratory control strategies or cognitive restructuring did not improve overall treatment effectiveness. It is possible that this technique may be helpful for certain patients;[37] however, further research is needed, including the identification of potential mechanisms of action.[38]

The effects of progressive muscle relaxation (PMR) techniques have been explored both in pure form and in combination with other treatments.[39,40] PMR involves training patients to tense and then relax specific muscle groups and to learn to discriminate tense from relaxed muscles. Attention to deep, diaphragmatic breathing is often included. Barlow and colleagues[39] compared exposure plus cognitive restructuring, PMR, PMR in combination with exposure and cognitive restructuring, and a wait-list control in the treatment of panic disorder with mild or no agoraphobia. Overall, results indicated that all three treatments were effective. However, although PMR better ameliorated psychosomatic symptomatology, it also had the greatest attrition. Craske et al[41] later examined the long-term effects of these treatments at 6-month and 24-month follow-up points. Their results indicated that individuals who received some form of exposure treatment tended to maintain their gains, whereas those who received relaxation treatment alone tended to be more unstable across the follow-up. Specifically, 81% of those individuals who received exposure plus cognitive restructuring were panic-free at the 24-month follow-up, compared with 43% in the combined group and 36% in the PMR group. Craske et al concluded that this may be suggestive of a damaging effect when PMR is added to exposure and cognitive therapy, perhaps due to the treatments being diluted when combined or to a negative effect of PMR.

More recently, Beck and colleagues[40] compared PMR and cognitive therapy (CT), both without any formal exposure training, in 64 patients with PDA. A minimal-contact control (MCC) condition was also included. Results indicated that CT and PMR were superior to MCC, and both were found to be moderately effective for the treatment of PDA (82% and 68% respectively were categorized as treatment responders). Interestingly, although exposure was not a formal part of any of the treatments, agoraphobic fear was reduced, suggesting that addressing patients' cognitions and physiologi-

cal arousal has an effect on agoraphobia.

In 1987, Öst[42] described a refinement to traditional PMR training called applied relaxation (AR), which extended PMR to include a hierarchy of in vivo exposure practices. AR was intended for use as an active coping skill to allow the patient to relax during episodes of anxiety and ultimately terminate the anxiety.

Öst[43] compared AR with PMR in 14 patients diagnosed with PDA. One hundred percent of the AR group was panic-free at both post-treatment and at 19-month follow-up. In comparison, 71% of individuals who underwent PMR were panic-free at post-treatment, and only 57% were panic-free at follow-up. Öst et al[44] later compared AR, in vivo exposure, and cognitive therapy in 45 individuals with PDA. Despite emphasizing different areas of panic-related anxiety (physiological arousal, behavioral avoidance and cognitions), the three treatments were comparable in efficacy, producing significant improvements at both post-treatment and a 1-year follow-up. Öst et al suggested that the equivalency among treatments may have been due to self-directed exposure by patients in the AR and CT groups.

In summary, there is some support for the use of relaxation treatments for panic disorder, particularly applied relaxation. However, further research is necessary to determine the mechanisms of action of this treatment, as well as variables that may be predictive of who will benefit from such relaxation techniques.

Cognitive and cognitive–behavioral treatment of panic disorder

The rationale for the cognitive and cognitive behavioral treatment of panic stem from the cognitive and cognitive–behavioral theories of panic respectively (see Chapter 7 in this volume). Individuals with panic disorder are thought to maintain the disorder via interpretation and amplification of the catastrophic meaning of the physical symptoms of panic and their potential consequences. Therefore treatment of panic disorder should address these cognitive distortions directly. Cognitive approaches to treatment assume that cognitions and cognitive schemata can be directly changed by teaching patients to examine and modify their cognitive misconceptions.

Components of treatment

The first part of cognitive therapy for panic is often informational, explaining the nature of panic and anxiety and providing scientific explanations of the feared anxiety-related symptoms. Next the therapist must identify, or help the patient to identify, 'automatic thoughts' – the central misinterpretations of panic symptoms and consequences of symptoms or panic attacks. The therapist may illustrate the importance of negative cognitions to mood states. The therapist then shows the patient any of a number of strategies for correcting or evaluating their cognitive errors: self-statement training, in which a neutral or more accurate statement is practiced in place of the former negative statement; probability re-evaluation, in which actual probabilities of catastrophic consequences are more realistically examined; and decatastrophizing, in which the feared impact of consequences of panic (e.g. fainting, being embarrassed, vomiting) are assessed more rationally. Homework assignments are designed to help patients first identify, and subsequently challenge, maladaptive cognitions. Consistent with the cognitive theory of panic, cognitive treatment of panic

disorder targets maladaptive cognitions surrounding the phenomenon of panic.

Few researchers utilize a 'pure' cognitive approach; most, like Clark, Beck and others, incorporate behavioral strategies such as interoceptive exposure, hypothesis testing or relaxation into a *predominantly* cognitive protocol. These predominantly cognitive approaches are distinguished conceptually from the cognitive–behavioral approaches, although there is often much overlap in the use of specific strategies. The cognitive approach contends that behavioral exposure is useful in treating panic because it provides opportunities to correctly evaluate fearful beliefs and predictions.

For example, in cognitive therapy, the patient is encouraged to experience feared situations, activities, or sensations so as to test specific panic-related predictions (e.g. 'If my heart pounds when I go into a grocery store, I will have a heart attack'). The cognitive–behavioral treatments utilize the same strategies, but as part of a broader treatment that also addresses conditioning and behavioral avoidance. In a cognitive–behavioral protocol, patients expose themselves to feared situations, activities and sensations, both to test out hypotheses *and* to promote physiological habituation to those sensations, activities and situations.

Interoceptive exposure is a repeated, systematic exposure to the feared physical sensations typical of panic; its purpose is to help the individual habituate to those symptoms, test hypotheses concerning symptoms, and practice coping strategies. In vivo exposure similarly helps individuals with panic to habituate to feared situations and activities, to test fearful (often unrealistic) predictions about anxiety, and to practice their panic control strategies. Changing or eliminating safety behaviors such as carrying a cellular phone, self-distraction or escape helps individuals learn that the panic will remit with or without these behaviors; such safety behaviors reinforce fear and avoidance. Additional strategies that may be included in cognitive and cognitive–behavioral treatment approaches include arousal reduction components such as breathing retraining or progressive muscle relaxation. Breathing retraining teaches individuals with panic to breathe diaphragmatically in a measured fashion, rather than hyperventilate or breath-hold.

Empirical studies

There have been a number of research studies evaluating the effectiveness of the cognitive treatment of panic disorder. Two influential treatment protocols are panic control treatment (PCT), developed by Barlow and his colleagues,[21,23,45] and the cognitive therapy (CT) approach developed by Clark and his colleagues.[46–48] These protocols have been evaluated in controlled treatment studies, often with impressive results.

Beck[49] conducted a treatment outcome study in which participants were given either or supportive psychotherapy. Those in the cognitive condition improved more than those in the supportive psychotherapy condition during the course of treatment and at 12-month follow-up. There were no dropouts in either condition. One confounding variable of the study was that CT participants received 12 weeks of treatment, whereas the other participants received 8 weeks of supportive psychotherapy. Although assessments at 4 and 8 weeks after beginning treatment showed an advantage for the cognitive condition, later studies tended to correct for such types of confound by providing comparison treatments that were more equivalent to the cognitive treatment.

Table 13.1 Clinical trials of cognitive behavioral treatments for panic disorder and intent-to-treat analysis* (Taken from Barlow et al[2])

Ref	Lengths of follow-up, months	Treatment no. of patients % panic free	Significant comparison, % panic free[†]	
			Other treatments	Wait lists
Craske et al	24	PCT/15/81	Yes: AR=36	...
			Yes: PCT and AR=43	...
Clark et al	12	CT/17/76§	Yes: AR=43§	...
			Yes IMI=43§	...
Klosko et al	PT	PCT/15/87	No: AL=50	Yes: 33
			Yes: PL=36	...
Newman et al	12	CTM/24/87	...	...
		CTNM/19/87	...	...
Côté et al	12	CBTM/13/92	...	...
		CBTNM/8/100	...	...
Beck et al	PT	CT/17/94	Yes: ST=25‖	...
Black et al	PT	CT25/32	Yes: FL=68	...
			No: PL=20	...
Margraf and Schneider	4 wk	CT/22/91	...	Yes: 5
Öst et al	12	CT/19/69§	No: AR=74§	...
Telch et al	PT	PCT/94/85	...	Yes: 30
Craske et al	PT	CBT/16/53	Yes: NPT=6	...
Shear et al	6	CBT/23/45	No: NPT=45	...

* AL indicates alprazoism; AR, applied relaxation; CBT, cognitive behavioral therapy; CBTM, cognitive behavioral therapy and medication; CBTNM, cognitive behavioral therapy without medication; CT, cognitive therapy; CTM, cognitive therapy and medication; CTNM, cognitive therapy without medication; FL, fluvoxamine maleate; IMI, imiprimine hydrochloride; NPT, nonprescription treatment; PL, pill placebo; PCT, panic control treatment (exposure and cognitive restructuring); PT, posttreatment; and ST, standard treatment.
[†]Yes indicates the comparison was significant; no, comparison not significant, and ellipses, no comparison made.
§Percentage of patients who were panic free at follow-up and who had received no additional treatment during the follow-up period.
At 8 weeks, which is the end of supportive therapy. At this time, 71% of patients undergoing CT were panic free.

Clark and his colleagues[50] compared the CT to imipramine, applied relaxation (developed by Öst) and 3-month wait-list. All participants in the therapy conditions were provided with 12 sessions of acute treatment with the option of up to three maintenance sessions in the subsequent 3-month period. Participants treated with imipramine were maintained on an active level of the drug for 6 months, and then tapered off. Unlike other studies, all participants were instructed to expose themselves to feared situations. All three active treatments were superior to wait-list. At 3-month assessment, the cognitive condition was superior to the other two active conditions. By 6-month follow-up, CT and imipramine-treated participants were doing better than those in the applied relaxation condition. Subsequent to being tapered off the imipramine, 40% of the imipramine-treated participants relapsed. By 15-month follow-up the participants in the cognitive condition were once again doing better than those in the other two treatment conditions.

Öst and Westling[51] also compared applied relaxation with CT. Both modalities produced significant improvement in the frequency of panic, panic-related distress and disability, and general anxiety. There were no between-group differences, however. Gains made in both groups persisted at 12-month follow-up. Clark[52] has suggested that a re-analysis of these data, controlling for experience level of the therapists, yields a significant advantage for CT over applied relaxation.

Similarly, Arntz and van den Hout[53] compared CT with applied relaxation. This particular study was conducted by researchers who did not participate in the development of Clark's cognitive therapy or of Öst's applied relaxation, which would tend to control for experimenter bias. Participants were assessed pre- and post-treatment and at 1- and 6-month follow-up. More participants receiving CT were classed as 'panic-free' by the end of treatment. At 1- and 6-month follow-up, participants from the cognitive group continued to be more likely to be panic-free.

In the study mentioned above in the context of evaluating PMR, Barlow and his colleagues[39] compared relaxation, cognitive therapy plus interoceptive exposure, a combination of all three components, and a wait-list control group. The three active treatments were superior to the wait-list control. The two conditions including cognitive therapy did better than the relaxation condition in yielding panic-free status by the post-treatment assessment. Interestingly, both conditions including relaxation showed relatively high dropout rates as compared with the other two groups. This study also described the combination of cognitive strategies, interoceptive exposure and breathing retraining that is now known as PCT.

Klosko et al[54] compared PCT, alprazolam, drug placebo and wait-list. By post-treatment follow-up, 87% of those in the PCT group were considered panic-free, whereas only 50% of those receiving alprazolam were panic-free. About a third of those on placebo and of those in the wait-list group were panic-free by post-treatment follow-up. PCT was significantly more effective than the other three conditions.[55]

Telch and colleagues[56] compared an 8-week PCT group treatment with a wait-list control. By post-treatment assessment, 85% of those in the PCT group were considered panic-free, versus less than a third of the wait-list group. A composite outcome measure involving panic frequency, general anxiety and behavioral avoidance also showed 63% of those in the PCT group as improved versus only 9% of those on the wait-list. By 6-month follow-up, nearly 80% of the PCT participants still met panic-free status, and 63% still met the composite improvement criteria.

Abbreviated and self-directed CBT

Recently, a few studies have investigated abbreviated or self-directed forms of CBT for panic disorder. Coté et al[57] found that 10 hours of in-person and telephone therapy was as effective as 20 hours of standard face-to-face cognitive behavior therapy administered over the same time period. More recently, Craske et al[58] found a four-session PCT protocol more effective than an equivalent amount of non-directive supportive therapy. Promising results have also been reported with self-help treatments involving minimal (e.g. 3 hours or less) therapist contract.[59–61] Those reports suggest that CBT can be delivered more efficiently than is currently done – at least for patients with mild levels of agoraphobia.

Cautionary findings

The above studies reflect some impressive results in the psychological treatment of panic disorder. Several caveats should be considered, however, and will be reviewed below. One important issue involves the natural course of panic and the necessity of appropriate follow-up procedures to assess more accurately the utility of proven treatments. A second significant factor in the treatment of panic is the presence of different levels of agoraphobic avoidance and its impact on psychological treatment of panic. The final topic discussed below is the state of research with racial and ethnic minority populations and the importance of basic empirical work in this area.

Panic course

As encouraging as the treatment literature is, it should be kept in mind that panic disorder is generally a chronic condition whose symptoms wax and wane over time. Studies that utilize single or widely spaced cross-sectional follow-up assessments are likely to underestimate the presence of infrequent panics and other fluctuating symptoms, and thus overestimate long-term improvement. This was clearly demonstrated in a recent follow-up study of 63 PD patients with not more than mild agoraphobia who were treated with CBT at our center in Albany.[62] In that sample, assessments conducted 3 months post-treatment found that 68% of patients were panic-free for the past month and 40% met criteria for high end-state functioning. By 24 months, the proportions had increased to 75% panic-free and 57% high end-state functioning. However, only 21% met criteria for high end-state functioning at both 3 and 24 months and were panic-free for the year preceding the 24-month assessment.

A similar finding was reported by Burns et al[63] for agoraphobic patients treated with in vivo exposure therapy. In that study, subjects as a group evidenced continued improvement at assessment points up to 8 years post-treatment, but longitudinal evaluations showed that their clinical courses were typically characterized by periods of setback. These studies illustrate the difficulty of accurately assessing the long-term outcomes of treatments for panic disorder.

Agoraphobic avoidance

Another important and cautionary issue in the treatment of panic disorder is that the presence of agoraphobic avoidance has repeatedly emerged as a predictor of poor outcome. In the Harvard/Brown Anxiety Research Program (HARP) study, for example, the presence of agoraphobia was associated with both a lower recovery rate and a higher relapse rate than the rates for panic disorder without agoraphobia.[64] Moreover, subjects with moderate to severe agoraphobia were less likely to remit than those with mild agoraphobia.

Other workers have reported similar findings.[65-68] When agoraphobic avoidance has been the specific focus of treatment, failure to eradicate it completely has been associated with a subsequent loss of improvement. For instance, in the Fava et al study reviewed above,[32] although the initial severity of agoraphobia did not predict long-term outcome, the presence of residual agoraphobia at post-treatment did. Two-thirds of the patients who were classified as treatment responders at post-treatment but who had some residual agoraphobic avoidance relapsed within 5 years.

Most studies of the efficacy of CBT for panic disorder have excluded patients with moderate or severe agoraphobia. Yet, despite such exclusions, patients often still have residual agoraphobic avoidance. For example, in the study conducted by Craske et al,[41] which excluded patients with moderate or severe agoraphobia, more than three-fourths of the subjects who received PCT were panic-free at 24-month follow-up. However, only half were classified as having high end-state functioning, mostly because of residual agoraphobic avoidance. Doubtless, the results would have been worse if patients with more severe agoraphobia had been included.

To address that problem, our group in Boston is currently experimenting with the addition of a brief, ungraded, situational exposure component to PCT. In a recently conducted uncontrolled trial, seven PD patients with moderate to severe agoraphobia were treated with 11 sessions of standard group PCT followed by 2–3 days of individually-administered exposure therapy. Therapist time for the exposure component averaged 6.5 hours per patient. Consistent with studies of mildly agoraphobic patients, subjects improved significantly across diverse measures during CBT; however, all seven continued to meet diagnostic criteria for PDA. The major reason was continued agoraphobic avoidance.

During the brief exposure component, further significant reductions occurred on all measures, and at post-treatment five of the seven subjects no longer met criteria for PDA. The two treatment components showed relative specificity of effect in that 80% of the total reduction in anxiety sensitivity occurred during PCT and approximately 60% of the reduction in agoraphobic avoidance occurred during the exposure component. This approach appears to be promising for markedly agoraphobic patients. Presently, we are also examining whether we can get similar results with shorter versions of PCT in combination with brief, ungraded exposure.

Treatment for racial and ethnic minorities

Our third caveat for consumers of the literature is that insufficient attention has been paid to treatment of panic disorder in racial/ethnic minority populations. In fact, no adequately controlled, large-scale treatment study has been reported evaluating the effectiveness of an empirically validated treatment of panic disorder in any racial/ethnic minority group.[69] The majority of the research that has examined panic disorder treatments in racial/ethnic minorities has used primarily African American samples. The results of these studies on panic disorder treatments in African Americans have not been promising.[70,71] These results are particularly troubling, considering the finding that African Americans are equally likely as Caucasians to experience panic disorder (1.2% and 1.4% respectively).[72,73] Therefore it is necessary to develop treatments that are empirically validated using samples of African Americans and persons from other racial/ethnic minority groups with panic disorder.

In our anxiety disorders clinic, we are enriching an empirically validated treatment of panic disorder, PCT,[74] to be more culturally sensitive with African American patients. The enrichments made to PCT are based on clinical/theoretical findings in the literature regarding culturally sensitive service delivery to African American clients.[75–79]

The enrichments made to PCT involve the following:

(1) adding an extensive pretreatment induction to orient African American patients to the cognitive–behavioral therapy approach;
(2) providing education about the prevalence and experience of panic disorder in African Americans;
(3) providing education about isolated sleep paralysis, a condition that seems to affect African Americans with panic disorder disproportionately;[80]
(4) using a casual rather than a formal learning approach;
(5) using audiovisual aids depicting other African Americans with panic disorder.

Furthermore, extended family members will be included in treatment as much as possible, issues of race and racism will be addressed as necessary in terms of how these factors interact with panic attacks and affect treatment, and specific focus will be placed on facilitating a positive therapeutic alliance with the African American clients and on treatment flexibility to decrease premature treatment dropouts.

The next logical stop after this treatment has been tested would be to conduct a large scale treatment study examining the comparative efficacy of enriched PCT against standard PCT with an African American sample. These treatments could also be compared with wait-list or minimal-treatment control conditions and with psychopharmacological interventions. However, until these large-scale treatment outcome studies can be conducted, researchers should continue to collect data evaluating the effectiveness of existing panic disorder treatments using samples of racial/ethnic minority persons.

Directions for further research

Overall, psychological approaches have been shown to be effective treatments for panic disorder and PDA. Behavioral, cognitive and cognitive–behavioral approaches in particular have been demonstrated to be useful in the treatment of panic disorder. Psychodynamic approaches have not been evaluated in controlled studies, and such work clearly needs to be done. Some additional directions for further research include disseminating and evaluating proven treatments within non-research populations. Current trends in managed care dictate investigation of success of psychological treatments at different types of sites, such as hospitals, clinics and health maintenance organizations (HMOs). Further research in the area of developing briefer versions of proven panic treatments is indicated, given ongoing pressure to decrease health-care costs. Predictors of successful outcome such as age, race, educational level, SES, level of agoraphobia, severity of panic, and motivation for change may also provide interesting areas for further study. Evaluation of combined psychological and pharmacological approaches to treatment should also continue to be pursued.

In conclusion, panic is one of the disorders for which psychological treatment has been demonstrated to be both feasible and potent, and further research should enhance the effectiveness and utility of psychological approaches, to the benefit of innumerable patients and treating clinicians.

References

1. Salvador-Carulla L, Segui J, Fernandez-Cano P, Canet J, Costs and offset effect in panic disorders. *Br J Psychiatry* 1995; **166**(Suppl 27): 23–8.
2. Barlow DH, Lehman CL, Advances in the psychosocial treatment of anxiety disorders: Implications for national health care. *Arch Gen Psychiatry* 1996; **53**: 727–35.
3. Gould RA, Otto MW, Pollack MH, A meta-analysis of treatment outcome for panic disorder. *Clin Psychol Rev* 1995; **15**: 819–44.
4. Shear MK, The psychodynamic approach in the treatment of panic disorder. In: *Panic Disorder and Agoraphobia: A Comprehensive Guide for the Practitioner* (Walker JR, Norton GR, Ross CA, eds). Pacific Grove, CA: Brooks/Cole, 1991.
5. Coté G, Barlow DH, Effective psychological treatment of panic disorder. In: *Handbook of Effective Psychotherapy* (Giles TR, ed.). New York: Plenum Press, 1993: 151–69.
6. Milrod B, Shear MK, Dynamic treatment of panic disorder: a review. *J Nervous Mental Dis* 1991; **179**: 741–3.
7. Fewtrell WD, Psychological approaches to panic attack – some recent developments. *Br J Exp Clin Hypnosis* 1984; **1**: 21–4.
8. Malan D, *The Frontier of Brief Psychotherapy*. New York: Plenum, 1976.
9. Mann J, *The Case of the Conquered Woman, in Time-Limited Psychotherapy*. Cambridge, MA: Harvard University Press, 1973.
10. McDougall J, *Theaters of the Mind*. New York: Basic Books, 1985.
11. Milrod B, The continuing usefulness of psychoanalysis in the treatment of panic disorder. *J Am Psychoanalytic Assoc* 1995; **43**: 151–62.
12. Sifneos PE, *Short-Term Psychotherapy and Emotional Crisis*. Cambridge, MA: Harvard University Press, 1972.
13. Silber A, Temporary disorganization facilitating recall and mastery: an analysis of a symptom. *Psychoanalytic Quart* 1984; **53**: 498–501.
14. Goisman RM, Warshaw MG, Peterson LG, Panic, agoraphobia, and panic disorder with agoraphobia: data from a multicenter anxiety disorders study. *J Nervous Mental Dis* 1994; **182**: 72–9.
15. Wiborg IM, Dahl AA, Does brief dynamic psychotherapy reduce the relapse rate of panic disorder? *Arch Gen Psychiatry* 1996; **53**: 689–94.
16. Shear MK, Cloitre M, Heckelman L, Emotion-focused treatment for panic disorder: A brief, dynamically informed therapy. In: *Dynamic Therapies for Psychiatric Disorders (AXIS I)* (Barber JP, Crits-Christoph P, eds). New York: Harper Collins, 1995.
17. Shear MK, Weiner K, Psychotherapy for panic disorder. *J Clin Psychiatry* 1997; **58**: 38–45.
18. Borkovec TD, Matthews AM, Treatment of nonphobic anxiety disorders: A comparison of nondirective, cognitive, and coping desensitization therapy. *J Consult Clin Psychol* 1988; **56**: 877–84.
19. Klein DF, Zitrin CM, Woerner MG, Ross DC, Treatment of phobias II. Behavioral therapy and supportive psychotherapy: Are there any specific ingredients? *Arch Gen Psychiatry* 1983; **40**: 139–45.
20. Shear MK, Pilkonis PA, Cloitre M, Leon AC, Cognitive behavioral treatment compared with nonprescriptive treatment of panic disorder. *Arch Gen Psychiatry* 1994; **51**: 395–401.
21. Barlow DH, Craske MG, *Mastery of Your Anxiety and Panic*. Albany, NY: Graywind Publications, 1989.
22. Milrod B, Busch F, Cooper A, Shapiro T, *Manual of Panic-Focused Psychodynamic Psychotherapy*. Washington, DC: American Psychiatric Press, 1997.
23. Barlow DH, *Anxiety and its Disorders: The Nature and treatment of Anxiety and Panic*. New York: Guilford Press, 1988.
24. McNally, *Panic Disorder: A Critical Analysis*. New York: Guilford Press, 1994.
25. Telch MJ, Singular and combined efficacy of in vivo exposure and CBT in the treatment of panic disorder with agoraphobia. Paper presented at the Meeting of the Association for Advancement of Behavior Therapy, New York, November 1996.
26. Telch MJ, Schmidt NB, Jaimez L et al, Singular and combined efficacy of in vivo exposure and CBT in the treatment of panic disorder with agoraphobia: interim results. Paper presented at the Meeting of the Association for

Advancement of Behavior Therapy, San Diego, CA, November 1994.

27. Telch MJ, Schmidt NB, Jaimez L et al, Singular and combined efficacy of in vivo exposure and CBT in the treatment of panic disorder with agoraphobia. Paper presented at the World Congress of Behavioural and Cognitive Therapies, Copenhagen, July 1995.

28. Marks IM, Swinson RP, Basoglu M et al, Alprazolam and exposure alone and combined in panic disorder with agoraphobia: a controlled study in London and Toronto. *Br J Psychiatry* 1993; **162**: 776–87.

29. Margraf J, Barlow DH, Clark DM, Telch MJ, Psychological treatment of panic: work in progress in outcome, active ingredients, and follow-up. *Behaviour Res Ther* 1993; **31**: 1–8.

30. Michelson LK, Marchione KE, Greenwald M et al, A comparative outcome and follow-up investigation of panic disorder with agoraphobia: the relative and combined efficacy of cognitive therapy, relaxation training, and therapist-assisted exposure. *J Anxiety Disorders* 1996; **10**: 297–330.

31. Bouchard S, Gauthier J, Laberge B et al, Exposure versus cognitive restructuring in the treatment of panic disorder with agoraphobia. *Behavior Res Ther* 1996; **34**: 213–24.

32. Fava GA, Zielezny M, Savron G, Grandi S, Long-term effects of behavioural treatment for panic disorder with agoraphobia. *Br J Psychiatry* 1995; **166**: 87–92.

33. Clark DM, Salkovskis P, Chalkley AJ, Respiratory control as a treatment for panic attacks. *J Behavior Ther Exp Psychiatry* 1985; **16**: 23–30.

34. Salkovskis PM, Jones DRO, Clark DM, Respiratory control in the treatment of panic attacks: replication and extension with concurrent measurement of behaviour and pCO_2. *Br J Psychiatry* 1986; **148**: 526–32.

35. de Ruiter C, Rijken H, Garssen B, Kraaimaat F, Breathing retraining, exposure and a combination of both, in the treatment of panic disorder with agoraphobia. *Behaviour Res Ther* 1989; **27**: 647–55.

36. Rijken H, Kraaimaat F, de Ruiter C, Garssen B, A follow-up study on short-term treatment of agoraphobia. *Behaviour Res Ther* 1992; **30**: 63–6.

37. Ley R, Breathing retraining in the treatment of

hyperventilatory panic attacks. *Clin Psychol Rev* 1993; **13**: 393–408.

38. Garssen B, de Ruiter C, van Dyck R, Breathing retraining: a rational placebo? *Clin Psychol Rev* 1992; **12**: 141–53.

39. Barlow DH, Craske MG, Cerny JA, Klosko JS, Behavioral treatment of panic disorder. *Behavior Ther* 1989; **20**: 261–82.

40. Beck JG, Stanley MA, Baldwin LE et al, Comparison of cognitive therapy and relaxation training for panic disorder. *J Consult Clin Psychol* 1994; **62**: 818–26.

41. Craske MG, Brown TA, Barlow DH, Behavioral treatment of panic disorder: a two-year follow-up. *Behavior Ther* 1991; **22**: 289–304.

42. Öst L, Applied relaxation: description of a coping technique and review of controlled studies. *Behaviour Res Ther* 1987; **25**: 397–409.

43. Öst L, Applied relaxation vs. progressive relaxation in the treatment of panic disorder. *Behaviour Res Ther* 1988; **26**: 13–22.

44. Öst L, Westling BE, Hellstrom K, Applied relaxation, exposure in vivo, and cognitive methods in the treatment of panic disorder with agoraphobia. *Behaviour Res Ther* 1993; **31**: 383–94.

45. Barlow DH, Cerny JA, *Psychological Treatment of Panic*. New York: Guilford Press, 1988.

46. Clark DM, A cognitive model of panic. In: *Panic: Psychological Perspectives* (Rachman S, Maser J, eds). Hillsdale: Erlbaum, 1988.

47. Clark DM, Anxiety states: Panic and generalized anxiety. In: *Cognitive Behaviour Therapy for Psychiatric Problems: A Practical Guide* (Hawton K, Salkovskis P, Kirk J, Clark DM eds). Oxford: Oxford University Press, 1989.

48. Salkovskis PM, Clark DM, Cognitive therapy for panic disorder. *J Cognitive Psychother* 1991; **5**: 215–26.

49. Beck AT, Cognitive approaches to panic disorder: theory and therapy. In: *Panic: Psychological Perspectives* (Rachman S, Maser J, eds). Hillsdale: Erlbaum, 1988.

50. Clark DM, Salkovskis PM, Hackmann A et al, A comparison of cognitive therapy, applied relaxation and imipramine in the treatment of panic disorder. *Br J Psychiatry* 1994; **164**: 759–69.

51. Öst LG, Westling B, Applied relaxation vs. cognitive therapy in the treatment of panic disorder. *Behaviour Res Ther* 1995; **33**: 145–58.

52. Clark DM, Panic disorder: from theory to therapy. In: *Frontiers of Cognitive Therapy* (Salkovskis P, ed.). New York: Guilford 1996.

53. Arntz A, van den Hout M, Psychological treatments of panic disorder without agoraphobia: cognitive therapy versus applied relaxation. *Behaviour Res Ther* 1996; **34:** 113–21.

54. Klosko JS, Barlow DH, Tassinari R, Cerny JA, A comparison of alprazolam and behavior therapy in treatment of panic disorder. *J Consult Clin Psychol* 1990; **58:** 77–84.

55. Barlow DH, Brown TA, Correction to Klosko et al. (1990). *J Consult Clin Psychol* 1995; **63:** 830.

56. Telch MJ, Lucas JA, Schmidt NB et al, Group cognitive–behavioral treatment of panic disorder. *Behaviour Res Ther* 1993; **31:** 279–87.

57. Coté G, Gauthier JG, Laberge B et al, Reduced therapist contact in the cognitive behavioral treatment of panic disorder. *Behavior Ther* 1994; **25:** 123–45.

58. Craske MG, Maidenberg E, Bystritsky A, Brief cognitive–behavioral versus non-directive therapy for panic disorder. *J Behavior Ther Exp Psychiatry* 1995; **26:** 113–20.

59. Gould RA, Clum GA, Self-help plus minimal therapist contact in the treatment of panic disorder: a replication and extension. *Behavior Ther* 1995; **26:** 533–46.

60. Lidren DM, Watkins PL, Gould RA et al, A comparison of bibliotherapy and group therapy in the treatment of panic disorder. *J Consult Clin Psychol* 1994; **62:** 865–9.

61. Hecker JE, Fritzler BK, Losee M, Fink CM, Mastery of your anxiety and panic: self-directed versus therapist-directed treatment of panic disorder. Paper presented at the 31st Annual Convention of the Association for Advancement of Behavior Therapy, Miami Beach, FL, November 1997.

62. Brown TA, Barlow DH, Long-term outcome in cognitive–behavioral treatment of panic disorder. *J Consult Clin Psychol* 1995; **63:** 754–65.

63. Burns LE, Thorpe GL, Cavallaro LA, Agoraphobia 8 years after behavioral treatment: a follow-up study with interview, self-report, and behavioral data. *Behavior Ther* 1986; **17:** 580–91.

64. Keller MB, Yonkers KA, Warshaw MG et al, Remission and relapse in subjects with panic disorder and agoraphobia. *J Nervous Mental Dis* 1994; **182:** 290–6.

65. Faravelli C, Albanesi G, Agoraphobia with panic attacks: 1-year prospective follow-up. *Comprehensive Psychiatry* 1987; **28:** 481–7.

66. Maier W, Buller R, One-year follow-up of panic disorder. *Eur Arch Psychiatric Neurol Sci* 1988; **238:** 105–9.

67. Noyes R, Reich J, Christiansen J et al, Outcome of panic disorder: relationship to diagnostic subtypes and comorbidity. *Arch Gen Psychiatry* 1990; **47:** 809–18.

68. Williams SL, Falbo J, Cognitive and performance-based treatments for panic attacks in people with varying degrees of agoraphobic disability. *Behaviour Res Ther* 1996; **34:** 253–64.

69. Chambless DL, Sanderson WC, Shoham V et al, An update on empirically validated therapies. *Clin Psychologist* 1996; **49:** 5–22.

70. Chambless DL, Williams KE, A preliminary study of African Americans with agoraphobia: Symptom severity and outcome of treatment with in-vivo exposure. *Behavior Ther* 1995; **26:** 501–15.

71. Friedman S, Paradis C, African American patients with panic disorder and agoraphobia. *J Anxiety Disorders* 1991; **5:** 35–41.

72. Eaton WW, Kessler LG, *Epidemiologic Field Methods in Psychiatry: The NIMH Epidemiologic Catchment Area Program.* Orlando: Academic Press. 1985.

73. Regier DA, Myers JK, Kramer LN et al, The NIMH Epidemiologic Catchment Area Program. *Arch Gen Psychiatry* 1984; **41:** 934–41.

74. Barlow DH, Craske MG, *Mastery of Your Anxiety and Panic*, 2nd edn (MAP II). Albany, NY: Graywind Publications, 1994.

75. Hatch ML, Paradis C, Panic disorder with agoraphobia: a focus on group treatment with African Americans. *Behavior Therapist* 1993; **16:** 240–1.

76. Sue DW, Arredondo P, McDavis RJ, Multicultural competencies and standards: a call to the professional. *J Counseling Dev* 1992; **70:** 477–86.

77. Sue DW, Bernier JE, Durran A et al, Position paper: cross-cultural counseling competencies. *Counseling Psychologist* 1982; **10:** 45–52.

78. Thorn GR, Hope DA, The therapeutic relationship with African-American male clients: separating myth from reality. Manuscript submitted for publication.

79. Thorn GR, Sarata BP, Psychotherapy with African American males: 'What we know and what we need to know'. Manuscript submitted for publication.

80. Neal AM, Turner SM, Anxiety disorders research with African Americans: current status. *Psychol Bull* 1991; **109**: 400–10.

14

Overview and future prospects

David J Nutt, James C Ballenger, Jean-Pierre Lépine

CONTENTS • **Diagnosis and epidemiology** • **Treatment** • **Which antidepressant?** • **How do drug treatments work?** • **New drugs for panic?** • **The future of psychological treatments** • **Biology**

The purpose of this book has been to provide a broad overview of current thinking on the basis, importance and treatment of panic disorder. We also wanted it to provide a strong foundation for clinical and research developments in panic disorder into the next millennium.

To what extent have we succeeded? That is for the reader to judge. However, we feel that the full spectrum of the illness has been covered. There are up-to-date chapters on all aspects of panic disorder – many with new research findings. Pointers to future basic and clinical research are readily apparent. In addition, the basis of the clinical management of the disorder has been clearly detailed, with the most comprehensive review of both drug and psychological treatments options ever pulled together in a single volume. We hope that the excitement that the authors of each chapter feel for the topic has been adequately conveyed to readers, whether they are psychiatrists or psychologists. Indeed, by bringing together the different perspectives on therapy in a single volume, we hope to facilitate cross-talk

between the disciplines to the benefit of research and, most importantly, patient care.

What of the future? Panic disorder is a rich source of new ideas, questions and challenges for treatment and research. Some of the key areas for development in the next decade are discussed below.

Diagnosis and epidemiology

Although in some areas close to teaching and research centres the diagnosis of panic is improving, there is still a great deal of ignorance about the disorder – not just amongst general practitioners (family physicians) but also amongst psychiatrists. Education needs to be improved and the central role of the panic attack in pointing to a diagnosis emphasized.

One area of clinical uncertainty is the prognosis and need for treatment of patients with limited symptom attacks. Another is the enhanced risk and poorer prognosis of patients with comorbid panic and depression. The evolving nature and interaction between these two syndromes is of great diagnostic and therapeutic concern.

Is panic disorder a unitary phenomenon? A number of pieces of evidence suggest that this is not so, yet little attempt has been made to properly address this question. For instance, challenge studies with the benzodiazepine antagonist flumazenil found that this mimicked naturally occurring panic in a realistic fashion, patients rating it as about 80% similar to their usual attacks,[1] yet it was clearly different in one way: flumazenil did not provoke as much in the way of respiratory symptoms.[2] There is some evidence from therapeutic trials that this finding may be mimicked clinically: differences have been reported between $GABA_A$ acting drugs (alprazolam) and antidepressants (imipramine).[3] In this analysis of a large multicentre panic study, respiratory symptoms were found to show some preference for response to imipramine, whereas alprazolam was better for somatic ones – particularly cardiovascular symptoms. It would be interesting to analyse the large SSRI databases to see if similar clinical differentiations are found. If they were, then this would be a good reason for investigating in more detail the subtyping of panic disorder.

Another area of research that is needed is into the interaction between stress and panic disorder. Here again, the relationship has been extensively studied in depression, but research in panic disorder lags several decades behind. This is particularly important, since our growing understanding of the brain basis of stress could lead to new approaches to therapy once the nature of the link has been clarified.

The issue of psychological set and its ability to predispose to panic attacks in panic disorder was touched upon in the chapter by Thorn and colleagues (Chapter 7). This area needs to be more fully explored with the view to interventions that might 'nip in the bud' the origins of such a propensity. Also, the basis of and reasons for different psychological forms of panic warrants some investment.

Treatment

A number of the chapters in this volume have been dedicated to the evidence base for drug treatment in panic disorder. A brief synopsis of their conclusions would be that there are two main classes of drugs that are effective in this condition (see Figure 14.1). The benzodiazepines act rapidly, often relieving anxiety in minutes, whereas the antidepressants work slowly, building up to a maximal therapeutic effect in weeks. These classes of drugs also differ in a number of other ways that have relevance to their clinical use. These are listed in Table 14.1.

In some countries, especially the UK, concern about the dependence and withdrawal aspects of the benzodiazepines has led to recommendations that their use be restricted to the short

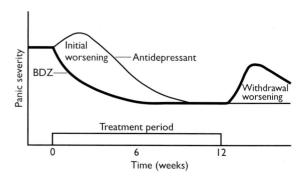

Figure 14.1 Time course of panic treatment (BDZ = benzodiazepine).

Table 14.1 Class differences in the drug treatment of panic disorder

	Benzodiazepines	Antidepressants
Speed of onset	Fast	Slow
Onset worsening	No	Yes
Withdrawal worsening	Yes	No
Dependence/abuse	Yes	No
Alcohol interactions	Yes	No
Therapeutic tolerance	Occasional	Rare
Treat associated depression	No	Yes
Safe in substance abusers	No	Yes

term, ideally less than four weeks, which presents problems when treating an enduring condition such as PD.

Onset worsening with antidepressants has been discussed in a number of preceding chapters. It occurs in about 20% of patients, and is clearly dose-related.[4] The easiest way of reducing its occurrence and impact is to start with a low dose of drug, conventionally half the lowest tablet die for the SSRIs and the lowest one for the tricyclic (e.g. 10 mg for imipramine), Generally, after one week, the dose may be doubled, in which case the therapeutic range is attained with the SSRI. In the case of tricyclics, it may take a month or more to titrate the dose up to the therapeutic range.

One of the pressing research needs is to properly explore the mechanisms underlying these differences in therapeutic action. Not only would such an understanding be of great intellectual value but it would also be a useful starting point for the development of new treatments.

Which antidepressant?

The choice of antidepressant is another area of both research and clinical interest. Although there are positive reports of the efficacy of MAOIs and RIMAs, these drugs have not been subject to sufficiently detailed study to allow them to be licensed for panic disorder. In practice, the choice then is limited to antidepressants of the uptake-blocking class, i.e. between the older tricyclics and the newer SSRIs. Both classes of drug are effective, and indeed panic disorder was discovered from observations on

Table 14.2 Differences between classes of antidepressant used to treat PD		
	Tricyclics	**SSRIs**
Efficacy	Very good	Very good
Side-effect burden:		
Early	High	Moderate
Late	Moderate	Low
Safety:		
in overdose	Poor	Very good
In cardiac patients	Poor	Good
Driving	Impairs	Neutral
Ease of dose titration	Difficult	Good

the actions of imipramine (See Chapter 1). However, at present, amongst the tricyclic class of drug, only clomipramine is relatively widely licensed for PD, but lofepramine also has this indication in Ireland. Paroxetine was the first SSRI to obtain an indication for panic disorder, and in this has recently been joined by citalopram in Europe. It seems likely that others in this class, especially sertraline, will obtain a licence in the near future.

Despite having similar efficacy in terms of the treatment of PD, tricyclics and the SSRIs do differ in ways that may have important clinical consequences (Table 14.2).

On the basis of these observations, the majority of experts in the field of clinical management of panic recommend that the SSRIs be considered the first-line treatment for PD. Their side-effect profile is relatively mild, especially when used in low doses at the start of treatment.

How do drug treatments work?

Perhaps the most burning questions in the pharmacotherapy of panic disorder are how do antidepressants work, and why do they take 3–6 weeks to produce their effects? In recent years, considerable progress has been made towards understanding these issues in the drug treatment of depression. Work from Charney and Heninger's group at Yale has replicated earlier findings that reducing brain 5-HT synthesis can obliterate the antidepressant effect of drugs such as the SSRIs and MAOIs.[5] This implies that tonically increased 5-HT synaptic activity is critical in the therapeutic response to the drugs. In contrast, the antidepressant action of noradrenergic agents such as desipramine was not affected by 5-HT depletion but was blocked by α-methylparqatyrosine (a tyrosine hydroxylase inhibitor) that decreases the synthesis of noradrenaline.

The situation in OCD, another condition responsive to the SSRIs, is rather different in that symptoms do not re-emerge on 5-HT depletion. In this case, the presumption is that receptors or other adaptations underlie the therapeutic action of the SSRIs in OCD.

The position in panic disorder is as yet unclear, although the easy availability of the 5-HT depletion paradigms mean that this should be easy to study. Such experiments are critically important for explaining the mechanisms of treatment efficacy. They also help direct the search for new forms of therapy.

The question of therapeutic delay in depression has also been the subject of much research in the past few years. The prevalent theory is that the increase in synaptic 5-HT concentration caused by drugs such as the SSRIs acts on pre-synaptic autoreceptors to inhibit cell firing and 5-HT release. This action offsets the uptake blocking properties, and over a period of weeks the inhibition wears off owing to receptor desensitization. Cell firing then increases, and synaptic levels of 5-HT rise into the range required to lift mood.

This theory has been tested in a number of centres in studies using pindolol in addition to SSRIs. Pindolol, though a beta-blocker, has significant 5-HT$_{1A}$ receptor antagonist properties, and in animal studies has been shown to prevent SSRI-induced reduction in cell firing, so allowing SSRIs to elevate cortical levels of 5-HT immediately.[6] Early clinical studies used pindolol to augment the therapeutic actions of antidepressants in patients who had made no or only a partial response. This was of limited success, and more recently efforts have been directed at accelerating the response to antidepressants by giving pindolol throughout a course of treatment.

Depression studies with both fluoxetine and paroxetine have found that in combination with pindolol there was a faster and in some cases a better response in the combination group.[7] It is possible that the therapeutic effects of SSRIs in panic disorder would also be accelerated by this approach, although another scenario is that, by increasing 5-HT release at the start of treatment, the anxiogenic actions of the SSRIs would be exaggerated. In either case, the results would be of great theoretical interest, and we would encourage these studies to be conducted soon.

The use of pindolol augmentation for panic disorder patients who have not fully responded has been suggested by some psychopharmacologists. There are no published data on this as yet, but it would seem another area worth exploring.

New drugs for panic?

Alprazolam is the only agent developed for a specific panic disorder indication. The SSRIs that are now becoming licensed for the treatment of panic disorder (paroxetine, citalopram and sertraline) are all established antidepressants that were later evaluated in panic disorder. A number of new antidepressants have been licensed since the SSRIs. These include venlafaxine (a mixed noradrenaline and 5-HT uptake blocker), nefazodone (a weak SSRI with potent 5-HT$_2$ receptor blocking properties), reboxetine (a pure noradrenaline uptake blocker) and mirtazapine (an α_2-adrenoceptor antagonist that also blocks 5-HT$_2$ and 5-HT$_3$ receptors). There have been case reports but no controlled trials on these drugs in panic disorder, although on the basis of their pharmacology both nefazodone and venlafaxine might be expected to show efficacy. It would also be interesting to test reboxetine, since the issue of the efficacy of noradrenergic agents is still unclear and this drug has the best side-effect profile of the available agents.

The future of psychological treatments

Panic disorder has proved to be one of the most active research areas of clinical psychology, providing a number of competing theories and new treatments. This exciting period seems set to continue as several of these theories can be tested in conventional psychological experiments or clinical trials. One important goal is to optimize the psychological package that is offered to patients – perhaps by distilling the most effective components from a number of the more clinically proven approaches.

The relation between psychological and physical treatments of panic disorder has often been an unnecessary source of tension and distrust. Both approaches have their merits and demerits (Table 14.3). In general, patients and therapists find that combining approaches seems to be the best in clinical practice, although formal tests of such combinations are only just being done. Certainly key elements in psychological approaches such as explanation and education and engaging the patient in a therapeutic alliance are critical in maximizing the value of drug treatment.

A number of other more specific research questions relating to psychological treatments require exploration. For instance, the brain circuits and neurochemical mechanisms underlying concepts such as 'catastrophic cognitions' are now amenable to study using neuroimaging techniques. Such studies should help determine whether these are real entities or just a useful shorthand for a more complex mix of experiences.

Another challenge in research on panic disorder is reconciling the commonalities and disimilarities that exist between drug and psychological treatments, and the mechanisms underlying them. Some research has shown that drug treatment will rectify certain psycho-

---

Table 14.3 Benefits and drawbacks of drug and psychological treatments

	Psychological	Drug
Ease of use for patients	Hard	Easy
Speed of onset	Slow	Faster
Availability	Low	High
Safety	Good	Good
Persistence of effects after treatment stops	Good	Moderate

logical aspects of panic disorder, such as the attentional bias towards threatening words.[8] Others have explored the effect that psychological treatments have on biological processes.[9] There is a great deal more to do, and we would hope that powerful new techniques such as brain imaging are brought to bear on this topic. Such research will greatly influence neuroscience as well as psychiatry/psychology, and could reveal unexpected findings that might lead to another revolution in treatment.

Biology

A unique feature of panic disorder is the ability for panic attacks to be provoked by a range of different pharmacological and non-pharmacological agents. The biological basis of the drug provocations is gradually being understood, although a major area of future research is in reconciling the different theories of action. Is there a single 'panicogenic' neural system into which a variety of different neurotransmitters feed, or are there independent pathways that can provoke panic by activation of a specific brain region or brain circuit?

The findings of decreased $GABA_A$ function detailed in Chapter 5 need to be incorporated into theories of action of treatments – both drug and psychological. For instance, does effective therapy with antidepressants upregulate the $GABA_A$ system and so offset the deficit found in our PET studies? Alternatively, it may be that the actions of antidepressants are 'downstream' of the $GABA_A$ system, potentially suppressing the outflow of a central hyperexcitable state, so blocking panics.

Further PET/SPECT studies may be able to address these issues, since there now exist good ligands for the 5-HT_{1A} and 5-HT_2 receptors, either of which may be involved in panic generation and its treatment.

Metabolic imaging offers the possibility of more clearly defining the brain circuits underlying panic attacks. It seems likely that this will be best achieved with either PET or SPECT, because fMRI is so claustrophobic that it is very unlikely that the average panic patient will agree to take part. Indeed, one of the real challenges is to be able to properly study the circuits activated by panicogenic challenges. In theory, this could clarify the issues raised earlier about commonalities in the mode of action of the various panicogens. In practice, this is very difficult in patients, since the anxiety induced by a challenge leads to large movement artefacts and in many cases a (quite understandable) desire of the patient to leave the scanner. Techniques that allow tracer injection outside the scanner with later imaging (e.g. HMPAO SPECT) may be the way forward, despite their poorer spatial resolution.

The brain circuits involved in other forms of anxiety have been approached by the use of imaginal activation of anxiety by, for instance, playing to patients' personal accounts of their own condition attacks. This has helped define the mechanisms of social phobia,[10] and in principle could be translated very easily to panic patients.

Mention of other anxiety disorders raises the issue of the biological specificity of challenge tests and neurobiological findings. For example, how specific are the findings of $GABA_A$ downregulation in panic disorder? Few such studies have been carried out in related conditions, so our ability to gauge the biological overlap of syndromes such as social phobia with panic is in its infancy. It is critical to evaluate these issues by conducting identical studies in the different anxiety disorders.

Undoubtedly, panic disorder is an area of psychiatry and psychology that is highly important in clinical practice; this importance is growing with the greater understanding of the disorder and better diagnosis, especially in primary care (family medicine). It is also a vibrant research area that is benefiting from the growth in new research technologies and terms. Moreover, in several areas, panic disorder research is very much leading the field in the development of new concepts of the brain mechanisms of psychiatric disorder. We hope that this chapter and the book as a whole serve to demonstrate these insights to the reader, so encouraging optimal clinical practice and driving further research.

References

1. Nutt DJ, Glue P, Lawson CW et al. Flumazenil provocation of panic attacks: Evidence for altered benzodiazepine receptor sensitivity in panic disorder. *Arch Gen Psychiatry* (1990) **47**: 917–25.

2. Nutt DJ, Glue P, Lawson C et al. Do benzodiazepine receptors have a causal role in panic disorder? In: *A BAP Monograph: Psychopharmacology of Panic.* Oxford: Oxford University Press, 1993: 74–90.

3. Briggs AC, Stretch DD, Brandon S, Subtyping of panic disorder by symptom profile. *Br J Psychiatry* 1993; **163**: 201–9.

4. Nutt DJ, Glue P, Clinical pharmacology of anxiolytics and antidepressants: a psychopharmacological perspective. *Pharmacol Ther* 1989; **44**: 309–34.

5. Salomon RM, Miller JL, Delgado PL et al. The use of tryptophan depletion to evaluate central serotonin function in depression and other neuropsychiatric disorders. *Int Clin Psychopharmacol* 1993; **8**: 41–6

6. Romero L, Bel N, Artigas F et al. Effect of pindolol on the function of pre- and postsynaptic 5-HT_{1A} receptors: in vivo microdialysis and electrophysiological studies in the rat brain. *Neuropsychopharmacology* 1996; **15**: 349–60

7. Perez V, Gilaberte I, Faries D et al. Randomised, double-blind, placebo-controlled trial of pindolol in combination with fluoxetine antidepressant treatment. *Lancet* 1997; **349**: 1594–7.

8. Weinstein AM, Nutt DJ, A cognitive dysfunction in anxiety and its amelioration by effective treatment with SSRIs. *J Psychopharmacology* **9**: 83–9.

9. Middleton HC, Ashby M, Clinical recovery from panic disorder is associated with evidence of changes in cardiovascular regulation. *Acta Psychiatr Scand* 1995; **91**: 108–13.

10. Bell CJ, Malizia AL, Nutt DJ, The neurobiology of social phobia. *Eur Arch Psychiatry and Clin Neurosci* (in press).

INDEX

Note: page numbers in *italics* refer to figures and tables